OXFORD
UNIVERSITY PRESS

Oxford University Press is a department of the University of Oxford.
It furthers the University's objective of excellence in research, scholarship,
and education by publishing worldwide.

Oxford   New York

Auckland   Cape Town   Dar es Salaam   Hong Kong   Karachi
Kuala Lumpur   Madrid   Melbourne   Mexico City   Nairobi
New Delhi   Shanghai   Taipei   Toronto

With offices in

Argentina   Austria   Brazil   Chile   Czech Republic   France   Greece
Guatemala   Hungary   Italy   Japan   Poland   Portugal   Singapore
South Korea   Switzerland   Thailand   Turkey   Ukraine   Vietnam

Oxford is a registered trademark of Oxford University Press
in the UK and certain other countries.

Published in the United States of America by
Oxford University Press
198 Madison Avenue, New York, NY 10016

Library of Congress Cataloging-in-Publication Data
Wray, Shirley H.
Eye movement disorders in clinical practice / Shirley H. Wray.
   p. ; cm.
ISBN 978–0–19–992180–5 (alk. paper)—ISBN 978–0–19–992181–2 (alk. paper)—
ISBN 978–0–19–998149–6 (alk. paper)
   I. Title.
[DNLM: 1. Ocular Motility Disorders—diagnosis—Case Reports.   2. Ocular Motility Disorders—etiology—Case
Reports.   3. Cranial Nerve Diseases—complications—Case Reports.   4. Cranial Nerve Diseases—diagnosis—Case
Reports.   5. Diagnosis, Differential—Case Reports.   6. Neuropsychological Tests—Case Reports. WW 410]
RE731
617.7′62—dc23
2013010302

3 5 7 9 8 6 4 2

Printed in China
on acid-free paper

For Anne
With All My Thanks

CONTENTS

PREFACE

This is a very personal book. It reflects my experience as a neurologist for more than 50 years. In the course of that time I knew and learned from the great neurologists at Queen Square, London, during my residency and fellowship in neurophysiology, and at the Massachusetts General Hospital when I arrived there in 1967. Their influence is part of this book and my specific indebtedness is to the late Raymond D. Adams and Charles Miller Fisher.

Eye movement disorders are common in clinical practice and yet they raise many difficult questions with respect to diagnosis, prognosis and management. The approach I have taken in this book is clinically oriented but the contents covers much of the relevant literature, and include many aspects of eye movement disorders. I realize that some of the views expressed, for example, my guides to clinical points to remember, are personal preferences but they have worked for me and I hope they may work for others. I have attempted as well to clarify the complex terminology and methods of ophthalmologists for neurologists and neurosurgeons, and to provide a comprehensive physiologic framework to aid in diagnosis.

While written with neurologists and neurosurgeons specifically in mind, I hope the students of other disciplines, among them ophthalmology, neuro-otology, neuro-pediatrics, neuro-oncology and internal medicine, will find my approach useful. Readers who would like to view additional videos of a variety of other eye movement disorders can access my website by accessing the NOVEL website of the North American Neuro-Ophthalmology Society: http://NOVEL. utah.edu or by accessing my collection at Harvard Medical School Countway Library: http:// Repository.Countway.Harvard.edu/Wray.

I am very grateful to many colleagues who have made the writing of this book possible. This especially applies to the late David Cogan at the Massachusetts Eye and Ear Infirmary who strongly encouraged me to film and video many unique cases for teaching purposes and I am especially grateful to my patients who contributed so much to my clinical experience and whose permission made possible the case studies published in this book. The expert help of Nancy Lombardo, Associate Director of Information Technology, and Ray Balhorn, M. Ed., Media Services Manager Spencer S. Eccles Health Sciences Library, University of Utah and of Stephen Smith, Department of Surgery, Massachusetts General Hospital made the DVD collection possible.

A number of people provided encouragement throughout this project and I would like to express my gratitude to John Leigh who critically reviewed the manuscript and David Zee who reviewed the case videos with me and to Agnes Wong and Hal Blumenfeld for their unfailing authorial generosity. Any errors that may remain are my own. I am also particularly indebted to Anne Jardim for her editing skill, helpful criticism and encouragement over the last several years, and to my secretary, Fran Christie, for her unstinting help in getting the manuscript ready for publication and who with Karen Hoenig and Marylou Moar typed draft after draft after draft until we were satisfied. My grateful thanks also go to members of the Massachusetts General Hospital Photographic Department, Michelle Rose and Paul Batista, for their remarkable professional competence and to the wonderful creative team at the CambridgeSide Galleria Apple Store for their support in creating the DVD. Thank you Tommy, Dan, Tony, Brook, and Akira.

Shirley H. Wray

HOW THE BRAIN MOVES THE EYES

THE CEREBRAL CORTEX

The brain sees what the eyes look at. Multiple, well-delineated visual areas analyze the visual scene, with each area having its own retinotopic map of the visual field. The visual areas act simultaneously to analyze the image on the retina, sending this information to the cortical areas controlling eye movements, where the image seen combines with internally stored neural information to produce a more comprehensive blueprint of the visual environment.

The speed with which this is accomplished is remarkable. The specialized extrastriate areas send output to satellite areas and to other regions of the cortex. There, potential targets for gaze are analyzed and selected and quick decisions made: whether or not to execute a saccadic eye movement from one target to another, for example, or whether to pursue a moving target in a field of moving and stationary potential targets or to stay fixed on a target waiting for it to move.

Once the decision is made, two major types of eye movements are generated by the cerebral cortex. *Volitional intentional saccades*, which are internally triggered to move the eyes toward a target, and *reflexive saccades*, which respond to the sudden appearance of a target on the retina. Both modes of saccadic generation act in concert and, once initiated, they cannot be stopped. They originate either in anterior cortical areas in the frontal cortex or in posterior cortical areas in the parietal lobe and superior temporal sulcus.

Stabilizing the Image Seen

For the clearest view of an image of interest, the image must be held within 0.5 degrees of the fovea, where photoreceptor density is greatest and visual acuity is at its best, and it must be stable and steady.[1] Unless movements of the eyes compensate for motion, images of interest cannot be held stable and steady and would slip off the fovea with every head movement. Retinal slip causes visual blur, nystagmus, and oscillopsia, an illusion that the visual world itself is moving.

Two types of reflex eye movements are needed to stabilize the image on the retina, the vestibulo-ocular reflex (VOR) and visually mediated reflexes. During brief head movements, the VOR stabilizes retinal images by counter-rotating the eyes at the same speed as the head but in the opposite direction. Head acceleration signals pass from the vestibular sensors in the labyrinth of the inner ear to VOR circuits in the brainstem that compute an appropriate eye velocity command to compensate for changes in position and orientation of the head; because the VOR is a vestibular-mediated reflex, it operates even in the dark.

Acting together with the VOR, three visually mediated classes of eye movements keep the image on the fovea: *visual fixation, optokinetic eye movements,* and *smooth pursuit. Fixation* opposes saccadic movement of the eyes away from a stationary target. When the eyes adjust to a visual scene during sustained self-rotation (e.g., being in a stationary vehicle next to one that is moving but feeling as if the stationary vehicle is moving and the moving vehicle is still), the eye movements needed to correct this are described as *optokinetic.* When the eye follows a moving object or maintains fixation on a near stationary target while one is oneself in motion, the movements are called *smooth pursuit.*

In each case, areas of cerebral cortex (the striate and extrastriate visual cortex) extract information about the direction and speed of retinal image-slip from each eye and send signals to the brainstem and cerebellar circuits to program an eye movement to correct image-slip as the image moves off the fovea. These visual areas all act together to stabilize the angle of gaze (eye position in space) so as to hold the image of interest fairly stationary on the fovea of each eye while the subject is in motion.

Still other eye movements are needed to look at a new object of interest because this requires shifting gaze and redirecting the line of sight to a new target. Saccades jump the fixation point from one feature to another during visual search, and most saccades are completed in less than 100 ms. During these brief eye movements the eye is apparently sightless.[2]

Parallel Visual Pathways

Cortical areas concerned with vision are organized into two parallel pathways: one, the ventral pathway, processes form and color; the other, the dorsal pathway, processes motion (Figure 1-1). This is a useful division, allowing disorders of color processing and object recognition to be grouped as ventral pathway disorders involving occipitotemporal structures and disorders of motor processing and spatial processing as dorsal pathway disorders involving lateral occipitoparietal structures. Colloquially, these have been dubbed the *"what and where"* pathways, although this easy mnemonic has been challenged by the suggestion that the dorsal pathway is configured for preparing responses to the environment and is better identified as an "action" pathway.

THE STRIATE CORTEX

The *striate cortex* (visual area V1) is of fundamental importance in controlling visually guided eye movements.[3]

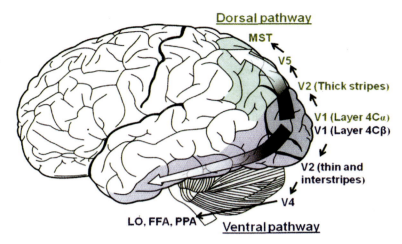

FIGURE 1-1 Schematic of the dorsal and ventral processing streams. MST, medial superior temporal area; LO, lateral occipital; FFA, fusiform face area; PPA, parahippocampal place area. The ventral stream begins in layer 4Cβ of area V1. The dorsal stream begins in motion-sensitive components of layer 4Cα in area V1.

Reproduced with permission.[3]

The *primary visual cortex* (the striate and extrastriate cortex V1 to V2) receives visual inputs from the retina. The attributes of the visual images received (color, motion, form, depth, and distance) are then distributed along the ventral and dorsal parallel pathways for further analysis by other visual association areas (V3–V4, color sensitive; V5, the middle temporal (MT) area sensitive to motion; and V6).

The dorsal motion detection pathway includes MT and the medial superior temporal (MST) area. MT contains neurons that encode the speed and direction of a target[4] and MST's neurons carry, in addition, eye movement signals that help to maintain smooth pursuit.[5,6]

THE FRONTAL CORTEX

There are four saccadic areas or eye fields in the frontal cortex: the frontal eye fields (FEFs), the supplementary eye field (SEF), the dorsolateral prefrontal cortex (DLPC), and the cingulate eye field (CEF) (Figure 1-2).

The FEFs generate all *voluntary intentional saccades* (memory-guided saccades, predictive saccades, antisaccades, and visually guided saccades) and help maintain smooth pursuit and vergence. They signal the brainstem circuits for immediate premotor saccade commands.

The SEF is important in generating saccades to respond to both visual and nonvisual cues.

The DLPC, also called the prefrontal eye field (PFEF), lies on the dorsal convexity of the frontal lobe and receives inputs from the FEF, SEF, and the posterior parietal cortex (PPC). This cortical area projects to the FEF, SEF, superior colliculus (SC), and the paramedian pontine

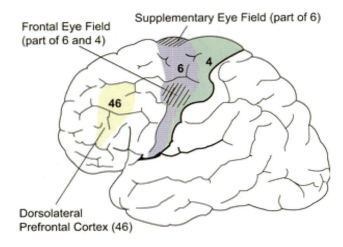

* Numbered areas denote corresponding Brodmann areas

FIGURE 1-2 Location of cortical visual areas in the frontal lobe.

Reproduced with permission.[7]

reticular formation (PPRF). It is important for programming memory-guided saccades and antisaccades.

The CEF in the anterior cingulate cortex is active during memory-guided saccades, antisaccades, and intentional saccades.[7,8]

■ **Clinical Points to Remember About Lesions of the Frontal Cortex**

- Acute FEF lesions produce a contralateral horizontal gaze palsy manifested by gaze deviation or gaze preference (the patient looks away from the hemiparesis to the opposite side). This resolves in time.
- Patients with chronic bilateral frontal lobe lesions have impaired initiation of voluntary saccades on command, a condition often called *acquired ocular motor apraxia*. A better term is *saccadic initiation defect*.
- Patients with frontocortical dementia have impaired ability to suppress a reflexive saccade in the antisaccade task (i.e., impaired reflexive saccadic inhibition[9,10]) and are unable to suppress inappropriate saccades to a novel visual stimulus.
- Lesions of the SEF result in a loss of ability to make a remembered sequence of saccades to an array of visible targets in the order that the targets appear (especially the case with left-sided lesions).
- Focal lesions of the DLPC cause errors in the antisaccade test.
- Focal unilateral lesions of the CEF cause hypometric memory-guided saccades.[11] Larger lesions, for example those due to resection of a tumor, cause deficits in the generation of antisaccades.[12] ■

In patients with frontal lobe neurodegeneration, deficits in the ability to suppress automatic behavior can lead to impaired decision making, aberrant motor behavior, and impaired social function, as seen in Case 1-1.

CASE 1-1 Pick's Disease: Frontotemporal Dementia

Video Display

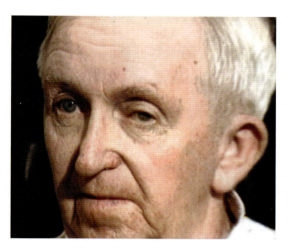

FIGURE 1-3 Sixty-eight-year-old man with echolalia.

The patient is a 68-year-old, retired, right-handed man who presented with a 1-year history of progressive behavioral change (Figure 1-3). His writing had become less legible, his speech slow and hesitant, and he was unable to balance his checkbook. When answering a question, he often had to repeat the question before giving the answer.

He denied any visual symptoms except trouble judging space and distance. He reported having had a minor car accident when he drove 100 feet in reverse, stopping only when he hit the garage door. He said he had no trouble with memory, no confusion, no difficulty finding words or understanding speech. He also denied weakness, stiffness, tremors, numbness, headache, or syncope.

He had experienced a progressive loss of balance, slowness walking, and difficulty climbing stairs, dressing, using a knife and fork, and getting in and out of a chair. Because of impaired balance, he needed to sit to put his trousers on.

Concerned that his "slowing up" might be due to Parkinson's disease (PD), his family consulted his primary care doctor who referred him to Dr. Raymond Adams for an opinion.

Family history was negative for degenerative central nervous system (CNS) disease. There was no past history of alcohol abuse or previous stroke or head trauma.

Analysis of the History

- What are the major presenting symptoms?
- Where are the CNS lesion(s) likely to be?

CASE 1-1 SYMPTOMS

Symptoms	Location Correlation
Progressive change in behavior	Frontotemporal lobe
Impaired executive function (unable to balance checkbook)	Frontal lobe
Loss of balance	Vestibular system

The analysis guides the clinical examination.

Examination

Neurological

- Fully oriented with good recall of public events
- Speech slow and hesitant with no paraphasic errors
- Echolalia—always repeating what was said to him
- Writing—tremulous, barely legible but with correct spelling
- Able to draw a clock and bisect a line correctly but had difficulty copying a complex drawing
- No limb apraxia; however, truncal movements seemed apraxic
- Motor strength 5/5 throughout
- Tendon reflexes 1+ symmetric, plantars flexor
- Frontal release signs with positive jaw and facial jerks
- Sensation normal throughout
- Gait slow; failed to swing his arms

Saccadic and Pursuit Eye Movements

- Infrequent full random eye movement
- Marked delayed initiation of horizontal saccades to look left
- Failed to look up or down on command
- Inability to make a refixation saccade on command to a target held on the left (including his own hand)
- Made reflexive saccades to loud hand clap and to sudden focal beam of light
- Impaired accuracy of memory-guided saccades when asked to look in the direction of a previously presented target—the examiner's finger held to the right side and also held to the left side
- Antisaccades—could not do the test
- Normal horizontal optokinetic nystagmus (fast phase)
- Normal oculocephalic reflex
- No saccadic intrusions or square-wave jerks
- Saccadic pursuit in all directions of gaze

Localization and Differential Diagnosis

This patient presented with a behavioral syndrome, disinhibition, agitation, and anger at times. He showed an extreme stimulus boundedness—for example, he picked up any object placed in front of him (including the examiner's coffee cup and pencil) but had difficulty releasing it. Tasks that were difficult for him he refused to do. The symptoms and signs localize to the frontotemporal lobe.

What Diagnostic Tests Should Follow?

- Neuroimaging of the brain
- Neuropsychological testing

Test Results

Noncontrast computerized tomography (CT) showed bilateral global generalized central and cortical atrophy affecting the frontal cortex and temporal lobes. (Magnetic resonance imaging [MRI] was not available; see Figure 1-4A–C).

Neuropsychological testing showed significantly depressed intellectual function and disturbance in spatial perception, orientation and perseverative movements, for example, going back and forth over already drawn lines.

Mental computing abilities were also significantly impaired:

- In addition to word finding difficulties, verbal and written fluency was significantly impaired
- Severely impaired abstract reasoning

This generalized depression of intellectual function and the patient's significant frontal lobe signs suggested circumscribed cortical atrophy. His memory impairment did not suggest Alzheimer's disease, in which memory impairment is usually an early feature.

The physician diagnosed Pick's disease,[13] and autopsy later showed frontotemporal lobar atrophy with argentophilic intranuclear inclusions—Pick bodies. (Among the neuropathic variants of frontotemporal dementia, some cases show neuronal inclusions containing the microtubule-associated protein *tau*.)[14,15]

Special Explanatory Note

The antisaccade test (which this patient failed) requires a subject to suppress a visually guided saccade and instead program a saccade to a nonexistent target in the opposite direction.[16,17] This test has been adopted as a model for understanding the impact of aging and brain disease on the ability to perform cognitive tests, and it is particularly revealing because the successful suppression of visually guided saccades, which the test requires, relies heavily on a neural network within the frontal cortex and DLPC.[18–22] Functional MRI studies of the brain have identified other areas involved within the antisaccade circuit, and structural MRI studies have shown a positive correlation between antisaccade performance and focal volume loss in the FEF.[23–25]

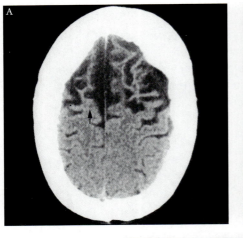
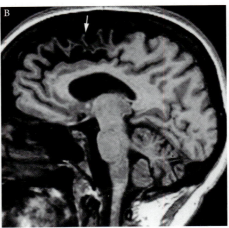
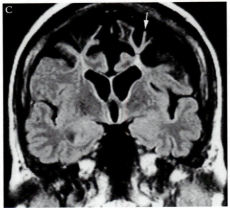

FIGURE 1-4 MRI images from a similar case: (A) Axial head CT scan shows striking frontal atrophy (*arrow*) with relative preservation of the parietal gyri. (B) Sagittal T1-MR shows the disproportionate enlargement of the frontal sulci (*arrow*). (C) Coronal fluid-attenuated inversion recovery (FLAIR) scan shows the frontal gyri are extremely atrophic and "knife-like." Note increased signal intensity in the affected gyri and underlying white matter (*arrow*).

Courtesy of Anne G. Osborn, M.D.

THE PARIETAL CORTEX

The parietal eye fields (PEFs) and parietal cortical areas—the medial parietal (MP) area, the posterior parietal cortical (PPC) area, and the lateral intraparietal (LIP) area play a pivotal role for all voluntary eye movements because of their importance in directing visual attention and generating *reflexive saccades* through direct projection to the SC.

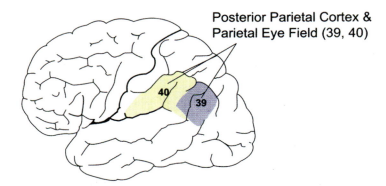

Posterior Parietal Cortex &
Parietal Eye Field (39, 40)

40

39

* Numbered areas denote corresponding Brodmann areas

FIGURE 1-5 Location of cortical visual areas in the parietal lobe.

Reproduced with permission.[7]

The PPC receives inputs from the MST sulcus, SC, cingulated cortex (CC), the pulvinar, and the intralaminar thalamic nuclei. It projects to the FEFs, lateral prefrontal cortex (LPC), and cingulated gyrus.

The PEFs are critically important in generating *reflexive saccades* in response to the sudden appearance of a novel visual stimulus (and to auditory or tactile stimuli as well). The PEF has a direct role in programming saccades.

Figure 1-5 shows the PEF as it lies in the intraparietal sulcus portion of Brodmann areas 39 and 40, where it receives input from the secondary visual areas and projects to the FEF and SC. The parietal cortical areas are particularly active during a variety of visuospatial and cognitive tasks, including spatial memory, reorienting gaze to novel visual stimuli, and shifting visual attention to new targets in external space. Neuronal activity in these areas triggers visually guided saccades.

■ **Clinical Points to Remember About Parietal Cortical Lesions**

- Unilateral posterior parietal lesions, especially right-sided, cause contralateral neglect, ipsilateral gaze deviation or preference, and impaired ability to make saccades and smooth pursuit in the contralateral hemifield of gaze.[26,27]
- During visual search, patients with parietal lobe lesions may show a double deficit consisting of hemispatial neglect (Figure 1-6) and impaired memory for previous targets.[28]
- In cases with mild dementia of the Alzheimer type, saccadic delay to a target moving unpredictably prevents the patient from following it. Alzheimer patients, like patients with Huntington's disease, are also unable to suppress reflexive saccades toward novel visual stimuli such as a suddenly appearing target. Pursuit eye movements in these cases are abnormal as well.
- Bilateral posterior parietal lesions cause Bálint's syndrome—a symptom triad consisting of disturbed visual attention (simultanagnosia), inaccurate arm pointing (optic ataxia), and difficulty initiating voluntary saccades to visual targets (ocular motor apraxia).[29]

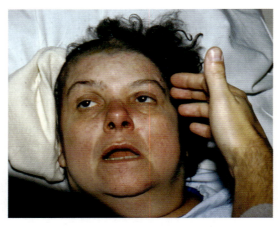

FIGURE 1-6 Elderly woman with a right hemisphere parietal lobe infarction, right conjugate horizontal gaze deviation and left hemi visual neglect. ■

An illustrative case of Alzheimer's dementia and Bálint's syndrome follows.

CASE 1-2 Alzheimer's Dementia: Bálint's Syndrome

Video Display

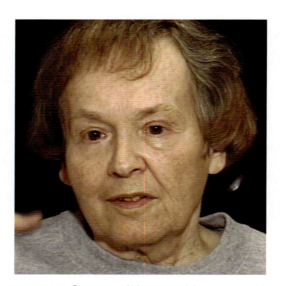

FIGURE 1-7 Seventy-eight-year-old woman with Alzheimer's dementia.

The patient is a 78-year-old, left-handed woman, a retired executive secretary and avid reader. Prior to the onset of psychiatric difficulties in 1996, she had enjoyed a high-functioning life and was always meticulously dressed. According to her caregiver, there had been a dramatic decline in behavior with the onset of confusion, forgetfulness, and inability to care for herself or remain independent (Figure 1-7).

She was admitted to a nursing facility, where she disturbed other patients by climbing into their beds.

Special Explanatory Note

Getting into another patient's bed is a sign of visual disorientation and spatial (topographic) localization. Patients with topographagnosia are unable to orient themselves in an abstract spatial setting. These patients cannot draw the floor plan of their home, describe a familiar route home, or find their way to their bedroom when at home. In short, such patients have lost *topographic memory.* This disorder is invariably due to lesions in the dorsal convexity of the right parietal lobe.

The patient was referred for a neurological evaluation and was found to be demented. A diagnosis of Alzheimer's disease was made. The neurologist noted that she failed to blink to threat and referred her to an ophthalmologist who, with difficulty, documented full visual fields on perimetry, a visual acuity of approximately 20/40 OU, and no abnormality on funduscopic examination. He referred her to the neurovisual clinic.

Analysis of the History

- What are the major presenting symptoms?
- Where are the CNS lesion(s) likely to be?

CASE 1-2 SYMPTOMS

Symptoms	Location Correlation
Dementia	Cerebral cortex
Topographagnosia	Parietal lobe

The analysis guides the clinical examination.

Examination

Saccadic and Pursuit Eye Movements

- Failed to blink to threat in both hemifields
- Infrequent full random eye movements
- Delayed initiation of horizontal and vertical saccades on command
- Hypometric horizontal saccades to a peripheral target
- Total inability to do the antisaccade test or make memory-guided saccades

- Absent reflexive saccades to novel target, hand clap, or focal beam of light
- Absent optokinetic nystagmus attributed to lack of attention fixating on the black stripes
- Normal oculocephalic reflex
- Saccadic pursuit in all directions of gaze

Localization and Differential Diagnosis

This patient has signs of biparietal lobe disease, the center of attention of the CNS. She failed to make reflexive saccades to the sudden appearance of a target or in response to a loud noise. She failed to blink to threat, a defect of visual attention that may underlie *simultanagnosia* (disturbed visual attention).

What Diagnostic Tests Should Follow?

- Test visual search by asking the patient to interpret a complex picture with multiple interrelated elements.
- Test coordination by asking her to reach for an object held in front of her (optic ataxia).
- Confirm that she is unable to initiate saccades to novel visual targets.

Test Results

When the patient was presented with the Cookie Theft Picture,[30] she failed to grasp the picture's story and had great difficulty reporting the items depicted.

To test object identification and selection, she was asked to pick up a paper clip from a tray holding seven objects (comb, coin, key, pen, ring, paper clip, spoon), but could not do so until four objects were removed one by one. With three left, she was able to see the paper clip and pick it up.

In a test of optic ataxia, she failed to touch the examiner's finger held at a short distance from her face, in both the left visual field and the right visual field. Lack of accuracy on this test is referred to as misreaching (optic ataxia), which probably reflects visuospatial misperception, since it can affect one arm more than the other and affect reaching to the patient's own body parts.

The patient could not initiate voluntary saccades to visual targets (ocular apraxia). A key feature of this condition is that reflexive saccades are absent to suddenly appearing visual targets and are usually absent to loud noises and sudden tactile stimuli.

Diagnosis: Alzheimer's Dementia and Bálint's Syndrome

Special Explanatory Note

The different elements of Bálint's syndrome and their relationships to each other have been debated over the years, and, in the past, simultanagnosia (disturbed visual attention) has been held responsible for both optic ataxia and ocular motor apraxia.[31] Other opinions consider each element of the triad as potentially dissociable,[32] and the relationships among them have been recently reviewed.[33]

The commonest cause of the syndrome is ischemia, particularly from watershed infarction,[34] and degenerative disorders such as subacute sclerosing panencephalitis[35] and posterior cortical atrophy.[36] Bálint himself thought that optic ataxia, or misreaching for an object, was independent of visual disturbances. However, there were interesting demurrers even at that time.[37]

VISUAL ASSOCIATION AREAS MT/MST

The visual areas concerned with motion, the MT and superior temporal sulcus (MST), lie adjacent at the occipitotemporal–parietal junction. Neurons sensitive to motion in the MT and MST participate in smooth pursuit eye movements and fixate a stationary target during self-motion. The MT is involved in motion perception and smooth pursuit initiation, whereas the MST receives inputs related to eye movements rather than to target movement and is involved in smooth pursuit maintenance. In functional imaging studies, these two regions are referred to as the MT/MST complex (Figure 1-8).

The MT has reciprocal connections to the MST and projects to the PEF. Descending pathways from the MT and MST target the dorsolateral pontine nuclei and optokinetic cell groups in the brainstem, such as the nucleus of the optic tract and the dorsal terminal nucleus.

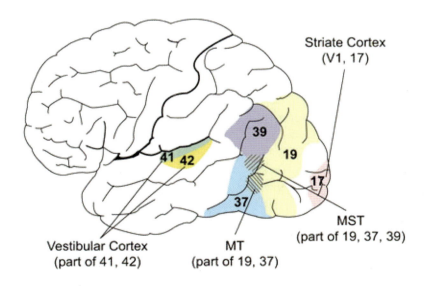

* Numbered areas denote corresponding Brodmann areas

FIGURE 1-8 Localization of visual association areas in the occipitotemporal region associated with motion.

Reproduced with permission.[7]

> **■ Clinical Points to Remember About Lesions of the MT/MST**
>
> - *Cerebral akinetopsia* is a selective impairment of motion perception.
> - Patients with unilateral lesions causing motion defects are either asymptomatic or have subtle complaints, such as "feeling disturbed" by the visually cluttered moving scene.[38,39]
> - Patients with bilateral MST lesions have trouble perceiving differences in speed, and their perception of direction is severely affected.[40] Symptomatically, they may have no impression of motion in depth or of rapid motion. Fast targets appear to jump rather than move.
> - The prognosis for motion perception deficits is not yet clear.   ■

THE SUPERIOR COLLICULUS

The SC acts in concert with the FEFs to trigger saccades, particularly saccades that redirect gaze to novel stimuli appearing on the periphery of the visual fields (the farthest extent of vision in the external world).

The SC is a multilayered structure.[41] Neurons in the dorsal layer are visual. The ventral layers contain a blueprint that predicts the size and direction of saccades.[42,43] Neurons at the rostral pole of the blueprint appear to be important for maintaining steady fixation and project to omnipause neurons (OPN) in the brainstem,[44,45] whereas more caudally located neurons project to burst neurons in the PPRF and to inhibitory burst neurons (IBN).[46,47] The SC may also make a contribution to smooth pursuit and vergence eye movements,[48] but principally it contributes to target selection and saccade initiation rather than to steering the eye accurately to the target.[49]

> **■ Clinical Points to Remember About Lesions of the Superior Colliculus**
>
> - Lesions of the SC cause an increase in saccadic latency, mild saccadic hypometria (undershoot), and a paucity of saccades when scanning a scene or responding to visual stimuli.
> - Clinical data suggest that the pulvinar (the largest posterior part of the thalamus) receives information from the retina and the SC and helps to shift visual attention and link visual stimuli through context-specific motor responses.[50]
> - Partial lesions of the striate visual cortex impair vision severely but may nonetheless leave unaffected the ability of the SC to produce saccades to novel stimuli in a portion of the visual field that is blind. This phenomenon—*blind sight*—is mediated by the SC, perhaps using extrastriatal pathways.   ■

THE SACCADIC SYSTEM

Each eye field is responsible for both saccadic and pursuit eye movements, but saccadic neurons preferentially interconnect with other saccadic neurons, and pursuit neurons preferentially interconnect with other pursuit neurons (Figure 1-9). Because of this, during normal ocular motor behavior, the frontal and parietal lobes complement each other.

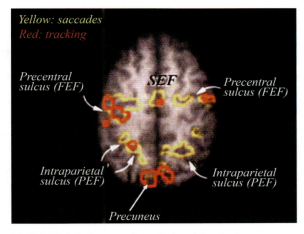

FIGURE 1-9 Increased cortical activity during a visual pursuit task (red outline) and a saccadic task (yellow outline) superimposed onto the subject's Talairach-normalized axial structural image.

Reproduced with permission.[56]

The FEF voluntarily directs the eyes toward an object or a location of interest, whereas the parietal lobes are more concerned with visual attention and generate reflexively induced saccades. Their combined activity is known to be modified by feedback information from the SC, the thalamus, the basal ganglia, and the cerebellum.

Descending Saccadic Pathway

The descending saccadic pathway shown in Figure 1-10 carries signals from the FEFs to premotor areas in the nucleus reticularis tegmenti pontis (NRTP) and rostral interstitial nucleus of the medial longitudinal fasciculus (riMLF) in the brainstem to generate saccadic eye movements. The pathway runs in the anterior limb of the internal capsule and then, below this level, the neural signals take their own separate pathways to many other structures involved in the production of saccades (Figure 1-10).

One pathway, the caudate and substantia nigra pars reticulata (SNpr), goes through the basal ganglia and generates saccades as part of more complex behavior that involves memory, expectations, and whether the behavior will be rewarded.[51,52] A transthalamic pathway projects to the intralaminar thalamic nuclei and provides a second basal ganglionic pathway by which the cortical eye fields may influence saccades.[53] For example, stimulation of the subthalamic nucleus in patients with PD causes improved accuracy of memory-guided saccades. Yet another pathway, the pedunculopontine, projects to the NRTP in the pons (see Figure 1-10).

All of these projections to the SC and NRTP in turn project to the cerebellum, the dorsal vermis, fastigial nucleus, flocculus, and ventral paraflocculus.[54]

Lesions of the pathway(s) through which the FEFs influence the SC can affect both the initiation and the suppression of saccades. Both deficits have been seen in patients with disorders affecting the basal ganglia, such as Huntington's disease (HD)[55] and other CAG triplet repeat disorders that may be mistaken for HD.

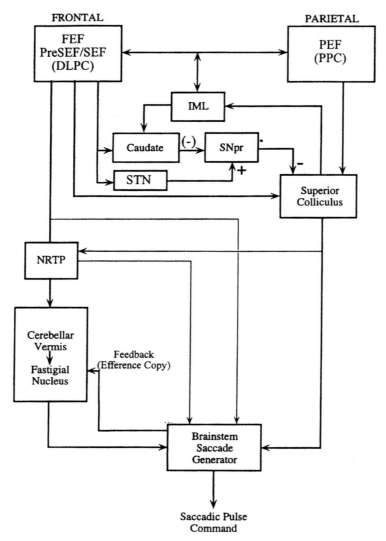

FIGURE 1-10 Block diagram of the major structures that project to the brainstem saccade generator (premotor, burst neurons in paramedian pontine reticular formation [PPRF] and rostral interstitial nucleus of the medial longitudinal fasciculus [riMLF]). Also shown are projections from cortical eye fields to superior colliculus. DLPC, dorsolateral prefrontal cortex; FEF, frontal eye fields; IML, intramedullary lamina of thalamus; NRTP, nucleus reticularis tegmenti pontis; PEF, partial eye fields; PPC, posterior parietal cortex; SEF, supplementary eye fields; SNpr, substantia nigra, pars reticulate; STN, subthalamic nucleus. Not shown are the pulvinar, which has connections with the superior colliculus and both the frontal and parietal lobes; projections from the caudate nucleus to the subthalamic nucleus via globus pallidus; and the pathway that conveys efference copy from brainstem and cerebellum, via thalamus, to cerebral cortex. –, inhibition, +, excitation.

Reproduced with permission.[2]

> ■ **Clinical Points to Remember About Saccades**
> - The saccadic subregion of the FEFs (FEFsac), as well as the saccadic region of the parietal eye field (PEFsac), participates in the control of saccades and shows increased cortical activity during pursuit eye movements.
> - The FEFsac initiates volitional intentional saccades.
> - The PEFsac initiates visually guided (reflexive) saccades.
> - The FEFsac projects to the SC directly and through the basal ganglia.
> - The FEFsac and SC project directly to the PPRF and riMLF.
> - A lesion of both the FEF and SC (not just one of them) causes defective generation of saccades.
> - A lesion of either of the FEFs or the SC alone causes subtle abnormalities—mildly hypometric and delayed (increased latency) initiation of saccades.
> - The cerebellum (dorsal oculomotor vermis and the fastigial nucleus) regulates the size of saccades and participates in the repair of saccade inaccuracy (flocculus and paraflocculus). ■

Classification of Saccades

Saccades can be classified in a decision hierarchy from high-level volitional, intentional saccades and memory-guided saccades, down to the simplest, quick phases of vestibular nystagmus (Table 1-1).

Diagnostic Signs

The hierarchy of saccades is important for diagnostic reasons. Saccadic impairment is a critical sign of underlying disease, and the progressive development of difficulty in generating saccades is often specific for the disease process and/or the cortical location.

TABLE 1-1: Hierarchy of Saccades

Classification Definition

Volitional, intentional saccades: Saccades made intentionally and for a specific purpose.

Reflexive saccades: Saccades generated to novel stimuli in the environment (visual, auditory, or tactile) that occur unexpectedly.

Predictive, anticipatory saccades: Saccades made in anticipation or in search of a target at a particular location.

Memory-guided saccades: Saccades made to a location in which a target has been previously seen.

Antisaccades: After being so instructed, saccades made in the direction opposite to the sudden appearance of a target.

On-command saccades: Saccades generated to a cue—for example, "look left."

Express saccades: Very short-latency saccades (documented on eye movement recordings) elicited when the novel stimulus is presented after the target for fixation has disappeared (gap stimulus).

Spontaneous saccades: Seemingly random saccades occurring without apparent purpose.

Quick-phase saccades: Quick phases of nystagmus generated during vestibular or optokinetic stimulation or as in an attempt to correct for spontaneous drift of the eyes.

To test *voluntary saccades to command,* simply ask the patient to make saccades rapidly between two stationary targets, for example two fingers held one to the right of center and one in the center for fixation with primary gaze. Loss of voluntary saccades with preservation of reflexive saccades is indicative of an initiation defect of saccades common in frontotemporal dementia.

To test *predictive, anticipatory saccades,* hold both hands up and ask the patient to make a saccade by looking at your finger when it moves. With predictable timing, move first a finger on your right hand and then a finger on your left hand and repeat this cycle several times, occasionally not moving one finger. By occasionally not moving one finger, you can determine if the patient makes a predictive saccade without a visual stimulus. A defect such as this is common in PD.

To test a *memory-guided saccade,* hold up a finger in the right hemifield and ask the patient to point to it. Do the same in the left half of the visual field. Then instruct the patient not to point at the finger when it is in view, but to point to where it was before it was removed. Defects in memory-guided saccades are common in Alzheimer's disease.

To test *reflexive saccades,* suddenly present an unusual visual object (e.g., a toy of some kind) in the periphery of the patient's visual field and note if there is a reflexive saccade to look at the toy. The same test can be repeated to a loud hand clap in one ear or a tactile stimulus touching one side of the head. Defects in reflexive saccades are an indication of lack of attention consistent with disease affecting the parietal lobe.

To test antisaccades, explain the test to the patient first and say what you are going to do and what he/she will be asked to do. Then hold both hands up in front of the patient and move a finger on one hand suddenly. Ask the patient to look *away from* the moving finger (i.e., look to the finger that does not move). Inattentive patients and patients with neurodegenerative disease, particularly those affecting the prefrontal cortex, will make many errors or completely fail the test. Errors on antisaccade tasks are common with lesions of the prefrontal cortex.

THE SMOOTH PURSUIT SYSTEM

Smooth pursuit eye movements allow for clear vision of moving objects. To succeed, their velocity must match the velocity of the target.[56,57] During head rotation, the smooth pursuit system must interact with the vestibular system, and these pathways are consequently important for mediating optokinetic nystagmus.

Descending Smooth Pursuit Pathway

The descending smooth pursuit pathway from the posterior parietal and extrastriate areas MT and MST is shown in Figure 1-11. This pathway runs ipsilaterally through the internal capsule and cerebral peduncle to reach the dorsolateral pontine nucleus (DLPN) and the NRTP, which projects to the dorsal cerebellar vermis, flocculus, and paraflocculus.[58–60]

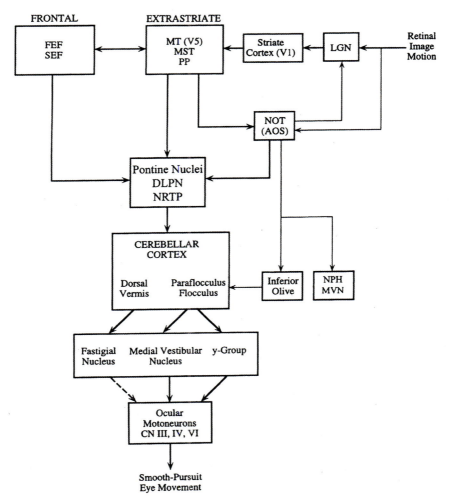

FIGURE 1-11 A hypothetical anatomic scheme for smooth pursuit eye movements. Signals encoding retinal image motion pass via the lateral geniculate nucleus (LGN) to striate cortex (V1) and extrastriate areas. MT (V5), middle temporal visual area; MST, medial superior temporal visual area; PP, posterior parietal cortex; FEF, frontal eye fields; SEF, supplementary eye fields. The nucleus of the optic tract (NOT) and accessory optic system (AOS) receive visual motion signals from the retina but also from extrastriate cortical areas. Cortical areas concerned with smooth pursuit project to the cerebellum via pontine nuclei, including the dorsolateral pontine nuclei (DLPN) and nucleus reticularis tegmenti pontis (NRTP). The cerebellar areas concerned with smooth pursuit project to ocular motor neurons via fastigial, vestibular, and y-group nuclei; the pursuit pathway for fastigial nucleus efferents has not yet been defined. The NOT projects back to LGN. The NOT and AOS may influence smooth pursuit through their projections to the pontine nuclei and, indirectly, via the inferior olive and the nucleus prepositus (NPH)-medial vestibular nucleus (MVN) region.

Reproduced with permission.[2]

modulate vergence movements by influencing which of many disparities in a complex visual scene are selected to provide the stimulus for depth.[74] There is also an underlying resting level of vergence tone—*tonic vergence*—that can cause changes in vergence induced by new sensory cues.[75]

Vergence eye movements usually occur without our being aware of them, in much the same way that we unconsciously shift our gaze across the visual field. However, vergence movements are under voluntary control, and three types of neurons are activated in the striate visual cortex (area VI) to produce them:

- *Tuned-zero/near-zero* neurons, which respond to binocular stimuli over a narrow range about the fixation point and which may be responsible for fine stereopsis.
- *Tuned-far neurons,* which respond to binocular stimuli farther from fixation and which may be responsible for coarse stereopsis.
- *Tuned-near neurons,* which respond to binocular stimuli nearer to fixation. Like tuned-far neurons, they may be responsible for coarse stereopsis.

Other cerebral cortical areas that participate in vergence include the frontal cortex within the pursuit subregion of the FEF, the LIP area in the parietal cortex, and MT and MST.

Vergence and the Midbrain

The supra-oculomotor area (SOA) within the mesencephalic reticular formation of the midbrain[76-78] contains neurons involved in generating vergence eye movements. These are:

- *Vergence tonic cells,* which discharge in relation to vergence angle
- *Vergence burst cells,* which discharge in relation to vergence velocity
- *Vergence burst-tonic cells,* which discharge in relation to both vergence velocity and angle

The elements of the vergence system and their relationships are shown in Figure 1-12.

Vergence and the Pons

Premotor commands for vergence in the pons are generated by the abducens internuclear neurons that activate the contralateral medial rectus subnucleus in the oculomotor nucleus. The projection from the abducens internuclear neurons runs in the medial longitudinal fasciculus (MLF). However, clinical lesions of the MLF (e.g., internuclear ophthalmoplegia) do not cause paralysis of vergence eye movements (see Chapter 6).

Vergence and the Cerebellum

The dorsal vermis, which projects to the fastigial oculomotor region, and the posterior interposed nuclei may also play a role in vergence.[79] Lesions of the dorsal vermis result in *esodeviation* (excess convergence), whereas lesions of the fastigial oculomotor region lead to *exodeviation* (excess divergence).

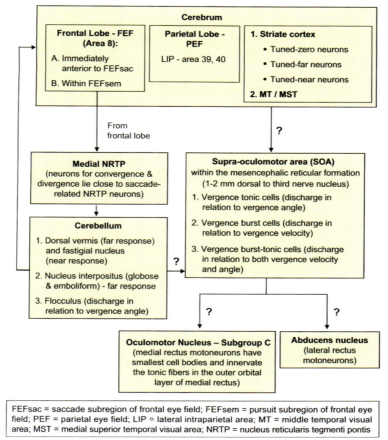

FEFsac = saccade subregion of frontal eye field; FEFsem = pursuit subregion of frontal eye field; PEF = parietal eye field; LIP = lateral intraparietal area; MT = middle temporal visual area; MST = medial superior temporal visual area; NRTP = nucleus reticularis tegmenti pontis

FIGURE 1-12 The neural substrate of vergence eye movements.

Reproduced with permission.[7]

Diagnostic Signs

The Near Triad

Vergence is part of the *near triad* characterized by convergence (when the eye abruptly changes focus from far to near), accommodation (the lens becomes more spherical and is accommodated for near vision), and pupillary constriction. Pupillary constriction probably plays only a minor role in focusing near objects, but the degree of pupillary constriction is useful clinical confirmation that the reflex is intact.

Near Point of Convergence

To test accommodative vergence (convergence/accommodation), measure the *near point of convergence (NPC)*. This is done by having the patient fix on a small target as it is brought toward the nose. The NPC is the point at which fusion can no longer be maintained and divergent movement of the eyes occurs.

Convergence Insufficiency

Convergence insufficiency is the commonest cause in elderly patients of blurred vision or diplopia when reading, and it occurs frequently in neurodegenerative disorders such as PD and progressive supranuclear palsy (PSP).

A disorder of the vergence system may contribute to convergence-retraction nystagmus associated with a supranuclear upward gaze palsy (Chapter 7).[80]

Spasm of convergence, or spasm of the near reflex, may be psychogenic. Psychogenic spasm of the near reflex may be misdiagnosed as a bilateral sixth nerve palsy because voluntary convergence gives the appearance of abduction weakness when the patient is asked to look to the left or to the right. However, it is the presence of miosis (constriction of the pupil) when these patients look laterally that establishes beyond doubt the diagnosis of spasm of the near reflex.[81]

Divergence Insufficiency and Divergence Paralysis

Divergence insufficiency and *divergence paralysis* are terms used to describe patients with *esotropia* (eyes deviated in) when they fix on a distant target but show no paresis of the lateral recti and normal amplitude and speed of horizontal saccades, which together rule out bilateral paresis of the abducens nerve.

Divergence insufficiency or divergence paralysis occurs in many different intracranial disorders, among them head trauma, obstructive hydrocephalus, midbrain or cerebellar tumors, thalamic hemorrhage, and raised intracranial pressure due to pseudotumor cerebri (Figure 1-13). Divergence insufficiency can also occur with intracranial hypotension from dural cerebrospinal fluid leak post lumbar puncture.[82]

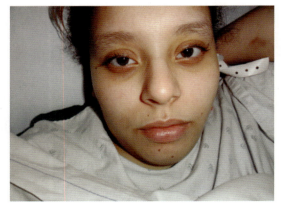

FIGURE 1-13 Twenty-six-year-old woman with divergence insufficiency with both eyes deviated inward (esotropic) due to raised intracranial pressure from pseudotumor cerebri.

> ■ **Clinical Points to Remember About Movements of the Eyes**
> - Saccades bring images of objects of interest onto the fovea.
> - Visual fixation holds the image of a stationary object on the fovea by minimizing ocular drift.
> - Smooth pursuit holds the image of a small moving target on the fovea or holds the image of a small near target on the retina during linear self-motion (this aids gaze stabilization during sustained head rotation).
> - Vergence eye movements rotate the eyes simultaneously in opposite directions so that images of a single object are placed or held simultaneously on the fovea of each eye.
> - The optokinetic system holds images on the retina during brief head rotations or translations.
> - Nystagmus quick phases reset the eyes during prolonged rotation and direct gaze toward the oncoming visual scene.   ■

THE FINAL COMMON PATHWAY

All functional classes of eye movements are governed by the brain, and, although each eye movement has a specific function, the same motor neurons and extraocular muscles are active for all. As a consequence, all eye movement signals entering the *final common path* in the brainstem reticular formation have the same two principal components: a *pulse* giving the torque needed to overcome the viscous drag of the orbital tissues, and a tonic component, the *step*, giving the torque needed to overcome the elasticity of the orbital tissues.[83–86]

Pulse-Step of Innervation

Saccades are initiated by trigger signals from the cerebral hemispheres and the SC. When the neural signal from the cortex reaches the pontine paramedian reticular formation and the rostral interstitial nucleus of the MLF in the mesencephalic reticular formation in the midbrain, a *pulse-step of innervation* is generated for a saccade to move the eyes. A simplified scheme of the brainstem pulse generator and the key classes of neurons involved is shown in Figure 1-14.

For horizontal saccades to be produced quickly and smoothly, the pulse (the eye velocity command) has to be integrated with the step (the eye position command) to hold the eyes in their new position of gaze. Integration is accomplished by neural integrators, which, for horizontal gaze, are the nucleus prepositus hypoglossi (NPH) in the pontine tegmentum and the MVN in the medulla. The interstitial nucleus of Cajal (INC) is the neural integrator for vertical and torsional eye movements. Inactivation of the INC, which is important for vertical gaze control, limits the range of vertical saccades without substantially affecting their velocity.

Excitatory burst neurons (EBN) that generate saccades also activate IBN, which inhibit antagonist motoneurons and OPN during the saccade. Once the actual eye position matches the desired eye position, the burst neurons cease firing, the omnipause cells resume their activity, and the saccade stops. Figure 1-15 illustrates this model of saccade generation.

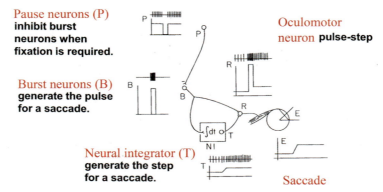

Pause neurons (P) inhibit burst neurons when fixation is required.

Burst neurons (B) generate the pulse for a saccade.

Oculomotor neuron pulse-step

Neural integrator (T) generate the step for a saccade.

Saccade

FIGURE 1-14 A simplified scheme of the brainstem pulse generator and the key classes of neurons involved. A saccade takes the eye to an eccentric position (E) and holds the eye steadily there. (R) A pulse of innervation (velocity command) is generated by burst neurons (B) that project to the ocular motor neurons. This same pulse signal is sent to neural integrator cells, (T) which generate the step of innervation.

Reproduced with permission.[86]

Pulse-Step Mismatch

A lesion of the NPH/MVN horizontal gaze integrator complex or the vertical gaze integrator (INC) results in a "leaky" integrator and inability to sustain eccentric eye position (the step) despite a normal eye velocity command (the pulse). This *pulse-step mismatch* results in saccadic hypometria manifested in slow saccades indicative of pontine or midbrain disease Impaired gaze holding in which eye position cannot be maintained, and the eyes drift back toward the primary

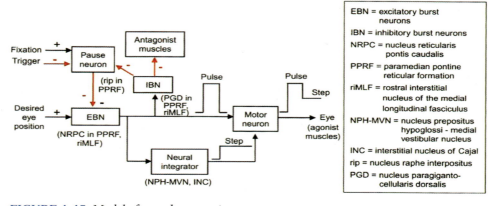

FIGURE 1-15 Model of saccade generation.

Reproduced with permission.[7]

or central position of gaze at the end of each eccentric saccade followed by a corrective saccade toward the eccentric position, results in gaze-evoked nystagmus.

Saccadic abnormalities due to pulse-step mismatch include:

- *Hypometric saccades* (due to decreased pulse amplitude)
- *Slow saccades* (due to decreased pulse height—i.e., firing rate)
- *Gaze-evoked nystagmus* (due to unsustained step)

Examples are shown in Figure 1-16.

■ **Clinical Points to Remember About the Pulse-Step**

- The pulse-step of innervation applies to all types of eye movements: saccades, pursuit, vergence, and nystagmus.
- The pulse (velocity command) and the step (position command) are integrated by neural integrators.
- The neural integrators for horizontal saccades are the NPH in the pons and the MVN in the medulla.
- The neural integrator for vertical and torsional saccades is the INC in the midbrain.
- "Leaky" neural integrators (which cannot sustain the step) cause gaze-evoked nystagmus.
- Pulse-step mismatch causes slow and hypometric saccades.
- Inactivation of the rostral interstitial nucleus of the MLF causes vertical saccades to become slow and small, whereas inactivation of the INC restricts the vertical range of saccades without affecting the speed. ■

Brainstem Generator

Three major groups of neurons in the PPRF are responsible for horizontal gaze: OPN, EBN, and IBN. *Omnipause neurons* are tonically active neurons that cease firing before a saccadic movement and remain quiet for a period equal to the duration of the saccadic movement. They are located in the nucleus raphe interpositus (rip).[87]

Excitatory burst neurons activate the motoneurons that innervate the appropriate agonist muscles; for example, the lateral rectus muscle to abduct the eye or the medial rectus muscle to adduct the eye.[88] The EBNs reside in the nucleus reticularis pontis caudalis (NRPC) in the PPRF for horizontal saccades and in the rostral interstitial nucleus of the MLF (riMLF) for vertical and torsional saccades. Each riMLF contains EBNs that discharge for torsional saccades in one direction only: the right riMLF generates conjugate clockwise saccades, and the left riMLF generates conjugate counterclockwise saccades.

Inhibitory burst neurons inhibit the motor neurons to antagonist muscles and discharge just before and during saccades.[89] Inhibitory burst neurons reside within the nucleus paragigantocellularis dorsalis (PGD) in the PPRF for horizontal saccades and in the riMLF for vertical and torsional saccades. Figure 1-17 shows a summary diagram of major pathways involved in horizontal and vertical saccade generation.[90]

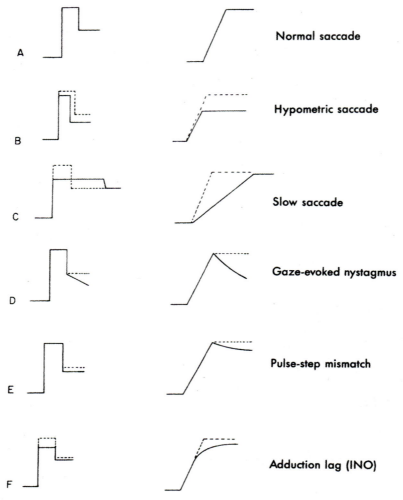

FIGURE 1-16 Saccadic abnormalities due to pulse–step mismatch. Innervation patterns are shown on the left, eye movements on the right. Dashed lines indicate the normal response. (A) Normal saccade. (B) Hypometric saccade: pulse amplitude (width × height) is too small, but pulse and step are matched appropriately. (C) Slow saccade: decreased pulse height with normal pulse amplitude and normal pulse-step match. (D) Gaze-evoked nystagmus: normal pulse, poorly sustained step. (E) Pulse-step mismatch (glissade): step is relatively smaller than pulse. (F) Pulse-step mismatch due to internuclear ophthalmoplegia (INO): the step is larger than the pulse, and so the eye drifts onward after the initial rapid movement.

Reproduced with permission.[2]

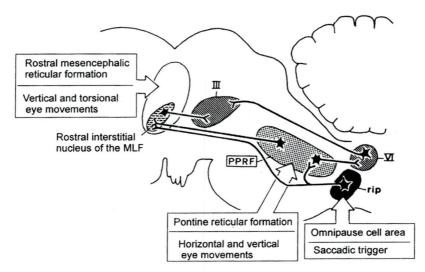

FIGURE 1-17 Summary diagram of major pathways involved in horizontal and vertical saccade generation.

Reproduced with permission.[90]

DIAGNOSTIC SIGNS

Saccadic Latency, Velocity, Duration, and Accuracy

Saccades should always be examined for saccadic latency (initiation time), speed (velocity), duration, and accuracy, bearing in mind that each saccadic disorder points to impaired function of a specific neurological structure.

- *Saccadic latency*: initiation time or the normal interval between the command to look left or the appearance of a target and the onset of the saccade. The normal interval is about 150–250 msec. Saccades are ballistic eye movements, and the brain can only use information received up to 70 msec before an upcoming saccade to modify it.
- *Velocity*: saccades are the fastest movements the body can make. Peak velocity increases with amplitude. The normal range is 30–700 degrees/sec for amplitude ranging from 0.5 to 40 degrees. The larger the saccade, the higher the peak velocity. Saccades are slower when made in darkness to a remembered target location and when in the opposite direction to a visual stimulus (the antisaccade test).
- When deciding if saccades are abnormally slow, it is always important to remember that elderly patients and patients who are drowsy, inattentive, or heavily medicated may have slow velocity but normal saccades. Super-fast saccades with a peak velocity greater than expected for the size of the saccade are a rarity. They occur in ocular myasthenia gravis (MG).
- Saccades that stall in mid-flight due to transient decelerations (difficult to detect clinically) occur in late-onset Tay-Sach's disease[91] and a number of CNS disorders.[92]

- *Saccadic duration:* the normal duration of a saccade is 30–100 msec for amplitude ranging from 0.5 to 40 degrees. The duration of saccades is decreased, and the velocity of small saccades may be increased in MG.
- *Saccadic accuracy:* the accuracy of a saccade is best judged by asking the patient to look to the right (at your hand) and back to the center (at your finger or nose). Small degrees of inaccuracy (saccadic dysmetria) are normal. A small overshoot (hypermetria) when the saccade returns the eyes back to center may occur with small-amplitude saccades, a small undershoot (hypometria) with larger amplitude saccades. Saccadic dysmetria becomes more prominent with age, fatigue, and inattention. Saccadic hypometria, a common abnormality in myasthenia, can be reversed by Tensilon, which will cause saccades to become hypermetric. Marked saccadic dysmetria is the hallmark of cerebellar disease (Chapter 9, Case 9-5).

Children with Gaucher's disease type 3 with selective slowing of horizontal or vertical saccades may have a characteristically curved trajectory for diagonal saccades that indicates that the vertical component of the saccade is faster than the horizontal component.

Saccades are inappropriate and intrusive if they interfere with steady foveal fixation of an object of interest. Several types of *saccadic intrusions* disrupt fixation: square-wave jerks, macrosaccadic oscillations, ocular flutter, and opsoclonus (see Chapter 10). Dyslexic children often show impairment of steady fixation, with excessive numbers of square-wave jerks and difficulty reading.

SACCADE SYNDROMES

Slow Saccade Syndrome

Saccade syndromes usually reflect abnormalities in the brainstem neural network, suggesting either intrinsic disturbances of burst neurons or omnipause cells, or failure to recruit an adequate population of burst neurons to generate the pulse velocity and a normal fast saccade. A decrease in the height of the saccadic pulse (which reflects discharge frequency) causes slow saccades.

Diseases of the CNS affecting the cerebral hemisphere, cerebellum, SC, or basal ganglia also lead to saccade slowing An illustrative case is presented here.

CASE 1-3 Slow Saccade Syndrome: Progressive Supranuclear Palsy

Video Display

The patient is a 60-year-old woman who, in 1992, realized that she was "slowing up": dragging her right foot, walking slowly, and falling (Figure 1-18). Her speech became slurred. She saw a number of physicians and was given a diagnosis of PD and started on Sinemet 50/200 t.i.d.

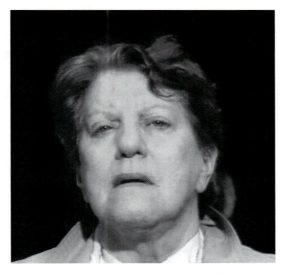

FIGURE 1-18 Sixty-year-old woman with neurodegenerative disease.

In January 1994, she was seen by a neurologist who noted the following:

Neurological Examination

- Age-related bilateral ptosis
- Dysarthria
- Flattened immobile facies
- Mild resting tremor of the hands
- Significant limitation of upgaze with normal downgaze
- No nystagmus
- No fibrillations of the tongue
- No bulbar weakness
- Mild decrease in spontaneous movements, with diminished arm swing and a stooped forward gait
- Mild decrease in strength bilaterally
- Marked hyperreflexia 3+ throughout, with ankle clonus and flexor plantar responses
- No cerebellar ataxia

The diagnosis of PD was confirmed and her medication changed to Permax. Nine months later, having failed to improve on this drug, she was referred for a third opinion.

When seen in October 1994, she said she had noted progressive difficulty reading. The print lines ran into each other, and she would have to rest from reading and start again. Occasionally, she noted double vision with horizontal separation of the image. She had no diplopia watching TV. She was afraid to go for her driving license exam because she thought she would fail it. She felt her memory was slipping. She forgot the names of people, and some numbers and distant events. She had no problem calculating her checkbook.

Analysis of the History

· What are the major presenting symptoms?
· Where are the CNS lesion(s) likely to be?

CASE 1-3 SYMPTOMS

Symptoms	Location Correlation
Memory slipping	Cerebral cortex
Bradykinesia	Extrapyramidal system
Hyperreflexia	Pyramidal system
Dysarthria	Pyramidal system
Double-vision reading	Convergence system

The analysis guides the clinical examination.

Examination

The neurological examination was essentially unchanged, but there were additional signs.

Additional Neurological Signs

· Disinhibited behavior—inappropriate laughing
· An expressionless akinetic face with her mouth half open
· Head hyperextended (nuchal dystonia)
· Inability to clap three times (the applause sign, frontal lobe sign)
· 1+ jaw jerk and facial jerks consistent with a mild pseudobulbar palsy
· Dysarthria
· Spastic tongue, normal palatal movements and gag reflex

Eyelids

· Infrequent blinking (decreased blink rate)
· Mild blepharoclonus
· Positive glabella tap
· Slow initiation of eyelid opening ("apraxia")

Ocular Motility

- Slow hypometric horizontal saccades—a mixture of extreme hypometria and slowing—slow saccade syndrome
- Supranuclear saccadic paresis of upward gaze with normal vertical pursuit
- Slow saccades on downgaze
- Square-wave jerks (small amplitude (0.5–5 degree) refixation eye movement)
- Absent vertical OKN and horizontal OKN
- Normal saccadic pursuit to a slow-moving target in all directions of gaze
- Normal Bell's reflex
- Normal oculocephalic reflex, horizontal and vertical
- Convergence insufficiency with exophoria at near
- Multiple errors on antisaccade test (frontal lobe function) and poor self-correction of errors

Localization and Differential Diagnosis

This patient has almost all of the ocular motor signs of PSP,[93] the most important of which is *slowing of vertical saccades,* either down, up, or both.[94] In a minority of PSP cases, this sign may fail to appear over the course of the disease,[95] and this should be kept in mind.

Other diagnostic features of PSP are slow hypometric horizontal saccades, selective defects of visual tracking,[96] loss of convergence, and disruption of steady gaze by square-wave jerks. Eyelid disorders include reduced blink rate, blepharospasm, repetitive blinking in response to flashlight stimulus (failure to habituate), and impaired initiation of eyelid opening (apraxia). Late in the disease, the ocular motor deficit may progress to complete ophthalmoplegia.

What Diagnostic Tests Should Follow?

- Brain MRI to evaluate cerebral atrophy

Special Explanatory Note

Atrophy of the rostral midbrain tegmentum (MT) when detected by mid-sagittal MRI looks like the bill of a hummingbird and is referred to as the "hummingbird" sign.[97] In PSP, the sign is due to atrophy of the rostral and caudal midbrain tegmentum and to a relative increase in the length of the interpeduncular fossa over that of the anteroposterior diameter of the midbrain tegmentum. Its presence on MRI helps establish the diagnosis (Figure 1-19).

Measurement of the midbrain tegmentum on midsagittal MRI section is also considered a reliable way of differentiating PSP from other Parkinsonian diseases.[98,99]

MRI

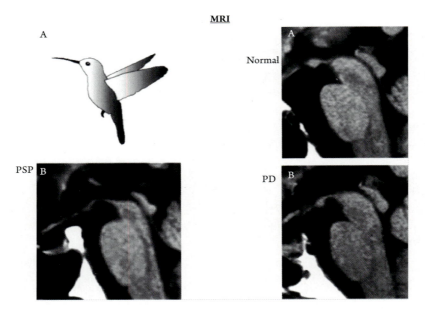

FIGURE 1-19 Brain MRI mid-sagittal plain. (A) Normal control. (B) PSP (Progressive supranuclear palsy), PD (Parkinson's Disease) The region including the most rostral midbrain, the midbrain tegmentum, the pontine base, and the cerebellum appears to correspond to the bill, crown, body, and wing, respectively, of a hummingbird (i.e., the "hummingbird sign").

Reproduced with permission.[98]

Test Results

Brain MRI showed atrophy of the rostral midbrain and tectal plate. A diagnosis of PSP was made.

Special Explanatory Note

Progressive supranuclear palsy is caused by a novel silent mutation in exon 10 of the tau gene and, like frontotemporal dementia, it is a tauopathy.[100] Two distinct phenotypes have been recognized in pathologically proven cases.[101] One is called Richardson's syndrome and is characterized by early falls, cognitive decline, and vertical gaze abnormalities. The second more closely resembles PD, with asymmetric findings, tremor, and some response to treatment with levodopa.

Spatial covariance analysis has been used with (18) F-fluorodeoxyglucose (FDG) positron emission tomography (PET) to identify the disease-related metabolic patterns that can serve as biomarkers in assessing PD, atypical PD, and PSP (Figure 1-20).[102]

FDG PET

PSP-Related Spatial Covariance Pattern

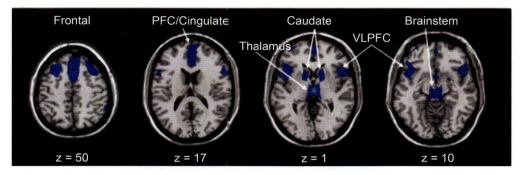

FIGURE 1-20 FDG positron emission tomography (PET): progressive supranuclear palsy (PSP)-related spatial covariance pattern.

Reproduced with permission.[102]

Selective causes of the slow saccade syndrome are shown in Table 1-3.

TABLE 1-3: Causes of the Slow Saccade Syndrome

Spinocerebellar ataxias (SCA) especially SCA2
Huntington's disease
Progressive supranuclear palsy
Parkinson's (advanced cases) and related diseases
Lytico-Bodig syndrome
Whipple's disease
Wilson's disease
Drug intoxications: anticonvulsants and benzodiazepines
Lesions of the paramedical pontine reticular formation
Paraneoplastic syndromes
Amyotrophic lateral sclerosis (some cases)

Reproduced with permission.[2]

Selective Saccadic Palsy

A comparatively rare saccade syndrome, selective saccadic palsy is an unexpected and unexplained complication of cardiac surgery, especially aortic valve replacement.

The case presented here is illustrative.

CASE 1-4 Selective Saccadic Palsy

Video Display

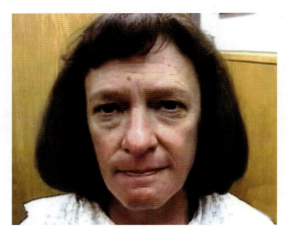

FIGURE 1-21 Fifty-year-old woman with selective saccadic palsy post cardiac surgery.

Courtesy of Scott Eggers, M.D.

The patient is a 50-year-old woman who underwent otherwise uncomplicated aortic valve replacement for an incidentally discovered ascending aortic aneurysm (Figure 1-21). On awakening from anesthesia, she noted difficulty directing her gaze and began using head movements to facilitate gaze shifts. She had no dysarthria, dysphagia, or gait instability. She was discharged and for 3 months had no problems other than her visual complaints. At this time, she developed complex partial seizures that responded to levetiracetam.

On examination 10 months postoperatively, a general neurological examination was notable only for diffuse hyporeflexia. Visual acuity, pupils, visual fields, and funduscopic examination were normal.

Analysis of the History

· What are the major presenting symptoms?
· Where are the CNS lesion(s) likely to be?

CASE 1-4 SYMPTOMS

Symptoms	Location Correlation
Paralysis of horizontal gaze	Pons
Complex partial seizures	Cerebral cortex

The analysis guides the clinical examination.

Examination

Saccadic and Pursuit Eye Movements

- Straight ahead fixation was steady, with no spontaneous saccadic intrusions, square-wave jerks, or nystagmus
- She made no fast volitional or reflexive saccades in any direction
- She made extremely slow eye movements to eventually reach a target, with slightly faster downward saccades
- Pursuit was smooth and of full range horizontally and vertically, even with high frequencies
- OKN testing, horizontal: the eyes pursued the lines and became fixed laterally in the orbits without any corrective quick phases
- OKN testing, vertical: the eyes pursued the lines up and made a few corrective downbeats of nystagmus
- Torsional head rolling produced excellent counter-rolling, but without any torsional quick phases
- With head-free gaze shifts, she had exaggerated head turns associated with blinks and contraversive vestibular slow-phase eye movements that drove the eyes into the corner of the orbits until the head was maximally rotated, and then the eyes continued to slowly drift toward the target
- With head fixed, the eyes made small, slow, hypometric saccades

Localization and Differential Diagnosis

The paralysis of saccadic eye movements following uncomplicated aortic valve replacement passed unnoticed by the clinician even though the patient noted immediately on awakening from anesthesia that she could not direct her gaze without moving her head. The patient had a selective defect of volitional and reflexive saccades with preservation of smooth-pursuit, vestibular, and vergence eye movements.

What Diagnostic Tests Should Follow?

- Brain MRI

Test Results

MRI of the brain showed a focus of increased fluid attenuated inversion recovery (FLAIR) signal and an increased T2 signal in the right dorsomedial pons. The diagnosis of selective saccadic palsy was confirmed. Prognosis for recovery is very poor.

Special Explanatory Note

A number of metabolic, toxic and degenerative disorders may cause selective paralysis of eye movements that suggest a selective cell vulnerabilty and loss of one popultion of key neurons in the brainstem involved in generating eye movements.

To recover from anesthesia unable to move the eyes without having to move the head as well is the signature symptom and sign of selective saccadic palsy following cardiac surgery.[103] It has frequently been missed. The attention paid to it in recent years reveals that few patients show any signs of recovery in the immediate postoperative period.

The clinical severity of the syndrome was documented in 2007 by Solomon et al.[104] who studied ten patients with visual complaints after cardiac or vascular surgery. Some patients' visual complaints were correctly identified as due to a selective saccadic palsy, but others were considered to be psychogenic, and a correct diagnosis was not reached for a year or more.

The extent and nature of the patients' deficits varied. Some were capable of generating slow saccades that carried the eye almost to the target. Others, when their eye movements were recorded using the magnetic search coil technique, made a "staircase" of ten or more small saccades to acquire the target, although clinically this appeared to be one slow, smooth movement. Most often, hypometria was combined with slowing.

The most severely affected patient of the ten had lost all ability to make saccades and quick phases. Nine patients showed slowing of both horizontal and vertical saccades, and slowing of vertical saccades occurred selectively in two. No patient showed slowing of just horizontal saccades. Like children with ocular motor apraxia, these patients developed a strategy of using eye blinks and head thrusts to shift their direction of gaze. Rapid gaze shifts that are achieved by combined, rapid eye-head movements (eye-head saccades or gaze saccades) act to bring the object of interest, detected in the retinal periphery to the fovea where it can be seen best.

The stereotypic clinical picture suggests brainstem ischemia, but Solomon detected no abnormalities in the patients reported. However, in a quite different patient with horizontal saccadic palsy following cardiac surgery who subsequently died of infection, ischemic changes were present in the paramedian pons.

Some of Solomon's patients had neurological findings such as ataxia, seizures, and a PSP-like syndrome in addition to saccadic palsy, and this suggests that other processes may also be involved, for example, intraoperative hypotension or hyperthermia.

SELECTED REFERENCES

1. Carpenter RHS. The visual origins of ocular motility. In: RHS Carpenter, ed. *Eye Movements*, vol. 8. London: Macmillan Press; 1991:1–10.
2. Leigh RJ, Zee DS. *The Neurology of Eye Movements*, 4th ed. New York: Oxford University Press, 2006.

3. Prasad S, Galetta SL. Anatomy and physiology of the afferent visual system. In: Kennard C, Leigh RJ, eds. *Handbook of Clinical Neurology*, chapter 1, 3rd series. Neuro-ophthalmology. New York: Elsevier. 2011;102:3–19.

4. Maunsell JHR, Van Essen DC. Functional properties of neurons in middle temporal visual area of the macaque monkey. I. Selectivity for stimulus direction, speed, and orientation. *J Neurophysiol.* 1983;49:1127–1147.

5. Newsome WT, Wurtz RH, Komatsu H. Relation of cortical areas MT and MST to pursuit eye movements. II. Differentiation of retinal from extraretinal inputs. *J Neurophysiol.* 1988;60:604–620.

6. Büttner U, Ono S, Glasauer S, Mustari MJ, Nuding U. MSTd neurons during ocular following and smooth pursuit perturbation. *Prog Brain Res.* 2008;171:253–260.

7. Wong AMF. *Eye Movement Disorders.* New York: Oxford University Press; 2008:165–177.

8. Paus T, Petrides M, Evans AC, Meyer E. Role of the human anterior cingulate cortex in the control of oculomotor, manual, and speech responses: a positron emission tomography study. *J Neurophysiol.* 1993;70:453–469.

9. Garbutt S, Matlin A, Hellmuth J, Schenk AK, Johnson JK, Rosen H, Dean D, Kramer J, Neuhaus J, Miller BL, Lisberger SG, Boxer AL. Oculomotor function in frontotemporal lobar degeneration, related disorders and Alzheimer's disease. *Brain.* 2008; 131:1268–1281.

10. Boxer AL, Garbutt S, Rankin KP, Hellmuth J, Neuhaus J, Miller BL, Lisberger SG. Medial versus lateral frontal lobe contributions to voluntary saccade control as revealed by the study of patients with frontal lobe degeneration. *J Neurosci.* 2006;26(23):6354–6363.

11. Gaymard B, Rivaud S, Cassarini JF, Ploner C, Pierrot-Deseilligny C. Effects of anterior cingulated cortex lesions on ocular saccades in humans. *Exp Brain Res.* 1998;120:173–183.

12. Milea D, Lehericy S, Rivaud-Pechoux S, Duffau H, Lobel E, Capelle L, Marsault C, Berthoz A, Pierrot-Deseilligny C. Antisaccade deficit after anterior cingulated cortex resection. *Neuroreport.* 2003;14:283–287.

13. Pick A. Uber die Beziehungen der senilen Hirnatrophie zur Aphasie. *Prag Med Wochenschr.* 1892; 17:165–167.

14. McKhann GM, Albert MS, Grossman M, Miller B, Dickson D, Trojanowski JQ. Clinical and pathological diagnosis of frontotemporal dementia: report of the work group on frontotemporal dementia and Pick's disease. *Arch Neurol.* 2001;58:1803–1809.

15. Kertesz A, Hillis A, Munoz DG. Frontotemporal dementia and Pick's disease. *Ann Neurol.* 2003;54(suppl 5):S1–S35.

16. Hallet PE. Primary and secondary saccades to goals defined by instructions. *Vis Res.* 1978;18:1279–1296.

17. Everling S, Fischer B. The antisaccade: a review of basic research and clinical studies. *Neuropsychologia.* 1998;36:885–899.

18. Munoz DP, Everling S. Look away: the anti-saccade task and the voluntary control of eye movements. *Nat Rev Neurosci.* 2004;5:218–228.

19. Guitton D, Buchtel HA, Douglas RM. Frontal lobe lesions in man cause difficulties in suppressing reflexive glances and in generating goal-directed saccades. *Exp Brain Res.* 1985;58:455–472.

20. Pierrot-Deseilligny C, Rivaud S, Gaymard B, Agid Y. Cortical control of reflexive visually-guided saccades. *Brain.* 1991;114:1473–1485.

21. Pierrot-Deseilligny C, Muri RM, Ploner CJ, Gaymard B, Demeret S, Rivaud-Pechoux S. Decisional role of the dorsolateral prefrontal cortex in ocular motor behaviour. *Brain.* 2003;126:1460–1473.

22. Walker R, Husain M, Hodgson TL, Harrison J, Kennard C. Saccadic eye movement and working memory deficits following damage to human prefrontal cortex. *Neuropsychologia.* 1998;36:1141–1159.

23. Connolly JD, Goodale MA, Menon RS, Munoz DP. Human fMRI evidence for the neural correlates of preparatory set. *Nat Neurosci.* 2002;5:1345–1352.

24. Curtis CE, D'Esposito M. Success and failure suppressing reflexive behavior. *J Cogn Neurosci.* 2003;15:409–418.

25. Ford KA, Goltz HC, Brown MR, Everling S. Neural processes associated with antisaccade task performance investigated with event-related fMRI. *J Neurophysiol.* 2005;94(1):429–440.

26. Bogousslavsky J, Regli F. Pursuit gaze defects in acute and chronic unilateral parieto-occipital lesions. *Eur Neurol.* 1986;25:10–18.

27. Morrow MJ. Craniotopic defects of smooth pursuit and saccadic eye movement. *Neurology.* 1996;46:514–521.

28. Husain M, Mannan S, Hodgson T, Wojciulik E, Driver J, Kennard C. Impaired spatial working memory across saccades contributes to abnormal search in parietal neglect. *Brain.* 2001;124:941–952.

29. Balint R. Seelenlahmung des "Schauens," optische Ataxie, raumliche Storung der Aufmerksamkeit. *Monatsschr Psychiatr Neurol.* 1909;25:51–181.

30. Goodglass H, Kaplan E. *The Assessment of Aphasia and Related Disorders,* 2nd ed. Philadelphia, PA: Lippincott Williams & Wilkins, Lea & Febiger; 1983.

31. Luria AR, Pravdina-Vinarskaya EN, Yarbus AL. Disturbances of ocular movement in a case of simultanagnosia. *Brain.* 1962;86:219–228.

32. Holmes G. Disturbances of visual orientation. *Br J Ophthalmol.* 1918;2:449–468, 506–516.

33. Bartin JJ. Disorders of higher visual processing. In: Kennard C, Leigh RJ, eds. *Handbook of Clinical Neurology,* chapter 9 (3rd series). Neuro-ophthalmology. New York: Elsevier; 2011:102:223–261.

34. Malcolm GL, Barton JJ. "Sequence agnosia" in Balint's syndrome: defects in visuotemporal processing after bilateral parietal damage. *J Cogn Neurosci.* 2007;19:102–108.

35. Yapici Z. Subacute sclerosing panencephalitis presenting with Balint's syndrome. *Brain Dev.* 2006;28:398–400.

36. Iizuka O, Soma Y, Otsuki M, Endo K, Tanno Y, Tsuji S. Posterior cortical atrophy with incomplete Balint's syndrome. *No To Shinkei.* 1997;49(9):841–845.

37. Holmes G, Horrax G. Disturbances of spatial orientation and visual attention, with loss of stereoscopic vision. *Arch Neurol Psychiat.* 1919;1:385–407.

38. Barton JJ, Sharpe JA, Raymond JE. Directional defects in pursuit and motion perception in humans with unilateral cerebral lesions. *Brain.* 1996;119:1535–1550.

39. Cooper SA, Joshi AC, Seenan PJ, Hadley DM, Muir KW, Leigh RJ, Metcalfe RA. Akinetopsia: acute presentation and evidence for persisting defects in motion vision. *J Neurol Neurosurg Psychiat.* 2012;83(2):229–230.

40. Shipp S, de Jong BM, Zihl J, Frackowiak RSJ, Zedi S. The brain activity related to residual motion vision in a patient with bilateral lesions of V5. *Brain.* 1994;117:1023–1038.

41. May PJ. The mammalian superior colliculus: laminar structure and connections. *Prog Brain Res.* 2006;151:321–380.

42. Moschovakis AK, Karabelas AB, Highstein SM. Structure-function relationships in the primate superior colliculus. I. Morphological classification of efferent neurons. *J Neurophysiol.* 1988;60:232–262.

43. Sparks DL, Hartwich-Young R. The deep layers of the superior colliculus. In: Wurtz RH, Goldberg ME, eds. *The Neurobiology of Saccadic Eye Movements.* Amsterdam: Elsevier; 1989:213–255.

44. Büttner-Ennever JA, Horn AK, Henn V, Cohen B. Projections from the superior colliculus motor map to omnipause neurons in monkey. *J Comp Neurol.* 1999;413:55–67.

45. Takahashi M, Sugiuchi Y, Izawa Y, Shinoda Y. Commissural excitation and inhibition by the superior colliculus in tectoreticular neurons projecting to omnipause neuron and inhibitory burst neuron regions. *J Neurophysiol.* 2005;94(3):1707–1726.

46. Sugiuchi Y, Izawa Y, Takahashi M, Na J, Shinoda Y. Physiological characterization of synaptic inputs to inhibitory burst neurons from the rostral and caudal superior colliculus. *J Neurophysiol.* 2005;93(2):697–712.

47. Shinoda Y, Sugiuchi Y, Izawa Y, Takahashi M. Neural circuits for triggering saccades in the brainstem. *Prog Brain Res.* 2008;171:79–85.

48. Walton MM, Mays LE. Discharge of saccade-related superior colliculus neurons during saccades accompanied by vergence. *J Neurophysiol.* 2003;90:1124–1139.

49. Optican LM. Sensorimotor transformation for visually guided saccades. *Ann NY Acad Sci.* 2005;1039:132–148.

50. Arend I, Machado L, Ward R, McGrath M, Ro T, Rafal RD. The role of the human pulvinar in visual attention and action: evidence from temporal-order judgment, saccade decision, and antisaccade tasks. *Prog Brain Res.* 2008;171:475–483.

51. Lauwereyns J, Takikawa Y, Kawagoe R, Kobayashi S, Koizumi M, Coe B, Sakagami M, Hikosaka O. Feature-based anticipation of cues that predict reward in monkey caudate nucleus. *Neuron.* 2002;33:463–473.

52. Takikawa Y, Kawagoe R, Hikosaka O. Reward-dependent spatial selectivity of anticipatory activity in monkey caudate neurons. *J Neurophysiol.* 2002;87:508–515.
53. Harting JK, Updyke BV. Oculomotor-related pathways of the basal ganglia. *Prog Brain Res.* 2006;151:441–460.
54. Rivaud-Pechoux S, Vermersch AI, Gaymard B, Ploner CJ, Bejjani BP, Damier P, Demeret S, Agid Y, Pierrot-Deseilligny C. Improvement of memory guided saccades in parkinsonian patients by high frequency subthalamic nucleus stimulation. *J Neurol Neurosurg Psychiat.* 2000;68(3):381–384.
55. Lasker AG, Zee DS, Hain TC, Folstein SE, Singer HS. Saccades in Huntington's disease: initiation defects and distractability. *Neurology.* 1987;37:364–370.
56. Petit L, Haxby JV. Functional anatomy of pursuit eye movements in humans as revealed by fMRI. *J Neurophysiol.* 1999;82:463–471.
57. Dürsteler MR, Wurtz RH. Pursuit and optokinetic deficits following chemical lesions of cortical areas MT and MST. *J Neurophysiol.* 1988;60:940–965.
58. Tusa RJ, Ungerleider L. Fiber pathways of cortical areas mediating smooth pursuit eye movements in monkeys. *Ann Neurol.* 1988;23:174–183.
59. Glickstein M, Gerrits N, Kralj-Hans I, Mercier B, Stein J, Voogd J. Visual pontocerebellar projections in the macaque. *J Comp Neurol.* 1994;349:51–72.
60. Langer T, Fuchs AF, Chubb MC, Scudder CA, Lisberger SG. Floccular efferents in the rhesus macaque as revealed by autoradiography and horseradish peroxidase. *J Comp Neurol.* 1985; 235:26–37.
61. Bittencourt PRM, Wade P, Smith AT, Richens A. Benzodiazepines impair smooth pursuit eye movements. *Br J Clin Pharmacol.* 1983;15:259–262.
62. Bittencourt PRM, Gresty MA, Richens A. Quantitative assessment of smooth-pursuit eye movements in healthy and epileptic subjects. *J Neurol Neurosurg Psychiat.* 1980;43:1119–1124.
63. DeKort PLM, Gielen G, Tijssen CC, Declerck AC. The influence of antiepileptic drugs on eye movements. *Neuro-ophthalmology.* 1990;10:59–68.
64. Schalen L, Pyykkö I, Korttila K, Magnusson M, Enbom H. Effects of intravenously given barbiturate and diazepam on eye motor performance in man. *Adv Oto-Rhino-Laryngol.* 1988;42:260–264.
65. Levy DL, Dorus E, Shaughnessy R Pharmacologic evidence for specificity of pursuit dysfunction to schizophrenia. Lithium carbonate associated with abnormal smooth pursuit. *Arch Gen Psychiat.* 1985;42:335–341.
66. Baloh RW, Sharma S, Moskowitz H, Griffith R. Effect of alcohol and marijuana on eye movements. *Aviat Space Environ Med.* 1979;50:18–23.
67. Avila MT, Sherr JD, Hong E, Myers CS, Thaker GK. Effects of nicotine on leading saccades during smooth pursuit eye movements in smokers and non-smokers with schizophrenia. *Neuropsychopharmacology.* 2003;28:2184–2191.
68. Rothenberg SJ, Shottenfeld S, Selkoe D, Gross K. Specific oculomotor deficit after acute methadone. II. Smooth pursuit eye movements. *Psychopharmacology.* 1980;67:229–234.
69. Levy DL, Lipton RB, Holzman PS. Smooth pursuit eye movements: effects of alcohol and chloral hydrate. *J Psychiat Res.* 1981;16:1–11.
70. Magnusson M, Padoan S, Ornhagen H. Evaluation of smooth pursuit and voluntary saccades in nitrous oxide induced narcosis. *Aviat Space Environ Med* 1989;60:977–982.
71. Enright JT. Perspective vergence: ocular motor responses to line drawings. *Vis Res.* 1987;27:1513–1526.
72. Wick B, Bedell HE. Magnitude and velocity of proximal vergence. *Invest Ophthalmol Vis Sci.* 1989;28:883–896.
73. McLin IN, Schor CM. Changing size (lumining) as a stimulus to accommodation and vergence. *Vis Res.* 1988;28:883–896.
74. Erkelens CJ, Collewijn H. Control of vergence: gaiting among disparity inputs by voluntary target selection. *Exp Brain Res.* 1991;87:671–678.
75. Owens DA, Leibowitz HW. Perceptual and motor consequences of tonic vergence. In: Schor CM, Ciuffreda KJ, eds. *Vergence Eye Movements: Basic and Clinical Aspects.* Boston: Butterworths; 1983:25–74.
76. Serra A, Chen AL, Leigh RJ. Disorders of vergence eye movements. [Review] *Curr Opin Neurol.* 2011;24(1):32–37.

77. Zhang Y, Gamlin PDR, Mays LE. Antidromic identification of midbrain near response cells projecting to the oculomotor nucleus. *Exp Brain Res.* 1991;84:525–528.

78. Gamlin PDR. Neural mechanisms for the control of vergence eye movements. *Ann NY Acad Sci.* 2002;956:264–272.

79. Zhang H, Gamlin PDR. Neurons in the posterior interposed nucleus of the cerebellum related to vergence and accommodation. I. Steady-state characteristics. *J Neurophysiol.* 1998;79:1255–1269.

80. Rambold H, Kompf D, Helmchen C. Convergence retraction nystagmus: a disorder of vergence? *Ann Neurol.* 2001;50:677–681.

81. Griffin JF, Wray SH, Anderson DP. Misdiagnosis of spasm of the near reflex. *Neurology.* 1976;26(11):1018–1020.

82. Horton JC, Fishman RA. Neurovisual findings in the syndrome of spontaneous intracranial hypotension from dural cerebrospinal fluid leak [abstract]. *Ophthalmology.* 1994;101:244–251.

83. Robinson DA. Models of the saccadic eye movement control system. *Kybernetik.* 1973;14:71–83.

84. Robinson DA. Oculomotor control signals. In: Lennerstrand G, Bach-y-Rita P, eds. *Basic Mechanisms of Ocular Motility and Their Clinical Implications.* Oxford: Pergamon; 1975:337–374.

85. Sharpe JA, Wong AM. Anatomy and physiology of ocular motor systems. In: Miller NR, Newman NJ, Biousse V, Kerrison JB, eds. *Walsh and Hoyt's Clinical Neuro-ophthalmology,* 6th ed. Philadelphia: Lippincott Williams & Wilkins; 2005:809–885.

86. Leigh RJ, Zee DS. With permission 2013.

87. Rucker JC, Ying SH, Moore W, Optican LM, Buttner-Ennever J, Keller EL, Shapiro BE, Leigh RJ. Do brainstem omnipause neurons terminate saccades? *Ann NY Acad Sci.* 2011;1233:48–57.

88. Strassman A, Highstein SM, McCrea RA. Anatomy and physiology of saccadic burst neurons in the alert squirrel monkey. I. Excitatory burst neurons. *J Comp Neurol.* 1986;249:337–357.

89. Keller EL, Heinen SJ. Generation of smooth pursuit eye movements: neuronal mechanisms and pathways. *Neurosci Res.* 1991;11:79–107.

90. Büttner U, Büttner-Ennever JA. Present concepts of oculomotor organization. In: Büttner-Ennever JA, ed. *Progress in Brain Research.* Chapter 1. Neuroanatomy of the Oculomotor System. Amsterdam: Elsevier BV 2006:151, 1–42.

91. Rucker JC, Shapiro BE, Han YH, Kumar AN, Garbutt S, Keller EL, Leigh RJ. Neuro-ophthalmology of late-onset Tay-Sach's disease (LOTS). *Neurology.* 2004;63(10):1918–1926.

92. Abel LA, Troost BT, Dell'Osso LF. Saccadic trajectories change with amplitude, not time. *Neuro-ophthalmology.* 1987;7:309–314.

93. Friedman DI, Jankovic J, McCrary JA. Neuro-ophthalmic findings in progressive supranuclear palsy. *J Clin Neuro-ophthalmol.* 1992;12(2):104–109.

94. Richardson JC, Steele J, Olszewski J. Supranuclear ophthalmoplegia, pseudobulbar palsy, nuchal dystonia and dementia. A clinical report on eight cases of heterogenous system degeneration. *Trans Am Neurol Assoc.* 1963;88:25–29.

95. Daniel SE, De Bruin VM, Lees AJ. The clinical and pathological spectrum of Steele-Richardson-Olszewski syndrome (progressive supranuclear palsy): a reappraisal. *Brain.* 1995;118:759–770.

96. Joshi AC, Riley DE, Mustari MJ, Cohen ML, Leigh RJ. Selective defects of visual tracking in progressive supranuclear palsy (PSP): implications for mechanisms of motion vision. *Vis Res.* 2010;50(8):761–771.

97. Iwata M. Humming-bird appearance of mid-brain in MRI of progressive supranuclear palsy. Annual Report of the Research Committee of CNS Degenerative Diseases. The Minister of Health and Welfare of Japan; Osaka University. 1994: 48–50.

98. Kato N, Arai K, Hattori T. Study of the rostral midbrain atrophy in progressive supranuclear palsy. *J Neurol Sci.* 2003;210(1–2):57–60.

99. Oba H, Yagishita A, Terada H, Barkovich AJ, Kutomi K, Yamauchi T, Furui S, Shimizu T, Uchigata M, Matsumura K, Sonoo M, Sakai M, Takada K, Harasawa A, Takeshita K, Kohtake H, Tanaka H, Suzuki S. New and reliable MRI diagnosis for progressive supranuclear palsy. *Neurology.* 2005;64(12):2050–2055.

100. Stanford PM, Halliday GM, Brooks WS, Kwok JB, Storey CE, Creasey H, Morris JG, Fulham MJ, Schofield PR. Progressive supranuclear palsy pathology caused by a novel silent mutation in exon 10 of the tau gene: expansion of the disease phenotype caused by tau gene mutations. *Brain.* 2000;123(Pt 5):880–893.

101. Williams DR, deSilva R, Paviour DC, Pittman A, Watt HC, Kilford L, Holton JL, Revesz T, Lees AJ. Characteristics of two distinct clinical phenotypes in pathologically proven progressive supranuclear palsy: Richardson's syndrome and PSP-parkinsonism. *Brain.* 2005;128(Pt 6):1247–1258.

102. Eckert T, Tang C, Ma Y, Brown N, Lin T, Frucht S, Feigin A, Eidelberg D. Abnormal metabolic networks in atypical parkinsonism. *Mov Disord.* 2008;23(5):727–733.

103. Eggers SD, Moster ML, Cranmer K. Selective saccadic palsy after cardiac surgery. *Neurology.* 2008;SA70(4):318–320.

104. Solomon D, Ramat S, Tomsak RL, Reich SG, Shin RK, Zee DS, Leigh RJ. Saccadic palsy after cardiac surgery: characteristics and pathogenesis. *Ann Neurol.* 2008;63(3):355–365.

| 2 |
THE EYELID AND ITS SIGNS

The muscles of the eyelid are the levator palpebrae (LP) superioris, Müller's muscles, and the orbicularis oculi (OOc). The LP a skeletal muscle, is responsible for upper eyelid opening. The LP contains red fast-twitch and intermediate-twitch muscle fibers, both of which exhibit high mitochondrial content and low intermediate fatigability, and it also contains a unique type of slow-twitch fiber.[1]

The fast-twitch fibers are well equipped for the rapid changes in lid position necessary at the end of a blink, whereas the slow-twitch fibers are capable of maintaining sustained eyelid elevation. Fast-twitch fibers probably play a role in the generation of lid saccades.

The LP is innervated by the superior branch of the third cranial nerve (the oculomotor nerve). Motoneurons activating the LP are located in a single unpaired midline central caudal nucleus (CCN) of the oculomotor complex in the midbrain. The CCN sits between the caudal pole of the oculomotor nucleus and the rostral pole of the fourth cranial nerve (trochlear) nucleus. The motoneurons of the LPs of both eyes intermingle within the unpaired CCN, hence a lesion of the CCN affects both eyelids (see Chapter 5).

The upper and lower lid tarsal muscles, more precisely *Müller's muscles*, are lid retractors and regulate the width of the palpebral fissure. They play only a minor role in lid opening. Müller's upper lid muscle inserts on the superior border of the upper tarsal plate and is innervated by the oculosympathetic pathway.[2] A similar, much smaller sympathetically innervated smooth muscle is located in the lower eyelid[3,4] (Figure 2-1).

Eyelid lowering during downgaze and gentle eyelid closure during sleep are mediated by passive downward forces. Ligaments and connective tissue, stretched during upgaze, are relaxed by inhibition of the LP.

Two further muscles innervated by the facial nerve act on the eyelid: *the frontalis muscle*, which helps to retract the lid in extreme upward gaze by elevation of the eyebrow, and the muscles.

The OOc is organized in concentric circles around the orbital margins of the eye and acts like a sphincter muscle. The muscle fiber of the OOc is designed for its principal functional task, which is rapid eye closure during blinking,[1] and it is the only muscle capable of eliciting eyelid closure. As such, it is a direct antagonist of the LP (Figure 2-2).[5-8] When the LP is synchronously inhibited, different parts of the OOc contract to control spontaneous and voluntary blinks, reflex blinking, and rapid vigorous eyelid closure in protective and expressive acts like sneezing.

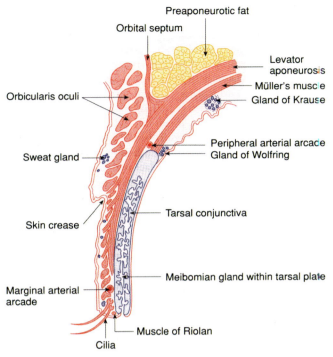

FIGURE 2-1 Cross-section of the upper eyelid.

Reproduced with permission.[4]

The motoneurons activating the frontalis and the OOc muscles reside in the dorsal subnucleus of the facial nerve nucleus. This nucleus lies within the caudal third of the pontine tegmentum, with the result that gentle eye closure and lid-eye coordination are unaffected by facial nerve palsy, whereas blinking and firm eye closure are impossible.

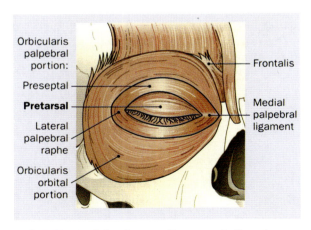

FIGURE 2-2 Orbicularis oculi anatomy in frontal view demonstrating the orbital, preseptal and pretarsal segments.

Reproduced with permission.[8]

The general organization of the lower lid is similar to that of the upper eyelid; however, there is no extraocular muscle for moving the lower lid as the LP specifically does for the upper. Sensory innervation of the eyelids is provided via the first (ophthalmic, VI) and second (maxillary, V2) division of the trigeminal nerve (cranial nerve [CN] V).

A synopsis of the innervation and action of eyelid muscles is shown in Table 2-1.

Voluntary lid opening and closure result from the reciprocal action of the LP and OOc muscles. Relaxation of the LP and contraction of the OOc cause closure and the reverse action of these muscles opens closed lids. Lid opening is also aided by Müller's muscle. Dysfunction of the LP and OOc can manifest itself as an inability to initiate lid opening or lid closure or difficulty in sustaining lid closure (motor impersistence).[9]

With fatigue, the lids lower involuntarily. During sleep, including rapid eye movement (REM) phases and in disorders such as myasthenia gravis, when the levator is severely affected, LP activity completely ceases and the eyes close.

This close relationship of lid position with the level of arousal suggests that the CCN receives additional input from other sources. For example, the periaqueductal gray (PAG) receives afferent input from the limbic system, and orexin-containing neurons in the lateral posterior hypothalamus are known to be involved in the maintenance of wakefulness.[10] These neurons may also play a role in levels of emotional arousal.

TABLE 2-1: Synopsis: Innervation and Action of Eyelid Muscles

	Motor Neurons	Nerve	Action
Levator palpebrae superioris (LP)	Single midline central caudal nucleus of the third cranial nerve (oculomotor) nucleus in the midbrain	Superior branch of the third nerve	Acts alone to elevate the eyelid
Superior tarsal muscle, Müller's muscle	Oculosympathetic neurons	Sympathetic efferents	Regulates the width of the palpebral fissure
Frontalis muscle	Dorsal subnucleus of the facial nerve nucleus within the caudal third of the pons	Facial nerve	Raises the eyebrow and, in extreme upward gaze, the upper eyelid
Orbicularis oculi (OOc)	Dorsal subnucleus of the facial nerve nucleus within the caudal third of the pons	Facial nerve	Actively closes the eyelids Different parts of the orbicularis oculi contract when the levator is synchronously inhibited to control spontaneous and voluntary blinks, reflex blinking, and rapid vigorous eyelid closure

Reproduced with permission.[36]

LID–EYE COORDINATION

Lid–eye coordination is an extremely fine-tuned movement controlled by a complex network of premotor neurons in the midbrain, connecting one with the other to enable a tight coupling of upward lid movements with upward saccadic eye movements. This *premotor area*, the *M-group*, is distinct from, and just medial to, the rostral interstitial nucleus of the medial longitudinal fasciculus (riMLF), the interstitial nucleus of Cajal (INC), the PAG, and the nuclei of the posterior commissure (nPC).[11,12] The M-group's location and the activating or inhibiting interconnecting pathways are important aids to the topographical localization of lesions (Figure 2-3).

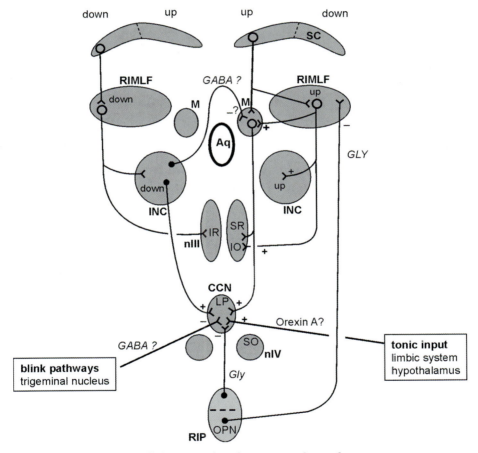

FIGURE 2-3 Pathways of lid-eye coupling during vertical saccades.

Reproduced with permission.[11]

The M-Group

The M-group cluster of cells in the mesencephalon receives excitatory projections from the superior colliculus (SC) and projects to the motoneurons of the LP in the CCN and to the superior rectus (SR) muscle and inferior oblique (IO) muscle in the third nerve nucleus.[13] It receives inputs from the areas in the SC that mediate upward saccades, and, in addition, the M-group receives afferent inputs from the vestibular nuclei, the INC, riMLF, and nPC. The INC neurons are activated by saccadic burst neurons from the riMLF and may convey an integrated position signal to motoneurons of the SR and IO, and to the LP motoneurons in the CCN.

This network of connections enables the M-group to excite the CCN to activate the LP to elevate the eyelid and to activate the motoneurons in the subnuclei of the SR and IO in the third-nerve nucleus to simultaneously contract and move the eye upward. Upward lid saccades, unlike eye saccades, do not occur in one smooth rapid motion. Rather, the initial lid movement is abrupt, reaching maximum velocity at the same time as the eye saccade, but it then slows down and glides to its final position in a movement visible at the termination of a saccade.[14,15]

Conjugate bilateral lid elevation on upgaze is achieved as a result of the intermingling of LP motoneurons for both eyes within the unpaired CCN and to single motoneurons in the CCN innervating both LPs. The CCN also receives additional input from the nPC, riMLF, and INC, and it is possible that during upgaze movements the M-group may receive a copy of the burst signal from excitatory up-burst neurons generating upward saccades in the riMLF. These reciprocal connections enable tight coordination of upward lid movements with upward saccades and supports the hypothesis that the M-group mediates lid–eye coordination during vertical upgaze.[11]

There are no parallel pathways from the M-group to motoneurons for downward-pulling eye muscles (the superior oblique [SO] and inferior rectus [IR] muscles). Thus, there must be a different premotor control of lid and eye movement during downward saccades. Horn suggests that inhibition of the M-group and LP motoneurons by neurons in the INC projecting to the M-group causes the passive relaxation of the LP that occurs with downward lid saccades during downward eye movements.*

■ **Clinical Points to Remember About Neuromuscular Control of the Eyelid**

- The LP acts alone to elevate the eye lid.
- Voluntary lid opening and closure results from the reciprocal action of the LP and OOc.
- The LP motoneurons are located in the single unpaired midline CCN of the third-nerve nuclear complex in the midbrain.
- Motoneurons activating the OOc muscles are located in the dorsal subnucleus of the facial nerve nucleus in the pons.
- The PAG receives afferent input from the limbic system and plays a role in the level of arousal.
- The M-group, a cluster of cells in the mesencephalon, is the site of premotor control of lid–eye coordination during upgaze.
- The M-group projects to the CCN to activate the LP to elevate the lid and to the subnuclei of the SR and IO muscles to move the eye upward.
- The M-group is inhibited during downgaze.
- Conjugate bilateral lid elevation is achieved by intermingling of LP motoneurons within the unpaired CCN. ■

---

* I am indebted to Dr. Anja K. E. Horn for her review of this section and permission to publish the anatomical figures, and to Dr. Jean A. Büttner-Ennever for permission to publish a number of anatomical figures in this book.

Bell's Phenomenon

Movement of the eyes, especially vertical movements, often accompany eye closure. This is *Bell's phenomenon* or *Bell's reflex*, first reported by Bell in 1823.[16] Bell's reflex is present in roughly 50% of the normal population, with the other 50% exhibiting slow tonic downward deviation during prolonged lid closure.[17,18] Bell's reflex does not occur with a blink because each eye typically rotates downward and nasally during a blink[19–20] and does so with a slower velocity than that of saccadic eye movements.[21,22] In the presence of a supranuclear upgaze palsy, Bell's reflex is intact and the eyes roll upward under tightly closed lids.[23] This is a valuable clinical diagnostic distinction because Bell's reflex is absent in patients with bilateral age-related upgaze palsy.

THE EYELID IN COMA

A new coma scale that takes the eyelid in coma into account is now used to grade the depth of coma. The Full Outline of Unresponsiveness (FOUR) score, has four testable components: eye responses (eye opening and eye movements), brainstem reflexes (pupil, corneal, and cough reflexes), motor responses, and respiration.[24–26]

The position of the eyelid in coma is determined by the tone of the LP muscle. In the unconscious state, the activity of the LP usually ceases (as in sleep), and the lids stay closed, although some unresponsive patients may occasionally continue to open and close their eyes and blink spontaneously. Terms used to describe this latter state include *akinetic mutism* and *coma vigil*. Akinetic mutism refers to a state in which the patient, although seemingly awake, remains silent and motionless[27] even though frontal release signs such as grasp or sucking may be present. The same term has been applied to the vegetative state, a rare state of apparent vigilance in an imperceptive and unresponsive patient.

Rarely, comatose patients maintain constantly open unblinking eyes (spastic eyes) due to failure of LP inhibition.[28] When manually closed, the lids promptly spring open and never close spontaneously, giving the impression of wakefulness. Spastic eyes can persist for as long as 6 months or until death finally intervenes. One reported case at autopsy showed massive infarction of almost all of the pontine tegmentum extending to the upper medulla. The midbrain tegmentum, pretectum, and diencephalon were normal.

The FOUR coma scale describing only the eyelid and brainstem reflexes is as follows

Eyelid response, grades 4–0:
- 4 = eyelids open or opened, tracking, or blinking to command
- 3 = eyelids open but not tracking
- 2 = eyelids closed but open to loud voice
- 1 = eyelids closed but open to pain
- 0 = eyelids remain closed to pain

Brainstem reflexes, grades 4–0:

- 4 = pupil and corneal reflexes present
- 3 = one pupil wide and fixed
- 2 = pupil or corneal reflexes absent
- 1 = pupil and corneal reflexes absent
- 0 = pupil, corneal, and cough reflexes absent

Locked-In Syndrome

A condition that can mimic coma, but which should be carefully distinguished from it, is the *locked-in syndrome*, a term introduced by Plum and Posner[29] to describe a condition characterized by anarthria, spastic quadriparesis, and intact consciousness. It is caused by complete occlusion of the basilar artery and destruction of the ventral portion of the pons. In these patients, useful voluntary blinks play an important role because a voluntary blink may be the patient's only means of communication.[30] In the everyday world of the intensive care unit, a patient suspected of possibly being "locked-in" should be instructed to blink once for Yes and twice for No in answer to direct questions, for instance, "Are you in pain"?

An extraordinary example of this condition is the story of Jean-Dominique Bauby, editor-in-chief of the French magazine *Elle*, who suffered a stroke with locked-in syndrome when he was 43 and was left with his right eye sutured closed but able to blink with his left. By blinking to identify letters, Bauby rearranged the alphabet, placing each letter according to its use-frequency in French. He called this alphabet his "chorus line," and started it with the letters E, S, A, R, I, N, T. Using this system, a visitor would read off the ESA alphabet (not ABC) until a blink of Bauby's eye stopped her at the letter to be noted. The process was repeated so that a whole word and then fragments of intelligible sentences were formed. Using this incredibly laborious technique, Bauby was able to compose a stunningly eloquent memoir, *Le Scaphandre et le Papillon* (The Diving Bell and the Butterfly).

Reports of locked-in syndromes due to infarcts of the midbrain are not common.[31–33] In one case, magnetic resonance imaging (MRI) showed bilateral infarcts in the middle and lateral portions of the cerebral peduncle that were attributed to thrombosis of the rostral basilar artery.

POSITION OF THE EYES IN COMA

The position of the comatose patient's eyes should always be documented by the examiner.

Sustained Upgaze

Sustained upward gaze in coma is a rare phenomenon that Miller Fisher regarded as indicating an intact upper brainstem. However, sustained upgaze in coma is a confusing sign that is, often interpreted as evidence of focal midbrain damage. In a report of 17 comatose patients with sustained upward gaze deviation (following cardiac arrest in 15 patients and prolonged systemic hypotension in 2 patients), autopsy findings confirmed the expected diffuse cerebral and cerebellar damage, with no focal lesions found in the upper midbrain or pretectum. The author concluded that persistent upgaze in coma is usually a result of severe hypoxic encephalopathy.[34]

Setting Sun Sign

Acute tonic deviation of the eyes downward—the "setting sun" sign—is an important sign of progressive and acute hydrocephalus. It is prominent in premature infants who have suffered intraventricular hemorrhage, and, in these cases, the sustained downward gaze cannot be driven above the horizontal meridian by the vertical doll's head maneuver. Sustained downgaze in coma is also seen in adult patients with thalamic hemorrhage complicated by hydrocephalus (Chapter 7).

Spontaneous eye movements, as well as eye movements induced by head rotation and cold-water calorics, are a documentable part of the examination of a comatose patient. The role of the oculocephalic or "doll's head" response and the vestibulo-ocular reflex (VOR) in determining the location and nature of the disease process causing coma are discussed in Chapter 6.

PERSISTENT EYELID CLOSURE

Patients with *persistent eye closure* are a diagnostic challenge—their eyes stay closed as if asleep and yet they are not. Two cases of persistent eye closure have been reported in patients with paraneoplastic anti-Ma2 associated encephalitis, and they provide insight into failure to open the eyes.[35]

Case 1 presented with lethargy, loss of libido, diabetes insipidus, and hypothyroidism progressing to a state of complete immobility and severe spasticity and rigidity. The patient stopped speaking and eating. He had prominent excessive daytime sleepiness (EDS). He was able to respond to thumbs up or down with good accuracy when answering autobiographic questions. Brain MRI showed bilateral abnormalities involving the hippocampi, amygdala, midbrain (substantia nigra), internal capsule, and globus pallidi.

Case 2 presented with loss of self-confidence, an unexplained sense of fear, diplopia, and EDS (with low cerebrospinal fluid hypocretin levels). He kept his eyes continually closed. Attempts by the examiner to open this patient's eyes elicited reflex blepharospasm. When prompted to speak, he barely moved his lips and spoke with inaudible hypophonia. Despite the appearance of being asleep, he was able to promptly follow commands such as raising his arms or standing up from a chair. He had the short-step gait seen in Parkinson's disease (PD). The initial MRI showed bilateral abnormalities involving the hippocampi, dorsal mesencephalon, and colliculi. Follow-up MRI revealed additional abnormalities in the medial thalami. He died as a result of progressive neurological deterioration 12 months after developing this neurological syndrome. No autopsy was obtained.

Interestingly, at the time of World War I (1914–1918), a unique epidemic of "encephalitis lethargica" was reported in which patients slept for long periods, sometimes until death. Examination of the brains of these patients at autopsy showed damage in the posterior hypothalamus.

Recent research has shown that neurons in the posterior lateral hypothalamus produce peptides called *orexins* (also known as hypocretins). These orexin neurons excite both the brainstem and hypothalamic arousal systems, which are crucial for the awake state. The ventrolateral perioptic area of the anterior hypothalamus inhibit neurons in the ascending activating systems, including posterior hypothalamic orexin neurons, reducing their activity in non-REM sleep and further depressing the activity of the brainstem and hypothalamic arousal systems (Figure 2-4).[36]

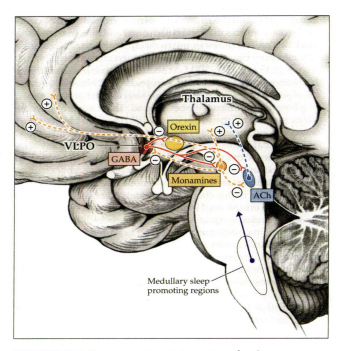

FIGURE 2-4 Brainstem circuits important for sleep regulation. During non-rapid eye movement (REM) sleep, GABAergic (and galanin) neurons in the ventral lateral preoptic area of the anterior hypothalamus inhibit neurons in the ascending activating systems, including posterior hypothalamic orexin neurons, monamines such as histamine (in the tuberomammillary nucleus, not shown), serotonin, noradrenalin, and dopamine, as well as brainstem cholinergics (Ach). Certain regions of the medulla may also play a role in promoting non-REM sleep. During REM sleep, monamine transmitters, particularly noradrenalin and serotonin, are further reduced. This contributes to increased cholinergic inputs to the thalamus and electroencephalographic appearance of arousal. Pontine circuits include mutually inhibitory REM-on and REM-off cells, as well as neurons that inhibit tonic muscle activity during REM dream states.

Reproduced with permission.[36]

BLINKS AND BLINK REFLEXES

Spontaneous, voluntary, and reflex blinks all arise from a common set of muscle activations and inactivations. Most types of blinks share the basic blink mechanisms in which the down phase of a blink, unassociated with gaze changes, is produced by abrupt inhibition of the LP motoneurons, which cease firing to allow the eyes to close. This is followed by a short burst of activity in the normally quiescent OOc—a pulse similar to that of a saccade—causing active OOc contraction and lid closure. Once momentary closure of the eyelids is over, OOc activity stops and the up-phase is produced by resumed tonic activity in the LP motoneurons with resulting lid opening. In firm eye closure, the OOc activity precedes and outlasts LP inhibition. During lid movement associated with gaze changes, the LP plays an active role and the OOc a passive role.

Spontaneous Blinking

Spontaneous blinking is controlled by the extrapyramidal system, specifically through the nigro-collicular pathway, and is highly dependent on dopaminergic transmission. The substantia nigra pars reticulata (SNR) in the basal ganglia provides tonic inhibition of the SC, and the SC provides tonic inhibition of blinking. The spontaneous blink rate on average is 19 blinks per minute in women and 11 blinks per minute in men. Normal individuals have an inherent rhythm and blink rate.

In PD, blink rates are decreased due to dopamine depletion, which decreases the inhibitory effect of the striatum on the SNR, which in turn increases SNR inhibition of the SC. This decreases the spontaneous blink rate while simultaneously increasing blink reflex excitability.[37] In schizophrenic patients with excessive levels of dopamine, the spontaneous blink rate is increased.

Voluntary Blinking

Voluntary blinking is the result of a conscious decision to close and open the eyes. Voluntary blinks can facilitate the ability to initiate saccades,[38] speed up slow saccades,[39] or induce saccadic oscillations.[40] The facilitation of a saccadic eye movement by a blink, an interaction termed *blink-saccadic synkineses*, is probably due to the modulation of omnipause neurons (OPNs) lying in the pontine reticular formation. Omnipause neurons are tonically active neurons that cease firing during a blink and before all saccadic movements for a period equal to the duration of the saccadic movement.[41]

The Corneal Reflex

The corneal reflex (CR) involves both the trigeminal nerve (CN V) and the facial nerve (CN VII). The afferent limb is mediated through the ophthalmic (VI) division of CN V. The CR is tested by stimulating the cornea with a drop of sterile saline or by touching each cornea with a wisp of cotton and observing any asymmetries in the blink response. The efferent limb of the reflex, mediated bilaterally through the facial nuclei and nerves, is evoked by a single burst of OOc activity lasting approximately 60 msec, and both lids blink within 49 msec of the stimulus.[42] Bilateral absent CR in comatose patients indicates pontine dysfunction.

■ **Clinical Points to Remember About the Corneal Reflex**

- The CR is elicited by stimulation of the cornea with a drop of sterile saline or with a cotton wisp—the response is eye closure.
- The CR is mediated by both monosynaptic and polysynaptic pathways.
- The afferent limb is mediated by the ophthalmic (VI) division of the trigeminal nerve to the chief sensory and spinal trigeminal nuclei in the brainstem.
- The efferent limb is mediated by the ipsilateral facial nerve to the OOc, causing eye closure.
- A decreased unilateral afferent CR (hypalgesia) is due to a lesion of the ipsilateral trigeminal sensory pathway.
- A decreased unilateral blink response (efferent CR) is due to a lesion of the facial nerve nucleus in the pons, the facial nerve, or their connections.
- A lesion of the sensorimotor cortex can cause a diminished CR in the eye contralateral to the lesion.
- Bilateral absent CR in a comatose patient indicates brainstem dysfunction. ■

Reflex Blinking

Reflex blinking is mediated through stimulation of all three divisions of the trigeminal nerve (CN V). Stimulation of the ophthalmic division (VI) is the most effective. Reflex blinks can also be evoked by stimulation of the supraorbital nerve through tactile stimulation of the eyelids or eyelashes or by tapping the forehead (glabella reflex). Feedback from the supraorbital nerve prevents a second blink by a reduction in trigeminal responsiveness and this inhibitory mechanism ensures that spasms of reflex blinks will not occur regardless of the stimulus used to produce the first blink. In patients with acute and usually large unilateral hemispheric strokes, the blink reflex may be transiently diminished when the contralateral cornea or forehead is stimulated.

Blink to Light

Reflex blink to bright light (dazzle or menace reflex) is a brainstem reflex mediated by central pathways other than the polysynaptic pathway for the CR. The blink-to-bright-light reflex is present even in neocortical death.[43] A single case reported is that of a 54-year-old woman in coma from cerebral anoxia, with an isoelectric electroencephalogram, absent visual evoked responses, and absent blink-to-visual-threat. The CR was intact and blink-to-light reflex persisted. At autopsy the brain showed almost complete cortical neuronal loss with preservation of the brainstem.

In progressive supranuclear palsy (PSP), some patients show an inability to inhibit a blink when a penlight is shone in their eyes, a phenomenon referred to as "visual glabella" or Myerson's sign.

Blink to Threat

Blink-to-threat is a cortically mediated reflex requiring an intact visual cortex and intact cortical association areas for visual attention in the parietal lobe and frontal eye fields. Blink-to-threat is a standard bedside method for testing the level of alertness in obtunded patients and for testing for a visual field defect or visual neglect in uncooperative patients or children. If the patient blinks in response to your hand moving rapidly toward the eyes from different directions, and if this results in either partial or complete closure of the lids, the reflex is considered intact. An absent blink-to-threat in both hemifields is present in cortically blind patients and in some Alzheimer's disease cases with severe dementia. Absent blink-to-threat to a hemifield stimulus is seen in patients with a homonymous hemianopsia or hemivisual neglect.

Auditory Blink Reflex

An auditory blink reflex, the *stapedius reflex*, is a startle response evoked by a sudden loud noise.[44] In infants, the persistence of the startle reaction to sound, *hyperacusis*, is associated with certain lipid storage diseases, for example, Tay-Sachs's disease and Sandhoff's disease due to GM2 ganglioside storage. A very similar startle response occurs in patients with Creutzfeldt-Jakob disease (CJD).

Blink Reflexes in Coma

The blink reflexes in coma are the most important source of information available to the clinician. The patient cannot speak or respond to touch, and the eyes are the last window left open to the brain.

■ **Clinical Points to Remember About the Eyelids and Blink Reflexes in Coma**

- Before touching the patient, observe the position of the eyelids and any spontaneous eyelid movements:
  - Are the lids resting closed as in sleep?
  - Do they continue to open and close and blink spontaneously (coma vigil)?
  - Do they remain constantly open and unblinking (spastic eyes)?
- Test reflex blink responses to:
  - Eyelash tickle.
  - Cotton swab stimulation of the nostril.
  - Corneal stimulation using 2 drops of sterile saline.

- Monocular bright light.
- Visual threat.
- Auditory stimulus (loud voice or hand clap).
- Painful stimulation (sternal rub).
- Watch for spontaneous lid movements synchronous with eye movements under closed lids—for example, ocular bobbing or ocular dipping.
- Periodic blinking of the eyelids should raise the suspicion of seizure activity.
- Check for reflex blepharospasm by manually opening closed eyelids—the patient may reflexively squeeze the lids shut, and this would indicate a lesion in the striatum.
- When the eyelids are held open, observe the position of the eyes at rest. Watch for random eye movements, and rotate the head from side to side or up and down to elicit the VOR. The absence of eye movements in the direction opposite to head movements (doll's eyes) suggests brainstem dysfunction (Chapter 6).
- When reflex responses are present they indicate normal brainstem function. When reflex responses are absent, particularly bilateral CR, they indicate dysfunction of the brainstem. ■

THE EYELID EXAMINATION

The eyelid examination is possibly one of the most overlooked aspects of the neurological examination yet it is straightforward provided the examiner knows: first, what to look for; second, the appropriate measurements to make; and third, how to test eyelid function. The sequence of the examination is as follows:

- Observe the eyelids and their positions at rest looking straight ahead.
  In adults the upper eyelid covers the top of the cornea.
  The lower eyelid lies at just below the limbus (junction of cornea and sclera).
  If the upper eyelid is above the limbus (scleral show) it implies disorders causing lid retraction or poor eye closure.
- Measure the width of the palpebral fissure (the opening between the upper and lower lids). In normal subjects, it is between 9 and 11 mm in height (in the middle) when the lids are open but relaxed (Figure 2-5).
- Palpebral fissure narrowing suggests ptosis or excessive contraction of the OOcs.
- Measure the marginal reflex distance (MRD)—the distance between the center of the pupil and the upper lid margin (Figure 2-5). The MRD is normally 3–4 mm. An MRD of greater than 4 mm suggests *lid retraction* and of less than 3 mm *ptosis*.
- Note the upper eyelid position during eye movements, particularly horizontal gaze.
- Normally, the palpebral fissure widens in the abducting eye in about 50% of normal subjects, and in about 15% of these, the lid elevates in adduction as well.
- Changes in the position of the eyelid occur with aberrant reinnervation of CN III, the oculomotor nerve (Case 5-4, Chapter 5).
- During upgaze, the tone of the levator muscle increases to lift the upper eyelid, and the eyelids should relax and follow the eyes smoothly looking down.

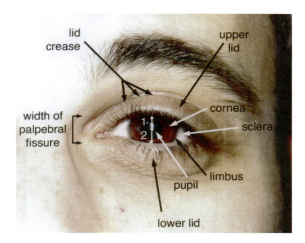

FIGURE 2-5 The normal left eye. (1) Marginal reflex distance (MRD 1). The distance between the upper eyelid edge and the corneal light reflex. (2) MRD 2 the distance between the lower eyelid edge and the corneal light reflex. The lid crease (*arrow*) follows the curvature of the upper lid approximately 10 mm from the lid margin.

Reproduced with permission.[45]

- Lid-lag on downgaze is present in a number of disorders; for example, the eye–lid relationship can be disrupted in dorsal midbrain lesions causing retracted eyelids to remain elevated while the eyes look down.
- LP function can be assessed by manually fixing the brow and asking the patient to look down. A ruler is then placed at the lid margin and the number of millimeters of lid elevation measured as the patient looks up.[45]
- To test eyelid closure, ask the patient to tightly close his eyes (as if he has soap in them). Failure to bury the eyelashes fully indicates weakness of the OOc. It occurs in patients with facial weakness, for example, dystrophia myotonica (Chapter 3).
- A review of old photographs is often very helpful since they can show an earlier presence of important signs, particularly ptosis.[46–50]

FUNCTIONAL EYELID DISORDERS

Cerebral (or Cortical) Ptosis

Ptosis, or drooping of the upper eyelid is commonly due to weakness of the levator or to weakness of Müller's muscles. Bilateral cerebral ptosis in an elderly stroke patient is a frequently underdiagnosed disorder that can often be dismissed as a sign of lethargy.[50,51] The case presented here was brought by a resident who was unable to get the patient to open her eyes.

CASE 2-1 Cerebral Ptosis

Video Display

The patient is an 82-year-old woman admitted to the ICU after being found down on the floor of her bathroom. She was alert and cooperative, and hemiplegic on the left side.

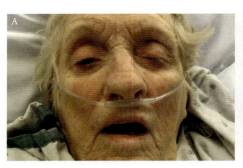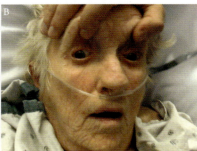

FIGURE 2-6 Eighty-two-year-old woman with (A) bilateral cerebral ptosis and (B) horizontal conjugate deviation of the eyes to the right.

Analysis of the History

· What are the major presenting symptoms?
· Where are the central nervous system (CNS) lesion(s) likely to be?

CASE 2-1 SYMPTOMS

Symptoms
Loss of consciousness
Left hemiplegia

Location Correlation
Right cerebral hemisphere

The analysis guides the clinical examination.

Examination

Neurological

· Alert and cooperative and able to follow two-step commands
· Rested in bed with eyes closed (Figure 2-6A)
· Failed to open her eyes on command
· Failed to blink with eyelash tickle
· No contralateral reflex blink on corneal stimulation
· Bilateral flaccid eyelids
· Unable to hold her eyes open once the eyes were manually opened for her (Patients with apraxia of eyelid opening can hold the eyes open once the eyes are manually opened)
· Conjugate deviation of the eyes to the right (Figure 2-6B)
· The eyes failed to cross the midline looking to the left
· Left visual neglect—failed to count correctly the number of people around her bed
· Left hemiparesis
· Left parietal sensory loss with impaired sensation to double simultaneous stimulation

Localization and Differential Diagnosis

The signs in this patient are those of a right parietal lobe syndrome: left hemiplegia (conjugate deviation of the eyes to the side of the lesion), left hemi-visual neglect, and impaired sensation to double simultaneous stimulation.

What Diagnostic Tests Should Follow?

· Non-contrast head computerised tomogram (CT)

Test Results

A non-contrast CT showed a right frontal lobe hemorrhage a subdural hemorrhage (Figure 2-7A) and a midline shift to the left of approximately 8 mm (Figure 2-7B).

Diagnosis: Right Frontal Lobe Hemmorhage and Subdural Hemorrhage

Treatment

A nonsurgical approach is the treatment of choice for clinically stable patients with small (up to 20–30 cm³ volume) lobar hematomas, and only supportive measures are appropriate for those in the poor prognosis category of large (>80 cm³) hematomas, especially if they have marked mass effect and midline shift on CT and/or brain magnetic imaging (MRI).

Special Explanatory Note

Bilateral cerebral ptosis is associated most often with extensive nondominant hemisphere lesions accompanied by ipsilateral conjugate gaze deviation. Lepore studied 13 patients after acute right frontotemporoparietal lobe lesions with bilateral cerebral ptosis, a condition he defined by the following characteristics: the

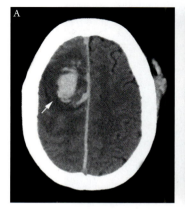
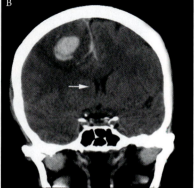

FIGURE 2-7 (A) Non-contrast axial head CT shows a right frontal lobe hemorrhage (*arrow*) and a subdural hemorrhage (B) Coronal image shows a midline shift to the left of approximately 8mm (*arrow*) due to a large right frontal hematoma.

which consists of paroxysmal eye pain somewhat like that of tic douloureux in the distribution of the ophthalmic division of the trigeminal nerve by neuroimaging of the orbit and cavernous sinus. Raeder syndrome may be idiopathic, especially in women, with no lesion found in or near the trigeminal ganglion.

Apraxia of Eyelid Opening and Closing

Apraxia of lid opening (ALO) is a supranuclear disorder characterized by a nonparalytic inability to open the eyes at will without visible contraction of the OOc muscle but with unaffected reflex blinking. (Use of the term *apraxia* is now under discussion, but it remains in the index of every textbook, and I have retained use of it here.) In 1965, Goldstein and Cogan reported four typical apraxic patients.[53] Involuntary lid closure was the presenting complaint of three of the four, although the actual difficulty involved lid opening. The first patient, a 77-year-old man with Huntington's chorea, took from 5 to 15 seconds to open his eyelids following either voluntary or involuntary eye closure. The lids then either opened normally or were facilitated to do so by the patient, either through contraction of the frontalis muscle, by thrusting his head backward, or by elevating the lids with his fingers. He could close his eyes readily on command and reopen them normally after blinking. The second case was a woman with PD who could read only by manually holding her eyelids open. Lid closure was precipitated by shining a light into her eyes or by touching her face. Urging her to open her eyes prolonged the period of lid closure, suggesting a block in frontal lobe or basal ganglia circuits initiating eyelid opening. In all four patients, a transient inability to open the eyelids followed voluntary closure, and in three it followed reflex closure as well. The lid closure was not accompanied by spasm of the OOc or by the lowered eyebrow (Charcot's sign), which is usually seen in blepharospasm.

Since then, reports emphasize the presence of this disorder in extrapyramidal and basal ganglia disease affecting the motor system, notably, in PD,[54] atypical parkinsonism, parkinsonism due to methyl-r-phenyl-1, 2, 3, 6-tetra hydrophyridine toxicity, PSP,[55-57] Huntington's disease, Wilson's disease,[58] and multisystem atrophy. In one PSP patient, difficulty opening the eyes was considered to be a type of akinesia,[59] and a similar case is presented here.

CASE 2-2 Apraxia of Lid Opening

Video Display

The patient is a 73-year-old man referred in 1973 because "my eyes are giving me trouble, they are my biggest complaint" (Figure 2-10). He said he had difficulty focusing close up, and his eyes kept shutting spontaneously much of the time. Bright sunlight provoked closure, and frequent closure made it difficult for him to hold a conversation with anybody. With his eyes open, he could see clearly.

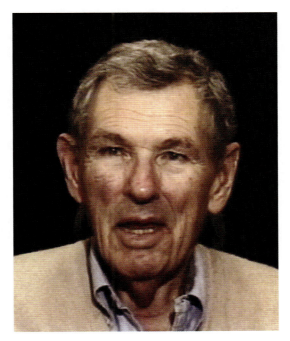

FIGURE 2-10 Seventy-three-year-old man with a chief complaint of "my eyes keep shutting."

Analysis of the History

· What are the major presenting symptoms?
· Where are the CNS lesion(s) likely to be?

CASE 2-2 SYMPTOMS

Symptoms	Location Correlation
Difficulty focusing at near	Convergence system
Eyes shut spontaneously	Orbicularis oculi muscles

The analysis guide the clinical examination.

Examination

Neurological

· A striking paucity of head, limb, and body movements
· Rigidity of the neck
· Difficulty getting up out of a chair, tending to topple backward

- Slowness walking and the need to make several small steps to turn
- His speech had become dysphonic more than dysarthric
- The tongue moved well
- Jaw jerk and facial jerks were absent

Ocular motility

- Age-related ptosis
- Infrequent blinking <11 per minute
- Positive glabella tap (bilateral eyelid closure tapping the forehead)
- Blepharoclonus (tremor of the lids with gentle eye closure)
- Impaired initiation of eye opening on command (apraxia)
- Supranuclear paralysis of up- and downgaze
- Impaired initiation of horizontal saccades on command
- Slow hypometric horizontal saccades
- Saccadic pursuit in all directions
- Square-wave jerks
- Absent convergence

Localization and Differential Diagnosis

A diagnosis of PSP (the Steele-Richardson-Olszewski syndrome) is primarily a clinical diagnosis, and, as in this case, based on signs of a supranuclear vertical gaze palsy, slow hypometric horizontal saccades, impaired initiation of eyelid opening and extrapyramidal eyelid signs—notably blepharoclonus, reduced blink rate, and a positive glabella tap.

What Diagnostic Tests Should Follow?

- Brain MRI

Test Results

PSP is characterized by atrophy of the upper brainstem and the midbrain is significantly diminished in size. In this case brain, MRI was not available, and the diagnosis of PSP was based on the constellation of clinical signs. The characteristic hummingbird sign of atrophy of the tectal plate in PSP, visible on brain MRI, is illustrated in Case 1-3 (Chapter 1).

Special Explanatory Note

Progressive supranuclear palsy is a tauopathy of unknown etiology. Core features of this disorder are a supranuclear gaze palsy that begins with slow hypometric saccades, an inability to voluntarily look down, axial rigidity, pseudobulbar palsy, and dementia. Delayed initiation of eyelid opening in PSP results from metabolic impairment of the motor network and cortical degeneration of the frontal lobes.[60,61]

Apraxia of lid closure (ALC) is a supranuclear defect in voluntary lid closure. ALC has been described in a small number of patients with pseudobulbar palsy and bilateral cortical infarcts of the Rolandic operculum, and in patients with diffuse hemispheric damage caused by diseases such as CJD. In the early stages of CJD, the patient may be unable to make a rapid series of blinks although a single sustained eye closure can be achieved. The patient may compensate with a rapid downward movement of the eyes or extension of the neck to initiate eyelid closure when he or she cannot voluntarily close the eyes. Associated neurological signs include facial akinesia, pseudobulbar palsy, spastic tetraparesis followed after some months by supranuclear gaze palsy, and dementia.

Apraxia of lid closure may occur in the late stages of amyotrophic lateral sclerosis (ALS), usually at the stage when the patient is intubated.

The case of familial ALS presented here is an example of this.

CASE 2-3 Apraxia of Lid Closure: Amyotrophic Lateral Sclerosis

Video Display

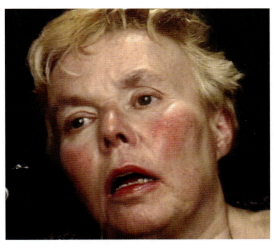

FIGURE 2-11 Fifty-eight-year-old woman unable to voluntarily close her eyes.

The patient is a 58-year-old woman who was referred to the neurology clinic in March 1995 with the recent onset of slurred speech and dysphagia (Figure 2-11). The disease progressed and, by November 1995, she could hardly speak and was no longer able to protrude her tongue or whistle. By April 1996, she had lost the ability to speak and was mute. She had difficulty chewing and swallowing, particularly liquids. In September 1996, a G-tube was placed, and by January 1997, she was confined to a wheelchair. She had no respiratory distress. At that time, the patient's husband sought advice because his wife had increasing difficulty closing her eyes, and the act required a conscious and sustained effort.

Analysis of the History

· What are the major presenting symptoms?
· Where are the CNS lesion(s) likely to be?

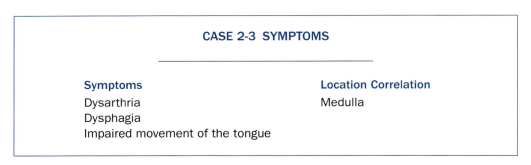

CASE 2-3 SYMPTOMS

Symptoms	Location Correlation
Dysarthria	Medulla
Dysphagia	
Impaired movement of the tongue	

The analysis guides the clinical examination.

Examination

Neurological

· Impaired palatal movement
· Positive gag bilaterally
· Diminished rapid movements of the tongue (spastic)
· No fasciculations
· Brisk jaw and facial jerks
· Increased muscle tone throughout
· Hyperreflexic deep tendon reflexes
· Bilateral extensor plantar response

Ocular motility

· Supranuclear paralysis of upgaze > downgaze
· Normal vertical pursuit
· Slow horizontal gaze to right and left; tends to move her head to look to either side
· Saccadic horizontal pursuit
· Absent convergence
· Slow initiating volitional eye closure
· Preserved spontaneous eyelid opening
· Blinks to threat and to loud noise
· Normal horizontal and vertical vestibular ocular reflex

Localization and Differential Diagnosis

The disease process in this patient involves the corticobulbar tracts bilaterally causing a spastic (pseudobulbar) *dysarthria* that is usually due to vascular, demyelinative, or motor system disease. ALS is the chief disorder in which signs of spasticity and atrophy (wasting and fasciculation) of the tongue are combined. *Dysphagia*—weakness or incoordination of swallowing—is attributable to weakness of the tongue. The presence of the gag reflex is quite limited in its importance as a neurologic sign since palatal elevation in response to touching the posterior pharynx only demonstrates that cranial nerves IX (glossopharyngeal) and X (vagus) are intact.

What Diagnostic Tests Should Follow?

· Electromyogram (EMG) looking for fasciculation of trunk and limb muscles
· Brain MRI

Test Results

EMG scanning of multiple muscles showed fasciculations, and brain MRI showed mild frontotemporal atrophy.

Diagnosis: Amyotrophic Lateral Sclerosis

In this patient, ALS continued to progress, with predominantly upper motoneuron bulbar signs and spasticity of the limbs. She died in 1998. No autopsy was performed.

Special Explanatory Note

Little attention has been paid to eyelid function in ALS because failure to initiate eye closure on command, in the presence of normal reflex closure is rarely encountered and, when present, is usually interpreted as an apraxia.[62,63] Lesions can be localized by neuroimaging and are localizable at autopsy.[64]

In a similar case of a 69-year-old woman with progressive bulbar palsy and ALS, the patient had noticed increasing difficulty closing her eyes and had developed the habit of closing them with her fingers. When examined, she was alert and cooperative with intact reflex blinking to bright light, visual threat, and corneal stimulation. Brain MRI disclosed mild cerebral atrophy in the frontal lobes and anterior temporal lobes. Single proton emission computed tomography (SPECT) showed reduced isotope intake in the frontal lobes. The patient died 2 years after the onset of these symptoms.

At autopsy, the brain showed diffuse cortical atrophy, maximal in the frontal lobes bilaterally. The entire area of the tegmentum of the pons and midbrain relevant to ocular motor function was normal. Moderate neuronal loss with astrocytosis was evident in the motor nuclei of the medulla oblongata and the anterior horn of the entire spinal cord. There was no relevant lesion in other parts of the brain, including the basal ganglia and the cerebellum, except for neuronal loss in the substantia nigra.

The selective loss of voluntary eyelid closure, with retention of normal eyelid reflexes, was attributed to atrophy of the frontal lobe or involvement of the frontopontine pathway, a localization and pathogenesis noted by others.[65,66]

Blepharospasm

Blepharospasm is a focal dystonia of the eyelids causing involuntary eyelid closure due to contraction of the OOc.[67] It occurs with ocular diseases such as dry eyes or in PD or focal brain lesions in the basal ganglia and thalami.[68]

In PD, the basal ganglia affect blink reflex excitability by altering the inhibitory drive from the substantia nigra to the SC. Dysfunction in this control system may also be involved in blepharospasm with impaired eyelid opening—apraxia of eyelid opening—which occurs in up to 10% of cases of blepharospasm. These patients not only show a significant delay in eyelid opening but an abnormal persistence of OOc activity.

Because dopamine acts through the same circuit, increases in striatal dopamine levels decrease nigral-collicular inhibition, resulting in a reduction in the excitability of trigeminal reflex blinks.

Other clinical settings in which blepharospasm may be observed are:

- Transiently after a stroke involving the striatopallidal system (mainly pallidum or the thalamus)
- After a small thalamomesencephalic infarct
- As part of a paraneoplastic midbrain encephalitis

Reflex blepharospasm is the involuntary contraction of the OOc with lid closure in response to stimulation from an examiner trying to pull open the eyelids. This phenomenon is associated with severe strokes (with a left rather than a right hemiplegia) and is more pronounced on the nonparalyzed side.[69] Case studies have further localized reflex blepharospasm to nondominant hemisphere lesions in the globus pallidum and putamen, also called the striatum.[70] Reflex blepharospasm occurs in both PD and PSP and usually also improves with dopaminergic drugs. When there are no associated underlying ocular or neurological disorders, the diagnosis is idiopathic or benign essential blepharospasm. Factitious (voluntary) blepharospasm is uncommon.[71]

Benign essential blepharospasm in an adult is a chronic progressive disease, as in the case presented here.

CASE 2-4 Essential Blepharospasm

Video Display

The patient is a 60-year-old manager with a history of retinal laser therapy, dry eyes, age-related bilateral ptosis, and cancer of the kidney (Figure 2-12). In 1995, he was referred with a 6-month history of frequent blinking and spasms of eye closure that he could not control. He reported driving cautiously because his eyes might shut completely

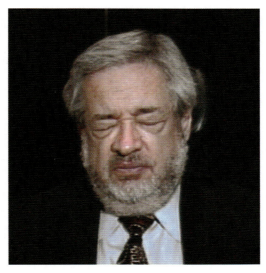

FIGURE 2-12 Sixty-year-old man with involuntary squeezing shut of his eyes.

during a spasm and interrupt his vision. He experienced difficulty watching television and reading, and his eye spasms were aggravated by stress, fatigue, sunlight, and bright room lighting. He declined social invitations because his "eyes were embarrassing." He had no involuntary movements of the lower face.

Analysis of the History

- What are the major presenting symptoms?
- Where are the CNS lesion(s) likely to be?

CASE 2-4 SYMPTOMS

Symptoms	Location Correlation
Frequent blinking	Orbicularis oculi
Spasm of eye closure	

The analysis guides the clinical examination.

Examination

Neurological

- Age-related ptosis
- Excess blinking—blink rate 20–30 per minute (normal 11 per minute)

- Frequent spasms of eye closure associated with difficulty initiating eyelid opening (apraxia)
- Blepharoclonus with gentle eye closure
- Blepharospasm suppressed when he counted the lines on a rotating optokinetic drum and subtracted 3 from 90 out loud
- Positive glabella tap
- Normal saccadic and pursuit eye movements
- Convergence insufficiency
- No involuntary movements of the face, jaw, tongue, or neck muscles
- Normal Bell's phenomenon (upward deviation of the eyes on tight eye closure)

Localization and Differential Diagnosis

The patient presented with progressive idiopathic blepharospasm. He had no involuntary movements of the face, jaw, tongue, or neck muscles to suggest Meige's syndrome—a cranial dystonia—no family history of neurological disease and no past history of depression or the use of narcoleptic drugs.

What Diagnostic Tests Should Follow?

- Brain MRI

Test Results

Brain MRI showed mild cortical atrophy.

Diagnosis: Benign Essential Blepharospasm

Treatment

The primary treatment option in this case is botulinum A toxin (Botox), which the patient declined. Instead, he received carbidopa-L-dopa 25/100 t.i.d., which markedly relieved the blepharospasm.

Special Explanatory Note

In patients free of underlying CNS disease, the treatment of choice for idiopathic benign essential blepharospasm is botulinum-A toxin (Botox) injected subcutaneously into several sites in the upper and lower eyelids and eyebrow to block acetylcholine at the neuromuscular junction and weaken the contraction of the OOc and adjacent facial muscles. Within 1 or 2 days, spasms of eye closure usually stop and, on average, the beneficial response lasts for 3 to 4 months before repeated cycles of treatment become necessary. Due to deep penetration of the toxin, complications may result. Ptosis occurs in about 8% of cases and diplopia in 2%, with the IO muscle being the commonest extraocular muscle affected.[72,73]

Many neurologists view responsiveness to L-dopa as a diagnostic marker for PD. The use of the drug is based on the finding that although striatal dopamine is depleted in Parkinson's patients, the remaining nigral cells can still be capable of producing some dopamine by taking up its precursor, L-dopa.

Blepharospasm is a sign of some significance, and a wide range of diseases of the brainstem and basal ganglia are associated with it. The list is shown in Table 2-2.

TABLE 2-2: Diseases of the Brainstem and Basal Ganglia Associated with Blepharospasm

---

Progressive supranuclear palsy
Parkinson's disease
Parkinsonism (including parkinsonism-dementia complex)
Shy-Drager syndrome
Hallervorden-Spatz disease
Huntington's chorea
Lytico-Bodig syndrome
Right hemisphere stroke
Wilson's disease
Olivopontocerebellar atrophy
Communicating hydrocephalus
Multiple sclerosis
Amyotrophic lateral sclerosis

Episodic Paroxysmal Eyebrow Spasms

Episodic paroxysmal eyebrow spasms are associated with serious epileptic seizures and are extremely rare. I have seen this disorder only once.

CASE 2-5 Episodic Paroxysmal Eyebrow Spasms: Tuberous Sclerosis Complex

Video Display

The patient is a 32-year-old man with tuberous sclerosis complex (TSC) characterized by medically intractable epilepsy, developmental delay, and structural brain abnormalities (cortical and subcortical tubers, subependymal nodules, and giant-cell astrocytomas). He also had cutaneous manifestations and retinal phakomas.

By age 32, when seen in consultation in the epilepsy clinic, he had developed highly stereotypic, periodic, involuntary, rotary movements of his eyes in a clockwise direction toward his left shoulder, accompanied by synchronous rhythmic elevation of both eyebrows at a frequency of about 2 to 3 Hz with facial grimacing similar to risus sardonicus.

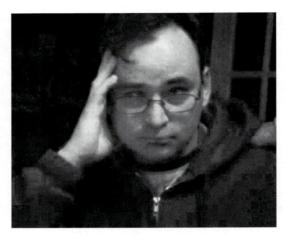

FIGURE 2-13 Thirty-two-year-old man with intractable epilepsy.

Courtesy of Daniel Costello, M.D.

He was unable to suppress eyebrow spasms by holding his brows down or by any other maneuver (Figure 2-13). The spasms lasted anywhere from 1 to 20 minutes but averaged 7–8 minutes, during which time he was able to converse normally and carry on with what he was doing. Eyebrow spasms were, however, very distressing for him.

What Diagnostic Test Should Follow?

· Brain MRI

Test Results

Brain MRI, with axial and coronal fluid attenuated inversion recovery (FLAIR) images showed numerous cortical tubers, the largest of which involved the left occipital cortex (Figure 2-14A–B).

Diagnosis: Tuberous Sclerosis Complex

Treatment

Tuberous sclerosis complex affects most organ systems, and treatment recommendations vary according to organ manifestations.[74] This patient continued on trials of anticonvulsant medications.

Special Explanatory Note

Tuberous sclerosis complex is a multisystem disorder that is transmitted as an autosomal-dominant trait. Two genes, *TSC1* and *TSC2*, and the gene products hamartin and tuberin have been identified.[75] The major pathologic features are in the brain and include cortical tubers, subependymal nodules, and giant-cell

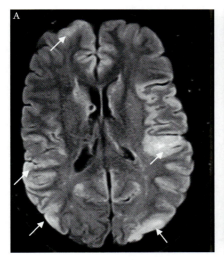
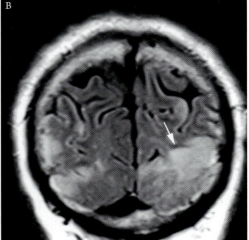

FIGURE 2-14 Magnetic resonance imaging (MRI) of a patient with tuberous sclerosis complex. (A) Axial fluid attenuated inversion recovery (FLAIR) image shows numerous cortical tubers, including a large lesion in the left occipital cortex (*arrows*). (B) Coronal FLAIR image shows cortical tubers again showing the left occipital cortex lesion (*arrow*).

Courtesy of Daniel Costello M.D.

tumors that cause mental retardation and early-onset epilepsy with infantile spasms.[76]

Eyelid twitching (or fluttering) may herald seizures[77] that begin with forceful, sustained horizontal deviation of the head and eyes, and sometimes the entire body to the side opposite the irritative seizure focus. These seizures are referred to as *versive* or *adversive* seizures.[78]

Hemifacial Spasm

CASE 2-6 Hemifacial Spasm

Neurovascular Compression Syndrome of the Right Facial Nerve Root

Video Display

Hemifacial spasm (HFS) is due to focal demyelination of facial nerve axons and the activation of adjacent nerve fibers by ephaptic transmission. Hemifacial spasm typically begins insidiously in the OOc muscle with eyelid twitching then progresses to involve the ipsilateral facial muscles with elevation of the corner of the mouth.[79] On occasion, eyelid twitching may be almost continuous, for example, requiring the patient to sit holding a hand over the eye in order to watch television. Hemifacial spasm is aggravated by emotional stress and fatigue and precipitated by active movement of any facial muscle, particularly when the patient is asked to show the teeth. The involuntary twitching of the cheek and the angle of the mouth are due to paroxysmal clonic and tonic synchronous contraction of the facial muscles caused by brief bursts of normal motor units firing at high frequency.

Neuroimaging of the brain is essential to rule out an ischemic lesion, pontine glioma,[80] multiple sclerosis,[81] or neurovascular compression of the facial nerve root near its exit from the brainstem by a basilar artery aneurysm or by an adjacent vascular loop or dolichoectatic artery.[82]

Botox is the treatment of choice for this disorder. Medication with carbamazepine (Tegretol) in a dose of 600–1,200 mg/day may control the spasm in up to two-thirds of patients. Baclofen or gabapentin is recommended if carbamazepine fails, but some patients cannot tolerate these drugs, have only brief remissions, or fail to respond.

Paraneoplastic Facial Spasm

Paraneoplastic facial spasm is a novel brainstem syndrome reported in two patients with adeno-carcinoma of the prostate.[83] It is characterized by progressive loss of voluntary horizontal eye movements and severe, persistent muscle spasms of the face, larynx, and pharynx, sparing the eyelids. Neither of the two patients reported had antineuronal antibodies in the blood. One patient developed continuous muscle spasms, beginning on the right side of the face and progressing to involve both sides of the face, the masseter muscles, and then the pharyngeal and laryngeal muscles. He complained of severe hyperacusis and noted that loud noises markedly aggravated the facial spasms. Magnetic resonance imaging of the brain with contrast was normal. At autopsy, neuronal loss was localized to the pontine tegmentum, the medullary sensory nuclei, and the cerebellum. Brainstem motor nuclei were preserved. The clinical and pathological findings suggest an autoimmune process (probably paraneoplastic) with selective damage to a sub-population of brainstem neurons critical for horizontal eye movements and recurrent inhibition of bulbar nuclei.

Eyelid Myokymia

Eyelid myokymia (orbicularis myokymia) is very common. The term refers to annoying twitches of the OOc of the lower eyelid or occasionally the upper eyelid on one side in otherwise normal persons. It is typically due to fatigue, stress, nicotine, or caffeine. The condition is benign, but patients become alarmed because they can feel the eyelid twitch and often complain that the lid or the eye is "jumping." Eyelid myokymia usually lasts for days or weeks, occurring intermittently for several hours at a time. It can also be treated with Botox, but the twitching characteristically resolves spontaneously once the patient is reassured.

Isolated eyelid myokymia lasting for more than 3 months and unilateral or bilateral facial myokymia are signs indicating brainstem disease. In these cases, an MRI of the brain is mandatory.

The Marcus Gunn Jaw-Winking Phenomenon

The Marcus Gunn jaw-winking phenomenon is an unusual synkinesis between the pterygoid muscles and the levator muscle, observed by Gunn in 1883,[84,85] in a 15-year-old girl with unilateral congenital ptosis who was able to elevate the ptotic lid by moving her jaw to the left.

CASE 2-7 Marcus-Gunn Jaw Winking

Video Display

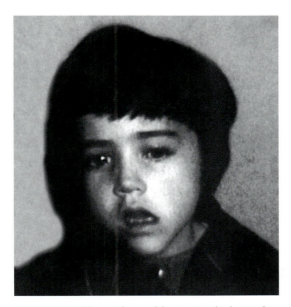

FIGURE 2-15 Young boy with congenital ptosis of the left eye.

A personally observed case of this rare synkinesis was in a young healthy boy with congenital ptosis of the left eyelid (Figure 2-15). His mother noticed that when he was sucking on a bottle the ptotic eyelid lifted.

Simultaneous contraction of the LP superioris with the external pterygoid muscle is the synkinesis seen in this child. The affected eyelid is usually ptotic and involuntary elevation of the lid can occur when:

- *the mandible is moved to the opposite side (contraction of the ipsilateral external pterygoid muscle),*
- *the mandible is projected forward or the tongue protruded (bilateral contraction of the external pterygoid muscles), or*
- *the mandible is strongly depressed on wide opening of the mouth).*

The lid remains elevated as long as the jaw muscle contracts.[86] The abnormal levator contraction is most evident when the patient is looking downward.

Eyelid surgery is the treatment of choice when age permits and when both parents and surgeon agree that the jaw-winking or ptosis or both are cosmetically objectionable.[87]

Children with the Marcus Gunn jaw-winking phenomenon commonly have associated ocular abnormalities including strabismus, amblyopia, anisometropia, and congenital nystagmus.

POSITIONAL EYELID DISORDERS

Lid Retraction with Thyroid Eye Disease

Thyroid-associated orbitopathy (TAO) or Graves' disease is the commonest cause of unilateral or bilateral lid retraction resulting in sclera showing above the limbus. Lid retraction may be the only ocular abnormality in TAO, or it may be accompanied by lagophthalmos (lid-lag looking down). These signs are present in more than 90% of patients[88] with Graves' disease, including the case presented here.

CASE 2-8 Graves' Disease: Thyroid-Associated Ophthalmopathy

Video Display

The patient is a 71-year-old woman with exophthalmos (forward protrusion of the globe) and ophthalmoplegia due to TAO (Graves' disease) (Figures 2-16). Her visual acuity was reduced to 20/200 OU (normal 20/20), and she was referred for urgent evaluation. She

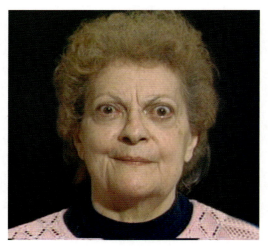

FIGURE 2-16 Seventy-one-year-old woman with lid retraction and exophthalmos.

had been treated for primary hyperthyroidism on three occasions with radioactive iodine and was taking Tapazole 5 mg/day.

Analysis of the History

- What are the major presenting symptoms?
- Where are the CNS lesion(s) likely to be?

CASE 2-8 SYMPTOMS

Symptoms	**Location Correlation**
Exophthalmos	Enlarged ocular muscles
Ophthalmoplegia	Orbit process
Reduced visual acuity	Optic nerves

The analysis guide the clinical examination.

Examination

Neuro-ophthalmic

- Visual acuity 20/200 (OU)
- Visual fields—bilateral central scotoma
- Fundus examination—mild optic disc hyperemia
- Retraction of all four eyelids with a prominent stare
- Lid-lag (persistent elevation of the upper eyelid in downgaze—von Graefe sign)
- A visible rim of sclera on gentle eye closure
- Prominent congested scleral blood vessels
- Bilateral exophthalmos
- Hertel exophthalmometer 25 OD, 28 OS, base 108 (normal 23)
- Tight orbits with reduced orbital resilience
- Restricted horizontal eye movements
- Marked limitation of upward gaze and mild limitation of downgaze
- Positive forced duction test
- Eyes failed to move upward under closed lids (absent Bell's reflex)
- Normal convergence

Localization and Differential Diagnosis

The classic ocular signs of Graves' disease—exophthalmos, lid retraction, tight orbit with reduced orbital resilience, and mechanical paresis of eye movements, especially vertically (restrictive orbitopathy)—are all illustrated by this case. Severe visual loss with bilateral central scotoma indicates compression of the optic nerves in the apex of the orbit.

What Diagnostic Tests Should Follow?

· Computed tomography (CT) of the head with attention to the orbit
· Orbital MRI

Computed tomography of the head with axial and coronal images is the best choice for imaging the orbit to look for the characteristic features of TAO, which are enlargement of the extraocular muscle belly with relative sparing of the tendon. Magnetic resonance imaging of the orbit with the recommended short tau inversion recovery (STIR) sequence highlights the extraocular muscles.

Test Results

Computed tomography of the head with attention to the orbits was diagnostic of TAO (Figure 2-17A–B).

Diagnosis: Thyroid-Associated Orbitopathy

The patient was diagnosed with advanced Graves' disease with bilateral compressive optic neuropathy.

Treatment

Treatment in this case consisted of steroid therapy and surgical decompression of the optic nerves. Bilateral orbital decompression and ethmoidectomy were performed.

A postoperative CT scan confirmed adequate removal of the medial orbital walls and the orbital floors over the maxillary sinuses. The surgeon partly divided the levator muscles because of severe upper lid retraction, which is rarely done. Vision recovered to 20/40 OD and 20/30 OS.

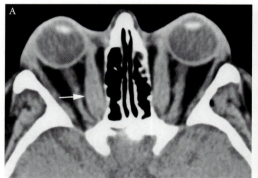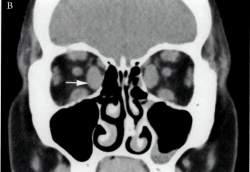

FIGURE 2-17 (A) Axial computed tomography (CT) through the orbit without contrast shows enlargement of the medial rectus muscle bilaterally (arrow). Note that the tendinous insertion is spared. (B) The coronal CT (reformatted from axial data set) without contrast shows enlargement of the medial rectus muscles,(arrow) inferior rectus muscles, and upper muscle complexes on both sides, crowding the apex of the orbit).

Courtesy of Hugh Curtin, M.D.

Special Explanatory Note

The precise mechanism of eyelid retraction in TAO is unclear, but it is possibly due not only to physical enlargement of the levator muscles but also to excessive neural stimulation and increased output to the SR in order to overcome the mechanical limitation of full upward gaze caused by restriction of the IR.[89,90]

Lagophthalmos, an inability to close the eye completely, and *von Graefe's sign*, a slowing of lid descent during eye movement from up- to downgaze, are diagnostic signs of thyroid eye disease. Thyroid eye disease, as in this case, is confirmed by orbital CT or MRI demonstrating enlarged extraocular muscles.

Neurogenic Causes of Lid Retraction

Bilateral lid retraction—Collier's "tucked" lid sign—is the clinical hallmark of the pretectal syndrome of the midbrain and is invariably accompanied by a supranuclear upgaze palsy. The pretectal syndrome due to vascular lesions, pineal region tumors, or hydrocephalus is fully discussed in Chapter 7.

Neurogenic causes of bilateral lid retraction include PSP which is characterized by a supranuclear vertical gaze palsy, typically affecting downward gaze ahead of upward gaze, within 3 years of symptom onset. Many PSP patients have a characteristic facies with lid retraction, slow blink rate, and staring. A personally observed case of PSP in a 72-year-old woman with dementia is shown in Figure 2-18. *Dementias associated with supranuclear gaze palsies are listed in Chapter 7* (Table 7-4).

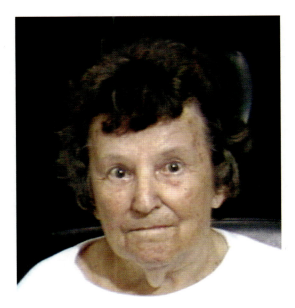

FIGURE 2-18 Elderly woman with progressive supranuclear palsy, bilateral lid retraction, and supranuclear paresis of upgaze.

SELECTED REFERENCES

1. Porter JD, Burns LA, May PJ. Morphological substrate for eyelid movements: innervation and structure of primate levator palpebrae superioris and orbicularis oculi muscles. *J Comp Neurol*. 1989;287:64–81.
2. Landolt E. A contribution to the histological and topographical anatomy of the aponeurosis of the levator palpebrae superioris and of the tarsal muscle in the normal lid and in blepharoptosis. *Int Ophthalmol*. 1985;7:249–253.
3. Kakizaki H, Zhao J, Nakano T, Asamoto K, Zako M, Iwaki M, Miyaishi O. The lower eyelid retractor consists of definite double layers. *Ophthalmology* 2006;113:2346–2350.
4. Dickinson AJ. Anatomy, physiology and malformations of the eyelids. In: Easty DL, Sparrow JM, eds. *Oxford Textbook of Ophthalmology*. New York: Oxford University Press; 1999:355–372.
5. Gordon G. Observations upon the movements of the eyelids. *Br J Ophthalmol*. 1951;35:339–351.
6. Bjork A, Kugelberg E. The electrical activity of the muscles of the eyes and eyelids in various positions and during movement. *Electroencephal Clin Neurophysiol*. 1953;5:595–602.
7. Evinger C, Manning KA, Sibony PA. Eyelid movements. Mechanisms and normal data. *Invest Ophthalmol Vis Sci*. 1991;32:387–400.
8. Sawle G. Dystonia. In: Sawle G, ed. *Movement Disorders in Clinical Practice*. Oxford: Isis Medical Media; 1999:93–118.
9. Fisher CM. Left hemiplegia and motor impersistence. *J Nerv Ment Dis*. 1956; 123:201–218.
10. Schreyer S, Buttner-Ennever JA, Tang X, Mustari MJ, Horn AKE. Orexin-A inputs onto visuomotor cell groups in the monkey brainstem. *Neuroscience*. 2009; 164:629–640.
11. Horn AKE, Buttner-Ennever JA, Gayde M, Messoudi A. Neuroanatomical identification of mesencephalic premotor neurons coordinating eyelid with upgaze in the monkey and man. *J Comparat Neurol*. 2000;420:19–34.
12. Chen B, May PJ. Premotor circuits controlling eyelid movements in conjunction with vertical saccades in the cat: II. Interstitial nucleus of Cajal. *J Comp Neurol*. 2007; 500:676–692.
13. Horn AKE, Buttner-Ennever JA. Brainstem circuits controlling lid-eye coordination in monkey. *Prog Brain Res*. 2008;171:87–95.
14. Weber RB, Daroff RB. Corrective movements following refixation saccades: type and control system analysis. *Vis Res*. 1972;12:467–475.
15. Becker W, Fuchs AF. Lid-eye coordination during vertical gaze changes in man and monkey. *J Neurophysiol*. 1988;60:1227–1252.
16. Bell C. On the motions of the eye, an illustration of the uses of muscles and nerves of the orbit. *Trans R Soc London*. 1823;111:166–186.
17. Collewijn H, van der Steen J. Steinman RM. Human eye movements associated with blinks and prolonged eyelid closure. *J Neurophysiol*. 1985;54:11–27.
18. Takagi M, Abe H, Hasegawa S, Usui T. Reconsideration of Bell's phenomenon using a magnetic search coil method. *Doc Ophthalmol*. 1992;80:343–352.
19. Evinger C, Shaw MD, Peck CK, Manning KA, Baker R. Blinking and associated eye movements in humans, guinea pigs, and rabbits. *J Neurophysiol*. 1984; 52:323–339.
20. Rottach KG, Das VE, Wohlgemuth W, Zivotofsky AZ, Leigh RJ. Properties of horizontal saccades accompanied by blinks. *J Neurophysiol*. 1998;79:2895–2902.
21. Riggs LA, Kelly JP, Manning KA, Moore RK. Blink-related eye movements. *Invest Ophthalmol*. 1987;28:334–342.
22. Bour LJ, Aramideh M, de Visser BW. Neurophysiological aspects of eye and eyelid movements during blinking in humans. *J Neurophysiol*. 2000;83:166–176.
23. Wray SH. The neuro-ophthalmic and neurologic manifestations of pinealomas. In: Schmidek H, ed. *Pineal Tumors*. Boston: Mason Publishing; 1977:21–59.
24. Wijdicks EFM. *The Practice of Emergency and Critical Care Neurology*. Oxford: Oxford University Press; 2010.
25. Iyer VN, Mandrekar JN, Danielson RD, Zubkov AY, Elmer JL, Wijdicks EFM. Validity of the FOUR score coma scale in the medical intensive care unit. *Mayo Clin Proc*. 2009;84:694–701.

26. Stead LG, Wijdicks EFM, Bhagra A, Kashyap A, Bellolio MF, Nash DL. Validation of a new coma scale, the FOUR score, in the emergency department. *Neurocrit Care.* 2009;10:50–54.

27. Kemper T, Romanul F. State resembling akinetic mutism in basilar artery occlusion. *Neurology.* 1967;17:74–80.

28. Keane JR. Spastic eyelids. Failure of levator inhibition in unconscious states. *Arch Neurol.* 1975;32:695–698.

29. Plum F, Posner JD. *The Diagnosis of Stupor and Coma.* 3rd ed. Philadelphia: FA Davis; 1980:1–30, 56–61.

30. Hawkes CH. "Locked-in" syndrome: report of seven cases. *Br Med J.* 1974;4:379–382.

31. Karp JS, Hurting HI. "Locked-in" state with bilateral midbrain infarcts. *Arch Neurol.* 1974;30:176–178.

32. Meienberg O, Mumenthaler M, Karbowski K. Quadriparesis and nuclear oculomotor palsy with total bilateral ptosis mimicking coma. *Arch Neurol.* 1979;36:708–710.

33. Chia L-G. Locked-in syndrome with bilateral ventral midbrain infarcts. *Neurology.* 1991;41(3):445–446.

34. Keane JR. Sustained upgaze in coma. *Ann Neurol.* 1981;9:409–412.

35. Dalmau J, Graus F, Villarejo A, Posner JB, Blumenthal D, Thiessen B, Saiz A, Meneses P, Rosenfeld MR. Clinical analysis of anti-ma2-associated encephalitis. *Brain.* 2004;127:1831–1844.

36. Blumenfeld H. *Neuroanatomy Through Clinical Cases.* 2nd ed. Sunderland, MA: Sinauer Associates; 2010.

37. Karson CN. Spontaneous eye-blink rates and dopaminergic systems. *Brain.* 1983; 106:643–653.

38. Leigh RJ, Newman SA, Folstein SE, Lasker AG. Abnormal ocular motor control in Huntington's disease. *Neurology.* 1983;33:1268–1275.

39. Zee DS, Chu FC, Leigh RJ, Savino PT, Schatz NJ, Reingold DB, Cogan DG. Blink-saccade synkinesis. *Neurology.* 1983;33:1233–1236.

40. Hain TC, Zee DS, Mordes M. Blink-induced saccadic oscillations. *Ann Neurol.* 1986; 19:299–301.

41. Mays LE, Morrissee DW. Activity of omnipause neurons during blinks. *Soc Neurosci Abstr.* 1993;19:1404.

42. Ongerboer de Visser BW, Moffie D. Effects of brainstem and thalamic lesions on the corneal reflex: an electrophysiological and anatomical study. *Brain.* 1979; 102:595–608.

43. Keane JR. Blinking to sudden illumination. A brain stem reflex present in neocortical death. *Arch Neurol.* 1979;36:52–53.

44. Tackmann W, Ettlin T, Barth R. Blink reflexes elicited by electrical, acoustic and visual stimuli. I. Normal values and possible anatomical pathways. *Eur Neurol.* 1982;21:210–216.

45. Galetta SL. The Neuro-ophthalmic Examination. In: Liu GT, Volpe NJ, Galetta SL, eds *Neuro-ophthalmology: Diagnosis and Management.* 2nd ed. Philadelphia, PA: Saunders/Elsevier; 2010;2:7–36.

46. Rucker JC. Normal and abnormal lid junction. In: Kennard C, Leigh RJ, eds. *Handbook of Clinical Neurology* 3rd series. Vol 102. *Neuro-ophthalmology.* Amsterdam: Elsevier Press; 2011;15:403–424.

47. Averbuch-Heller L. Neurology of the eyelids. *Curr Opin Ophthalmol.* 1997;8(6):27–34.

48. Averbuch-Heller L, Stahl JS, Reich SG. Lid-eye incoordination in Parkinson's disease. *Soc Neurosci Abstr.* 1997;23:297.6.

49. Helmchen C, Rambold H. The eyelid and its contribution to eye movements. In: Straube A, Buttner U, eds. *Neuro-ophthalmology, Developmental Ophthalmology.* Vol 40. Basel: Karger; 2007:110–131.

50. Lowenstein DH, Koch TK, Edwards MS. Cerebral ptosis with contralateral arteriovenous malformation: A report of two cases. *Ann Neurol.* 1987;21:404–407.

51. Lepore FE. Bilateral cerebral ptosis. *Neurology.* 1987;37:1043–1046.

52. Kerstein RC, de Concilis C, Kulwin DR. Acquired ptosis in the young and middle- aged adult population. *Ophthalmology.* 1995;102:924–928.

53. Goldstein JE, Cogan DG. Apraxia of lid opening. *Arch Ophthalmol.* 1965;73:155–159.

54. Brusa A, Mancardi G, Meneghini S, Piccardo A, Brusa G. "Apraxia" of eye opening in idiopathic Parkinson's disease [letter]. *Neurology.* 1986;36:134–136.

55. Dehaene I. Apraxia of eyelid-opening in progressive supranuclear palsy. *Ann Neurol.* 1984;15:115–116.

56. Jankovic J. Apraxia of eyelid opening in progressive supranuclear palsy [reply]. *Ann Neurol.* 1984;15:115–116.

57. Golbe LI, Davis PA, Lepore FE. Eyelid movement abnormalities in progressive supranuclear palsy. *Mov Disord.* 1989;4:297–302.

58. Keane JE. Lid-opening apraxia in Wilson's disease. *J Clin Neuro-ophthalmol.* 1988; 8:31–33.

59. Case records of the Massachusetts General Hospital. Case 32–1975. *N Engl J Med.* 1975;293:346–352.

60. Smith D, Ishikawa T, Dhawan V, Winterkorn JS, Eidelberg D. Lid opening apraxia is associated with medial frontal hypometabolism. *Mov Disord.* 1995;10:341–344.

61. Adair JC, Williamson DJG, Heilman KM. Eyelid opening apraxia in focal cortical degeneration [letter]. *J Neurol Neurosurg Psychiat.* 1995;58:508–509.

62. Lewandowsky M. Ueber Apraxie des lid-schlusses. *Berl Klin Wschr.* 1907;44:921–923.

63. Hoyt WF, Loeffler JD. Neurology of the orbicularis oculi: Anatomic, physiologic, and clinical aspects of lid closure. In: Smith JL, ed. *Neuro-ophthalmology.* Vol 2. St. Louis: CV Mosby; 1965:167–205.

64. Abe K, Fujimura H, Tatsumi C, Toyooka K, Yorifuji S, Yanagihara T. Eyelid "apraxia" in patients with motor neuron disease. *J Neurol Neurosurg Psychiat.* 1995;59:629–632.

65. Lessell S. Supranuclear paralysis of voluntary lid closure. *Arch Ophthalmol.* 1972; 88:241–244.

66. Ross Russell RW. Supranuclear palsy of eyelid closure. *Brain.* 1980;103:71–82.

67. Fahn S. Blepharospasm: a form of focal dystonia. *Adv Neurol.* 1988;49:125–133.

68. Miranda M, Millar A. Blepharospasm associated with bilateral infarts confined to the thalamus: case report. *Mov Disord.* 1998;13:616–617.

69. Fisher CM. Reflex blepharospasm. *Neurology.* 1963;13:77–78.

70. Grandas F, Lopez-Manzanares L, Traba A. Transient blepharospasm secondary to unilateral striatal infarction. *Mov Disord.* 2004;19:1100–1102.

71. Volow MR, Cavenar JO Jr, Grosch WN, Shipley RH, Myers M. The diagnostic dilemma of blepharospasm. *Am J Psychiat.* 1980;137:620–621.

72. Price J, O'Day J. Efficacy and side effects of botulinum toxin treatment for blepharospasm and hemifacial spasm. *Aust N Z J Ophthalmol.* 1994;22(4):255–260.

73. Ainsworth JR, Kraft SP. Long-term changes in duration of relief with botulinum toxin treatment of essential blepharospasm and hemifacial spasm. *Ophthalmology.* 1995;102:2036–2040.

74. Roach ES, DiMario FJ, Kandt RS, Northrup H. Tuberous sclerosis consensus conference: Recommendations for diagnostic evaluation. *J Child Neurol.* 1999; 14(6):401–407.

75. Kwiatkowski DJ, Reeve MP, Cheadle JP, Sampson JR. Molecular genetics. In: Curatolo P, ed. *Tuberous Sclerosis Complex: From Basic Science to Clinical Phenotypes.* International Child Neurology Association. London: MacKeith Press; 2003:228–263.

76. Horita H, Hoashi E, Okuyama Y, Kumagai K, Endo S. The studies of the attacks of abnormal eye movements in a case of infantile spasms. *Folia Psychiatrica Neurologica Japonica.* 1977;31:393–402.

77. Miller JW, Ferrendelli JA. Eyelid twitching seizures and generalized tonic-clonic convulsions: a syndrome of idiopathic generalized epilepsy. *Ann Neurol.* 1990; 27:334–336.

78. Wyllie E, Luders H, Morris HH, Lesser RP, Dinner DS. The lateralizing significance of versive head and eye movements during epileptic seizures. *Neurology.* 1986; 36:606–611.

79. Janetta PJ. Typical or atypical hemifacial spasm. *J Neurosurg.* 1998;89:346–347.

80. Westra I, Drummond GT. Occult pontine glioma in a patient with hemifacial spasm. *Can J Ophthalmol.* 1991;26:148–151.

81. Koutsis G, Kokotis P, Sarrigiannis P, Anagnostouli M, Sfagos C, Karandreas N. Spastic paretic hemifacial contracture in multiple sclerosis: a neglected clinical and EMG entity. *Mult Scler.* 2008;14:927–932.

82. Campos-Benitez M, Kaufmann AM. Neurovascular compression findings in hemifacial spasms. *J Neurosurg.* 2008;109:416–420.

83. Baloh RW, DeRossett SE, Cloughesy TF, Kuncl RW, Miller NR, Merrill J, Posner JB. Novel brainstem syndrome associated with prostate carcinoma. *Neurology.* 1993;43:2591–2596.

84. Gunn RM. Congenital ptosis with peculiar associated movements of the affected lid. *Trans Ophthalmol Soc UK.* 1883;3:283–287.

85. Sinclair WW. Abnormal associated movements of the lids. *Ophthalmol Rev.* 1895; 14:307–319.

86. Sano K. Trigemino-oculomotor synkinesis. *Neurologica.* 1959;1:29–51.

87. Bullock JD. Marcus-Gunn jaw-winking ptosis: Classification and surgical management. *J Ped Ophthalmol Strabismus.* 1980;17:375–379.

88. Bartley GB, Gorman CA. Diagnostic criteria for Graves' ophthalmopathy. *Am J Ophthalmol.* 1995;119:792–795.

89. Ohnishi T, Noguchi S, Murakami N, Nakahara H, Hoshi H, Jinnouchi S, Futami S, Nagamachi S, Watanabe K. Levator palpebrae superioris muscle: MR evaluation of enlargement as a cause of upper eyelid retraction in Graves' disease. *Radiology.* 1993;188:115–118.

90. Hamed LM, Lessner AM. Fixation duress in the pathogenesis of upper eyelid retraction in thyroid orbitopathy. A prospective study. *Ophthalmology.* 1994; 101:1608–1613.

| 3 |
PTOSIS AND NEUROMUSCULAR SYNDROMES

PTOSIS

Ptosis, or drooping of the upper eyelid, is due to weakness of the levator palpebrae superioris muscle. Patients with ptosis often have a long history of droopy lids, with non-neurogenic problems such as levator dehiscence and age-related involutional ptosis among the most common causes (Chapter 2). This said, ptosis can be a sign of considerable significance, and its development over time, which a careful patient history can reveal, is often essential to final diagnosis. These questions are helpful in getting the history process started:

- When did you first notice drooping of your eyelid?
- Was the onset acute?
- Did you notice the lid droop, or did a friend draw your attention to it?
- Has the ptosis increased in severity or improved since it started?
- Do you find it is better after a good night's sleep?
- Is it worse at the end of the day when you are tired?
- Does anything make it better—for example, gently closing your eyes for a few seconds and then opening them?
- Can you close your eyes tightly?
- When you hold the eyelid up are you seeing double?
- Have you ever had ptosis or double vision before?
- What medications are you taking?

Sudden-onset ptosis strongly suggests a vascular etiology, for example acute unilateral ptosis due to microinfarction of the oculomotor nerve (cranial nerve [CN] III) (Chapter 5, Case 5-3).

Sudden-onset bilateral ptosis suggests acute infarction of the central caudal nucleus (CCN) of (Case 5-1, Chapter 5) the oculomotor nuclear complex which can cause isolated bilateral ptosis (selective CCN palsy) or bilateral ptosis, an ipsilateral CN III palsy and contralateral superior rectus weakness.

A pattern of ocular and generalized muscle weakness is a central diagnostic attribute of neuromuscular disease, and the following questions help differentiate between a disorder of neuromuscular transmission such as myasthenia gravis [MG] and a mitochondrial myopathy such as progressive external ophthalmoplegia:

- Do you feel generally fatigued and/or weak?
- Do you have any difficulty chewing or swallowing?
- Can you whistle and blow out your cheeks?
- Can you drink liquids without drooling?
- Is it difficult for you to hold your head up?
- Can you get up out of a low chair without using your arms?
- Do you have weakness of your legs and difficulty running?
- Do you have any muscle pain or tenderness?
- Do you get shortness of breath when you exercise or run?

A topographic pattern of weakness will become apparent from the patient's answers.

Myasthenic patients commonly complain of an inability to hold up their heads late in the day, and both flexors and extensors of the neck will be weak. Proximal limb weakness is also a common feature but, in most cases, only after ocular or pharyngeal involvement has begun. Although these topographic patterns of weakness suggest certain neuromuscular diseases and exclude others, the differential diagnosis of ptosis depends on additional considerations—the age of the patient at the time of onset, the tempo of progression, the severity of the ptosis, and the coexistence of medical and neurological disorders.

DIAGNOSTIC PTOSIS SIGNS

Ptosis Measurements

The width of the palpebral fissure (the opening between the upper and lower lids) is essential to the clinical assessment of ptosis. In normal subjects, the fissure is between 9 and 11 mm in height (in the middle) when the lids are open and relaxed. Palpebral fissure narrowing suggests ptosis or excessive contraction of the orbicularis oculi muscles. Measurement of the marginal reflex distance (MRD—the distance between the center of the pupil and the upper lid margin) should be documented (Figure 2-5). The MRD is normally 3–4 mm. An MRD of greater than 4 mm suggests lid retraction. Less than 3 mm suggests ptosis. When possible, photograph the patient and ask to see old photographs. A review of old photographs or even a driver's license or other picture I.D. may show the early presence of ptosis in patients with an insidious, progressive disorder.

Measurement of levator function (the number of millimeters of lid elevation as the patient looks up) is equally important. Normal levator function is greater than 12 mm, and patients with ptosis due to levator dehiscence or Horner's syndrome usually have normal function. However, levator function is reduced in congenital ptosis, ptosis associated with third-nerve palsies, MG, and myopathic conditions such as chronic progressive ophthalmoplegia and myotonic dystrophy.

Fatigue ptosis, or drooping of the eyelids after an extended period of upgaze, and *curtaining* (elevation of a ptotic eyelid causing drooping of the other eyelid), are characteristic of myasthenic ptosis, although they may also be present in other ptotic disorders.

Enhanced ptosis refers to increased (or unmasked) ptosis in a lid that is nonptotic or less ptotic than the contralateral lid on manual elevation of the nonptotic lid.[1] Hering's law of equal neural innervation of both eyelids explains this sign: for conjugate eye movements, the yoked muscle pair must receive equal innervation if the eyes are to move together.[2]

Ptosis recovery on eye closure—ptosis that recovers on gentle eye closure—is a reflection of decreased activity of acetylcholinesterase (AChE) at the motor end plate and is seen in MG.

Cogan's lid twitch sign is characterized by an overshoot of the ptotic lid after the patient looks down for 3–5 seconds, then looks up quickly. Several small lid twitches may occur before the lid comes to rest.[3] A build-up of acetylcholine (ACh) in the neuromuscular junctions (NMJ) of the levator muscle fibers while the eyelid rests in downgaze is thought to be the explanation for the lid twitch. Following the upward twitch and refixation, the levator quickly fatigues and the eyelid droops. This sign is not pathognomonic of ocular MG; it can occur in other myopathic disorders.

Weakness of eyelid closure and inability to bury the eyelashes fully is a sign of weakness of the orbicularis oculi. It is present in nearly all patients with myasthenia, mitochondrial myopathy, and myotonic dystrophy (in which it is associated with weakness of lid closure).

The *lid peek sign* is positive when a patient with MG is asked to close his or her eyes tightly and maintain them tightly closed for 3–5 seconds. This increases the weakness of the orbicularis oculi, and fatigue allows the lids to separate and the palpebral fissures to open and expose the globe despite initial complete eye closure.[4]

Pseudo-lid retraction is a phenomenon attributable to Hering's law that is seen with myasthenic ptosis. Maximum innervation to keep a ptotic lid open may result in excess lid retraction of the other eye (Case 3-1).[5–7]

Lid retraction in myasthenia should raise the possibility of coexisting thyroid eye disease, especially if proptosis (exophthalmos or forward projection of the eyeball) is present. Thyroid disease occurs with a higher incidence in MG (particularly in patients with antiacetylcholine antibodies) and is more likely to occur in those with ocular MG.[8,9]

The strength of myasthenic muscles often improves when the muscles are cooled—the *ice pack test*—due to suppression of the enzyme AChE.[10–12] This test requires the examiner to first measure the MRD of the upper lid and then hold an ice pack (crushed ice in a surgical glove is effective) over the most obviously ptotic lid for 2 minutes. The test is positive if the MRD (measuring <4 mm) has increased by greater than 2 mm, with visible improvement lasting about 1 minute. This test has a 95% sensitivity and is 100% specific for the diagnosis of MG, making it the fastest, simplest, most risk-free clinical test. However, a *false-negative ice test* can occur in myasthenic patients with complete or nearly complete ptosis, and the ice test is not clinically useful in patients with ophthalmoplegia (weakness of the extraocular muscles) but no ptosis.

The *Tensilon test* is the most serious diagnostic ptosis test for MG. Tensilon (intravenous (IV) edrophonium chloride) is an AChE inhibitor with rapid onset, short duration, a sensitivity of 80–90%—and many false-negative and false-positive results. It is also not without risk. About 5% of clinicians in one series involving IV Tensilon reported serious complications.[12–14] Elderly patients on medication for cardiac disease must be tested in the safety of an emergency room, and the test should never be performed in offices with no emergency facilities close by.

The Tensilon test is recommended for patients with obvious ptosis or paresis of the extraocular muscles since it allows the examiner to easily detect an improvement in function. A modified small-incremental method of giving IV Tensilon is the most effective.[15] The following precautions must be taken:

1. Start by asking the patient if he or she has ever had Tensilon before and whether there were any side effects.

2. Make a list of current medications and any known allergies. *Do not give Tensilon if the patient is taking anticholinesterase drugs.*

3. If possible, never do a Tensilon test alone—preferably have another doctor present to monitor blood pressure (BP), take the pulse rate, and, when necessary, hold the eyebrow(s) down since spontaneous recruitment of the frontalis muscles during the test can elevate the eyebrows and eyelids, and this reaction can be misinterpreted as a positive Tensilon response.

4. Insert a butterfly infusion set into a vein and attach a two-way stop cock. Fill a 2-mL syringe with normal saline, and a 1-mL tuberculin syringe with 10 mg (1 mL) of Tensilon. It is important to have atropine and adrenalin available, but I do not routinely administer atropine prior to Tensilon testing since side effects are quite uncommon with the use of slowly increasing doses of Tensilon.

5. Take a baseline BP and pulse rate and select the endpoint(s); e.g., recovery of ptosis and/ or limb weakness.

6. Advise the patient that Tensilon may cause increased salivation, tearing, mild sweating, twitching of the eyelids, and mild nausea and that if other symptoms are experienced to alert you. (More distressing side effects such as hypotension and bradycardia are extremely rare.)

7. *Always give a 0.2 mL test dose of Tensilon first*, flushed in with normal saline. Recheck BP and pulse rate and observe the patient for 1.5 minutes. If no bradycardia or drop in BP or other symptoms occur, proceed with a dose of 0.3 mL Tensilon and again observe the patient for 1.5 minutes. If no response, give a further dose of 0.5 mL Tensilon, slowly completing a full dose of 1 mL (10 mg) Tensilon. Most myasthenic muscles will respond to 2–3 mg of Tensilon within 30–45 seconds.

8. Improved elevation of the eyelid is a positive response. The eye need not be fully open. Direct observation of significant improvement in the movement of paretic extraocular muscles also represents a positive response. Because Tensilon continues to act for 3–5 minutes, the examiner will have time to watch the positive response fade and ptosis return.

Once the test has been completed, the examiner should observe the patient's eye movements immediately post Tensilon. As impaired motility responds to Tensilon, it unmasks the effects of central adaptation and exposes an increased saccadic innervation resulting in saccadic hypermetria. Sometimes the patient is not able to hold steady fixation post-Tensilon because of repetitive hypermetric saccades that overshoot the target in both directions—these movements are called *macrosaccadic oscillations.*[16]

The alternative to Tensilon as a diagnostic test is neostigmine (Prostigmin; 15 mg po), a longer acting drug that permits more time for detailed evaluation of muscle strength. Neostigmine intramuscularly is the diagnostic test of choice in children and in suspected myasthenic adults with diplopia without ptosis. The appropriate dose for an adult is a mix of 0.6 mg of atropine sulfate with 0.5–1.5 mg of neostigmine in a 3 cc syringe injected into the deltoid muscle. A response is usually apparent within 15 minutes and more obvious 30–45 minutes post-injection. The sensitivity of the neostigmine test ranges from 70% to 94%.

THE NEUROMUSCULAR JUNCTION

The NMJ is a specialized chemical synapse that consists of a terminal Schwann cell process, motor nerve terminal, synaptic space, and a postsynaptic region containing receptors and junctional sarcoplasm. Each nerve terminal contains thousands of vesicles aligned near the presynaptic membrane, some of which cluster around slight thickenings in the membrane called *release sites* or *active zones*. The vesicles contain packets or quanta of ACh, the neurotransmitter released by a calcium-dependent process of excitation that occurs both spontaneously and in response to nerve impulses. The arrival of a nerve impulse results in neuronal depolarization, and this causes voltage-gated calcium channels in the presynaptic membrane to open and allow calcium ions to enter. This process triggers fusion of the vesicles with the presynaptic membrane, releasing ACh into the synaptic cleft. Acetylcholine then crosses the synaptic space to reach receptors on the muscle sarcolemma, which are concentrated in the peaks of the junctional folds opposite the release sites. When ACh binds to the ACh receptor (AChR), the receptor's ion channel opens transiently and cations, mainly sodium, enter the muscle cell, producing a localized endplate potential (EPP). If the amplitude of this potential is sufficient, it generates an action potential that spreads along the length of the muscle fiber, triggering the release of calcium from internal stores, which leads to muscle contraction.[17]

The EPPs are normally more than sufficient to generate consistent muscle action potentials with no failures—the EPP excess is the "safety margin" of neuromuscular transmission. The transmission process is extremely rapid, measured in milliseconds, and terminates through hydrolysis of ACh by AChE. When transmission fails at multiple junctions, muscle power progressively declines into clinically evident weakness.

This principle is basic to an understanding of the pathophysiology of disorders of neuromuscular transmission, and it is particularly relevant to the pathogenesis of MG. Not surprisingly, researchers have considered the NMJ the Achilles heel of the motor system since virtually every step of the transmission process is vulnerable to disease, plant and animal toxins, and weapons of biological warfare.

DISORDERS OF NEUROMUSCULAR TRANSMISSION

Myasthenia Gravis

Myasthenia gravis is a disease of the postsynaptic region of the NMJ. The Lambert-Eaton myasthenic syndrome, in contrast, affects the presynaptic region, yet both diseases share an unmistakable symptom: they are both characterized by fatigable muscle weakness due to failure of neuromuscular transmission at the critical junction where muscle contraction must begin. Of the two diseases, MG (from the Latin for "serious muscle disease") is by far the most significant.

In MG, failure of neuromuscular transmission is due to an autoantibody-mediated process. The nicotinic AChR is the principal antigenic target, and AChR antibodies (AChR-ab) access the NMJ (which is outside the blood–nerve barrier) and bind to the AChRs.

It is still not clear which properties of extraocular muscles predispose them to symptomatic involvement in MG since extraocular muscles differ anatomically, physiologically, and immunologically from limb muscles. One explanation may be that the safety margin in the neuromuscular transmission process is smaller in extraocular muscles than in skeletal muscles because of less prominent synaptic folds and fewer AChRs on the postsynaptic membrane.

In pure ocular myasthenia, in contrast to the generalized form, onset is with extraocular muscle weakness, and generalized muscle weakness may not follow for up to 2 years.[18–20]

The peak age of onset of MG is between 20 and 30 years in women and between 50 and 60 years in men. Under the age of 40, women are affected two to three times as often as men. In later life, the incidence in men is higher, and there is evidence of underdiagnosis.[21]

Criteria for ocular MG (OMG) include demonstration of:

- Uni- or bilateral ptosis
- Uni- or bilateral extraocular weakness—if only lateral rectus muscle weakness is present, clear-cut fatigability or demonstrable response to treatment are required
- Uni- or bilateral orbicularis oculi weakness, but no other weakness of head and neck muscles
- No pupillary abnormality
- Fatigue of affected muscles with clear-cut ptosis after sustained upward gaze[22]

The most important characteristic of MG is variable weakness and fatigability, and this needs to be identified in the patient's clinical history, as well as in the examination of both symptomatic and nonsymptomatic muscle groups. Most often, normal strength is experienced on waking in the morning, and fatigue becomes more obvious toward the end of the day, resulting in noticeable ptosis with or without diplopia.

In generalized MG (GMG), the gradual reduction in motor function throughout the day may result in frequent falls and difficulty negotiating stairs. Weakness chewing and swallowing and sometimes choking episodes at an evening meal can occur. Lower limb involvement is often relatively delayed or minimal.

In pure ocular adult myasthenia, 50% of patients have AChR-ab and the remainder have antibody-negative disease. In generalized myasthenia, 85% of patients have AChR-ab. As already noted, these antibodies access the NMJ and bind to the AChRs, leading to loss of receptors and impaired function[23] (Figure 3-1). A genetic basis for MG is suggested by the association of human leukocyte antigen (HLA) groups, such as HLA-B8 and HLA-DR3, in approximately 60% of the white population. Genetic susceptibility is also suggested by the association of MG with other autoimmune disorders, such as type 1 diabetes, thyroid disease, systemic lupus erythematosus, and rheumatoid arthritis.[24]

In the case presented here, ptosis is a principal presenting sign—and it is a clinical alert to the severity with which MG can develop over time.

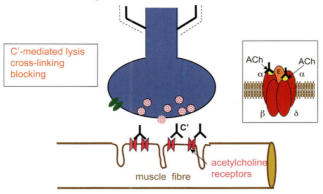

acetylcholine receptor antibodies are present in 85% of MG patients and cause AChR loss

FIGURE 3-1 The neuromuscular junction and myasthenia gravis. The normal junction is shown with the pre- and postsynaptic ion channels and acetylcholine receptors (AchRs). In myasthenia gravis, antibodies from the circulation bind to the AchRs, leading to AchR loss and complement-mediated damage to the postsynaptic membrane. The nerve terminal is unaffected.

Courtesy of Professor John Newsom-Davis.

CASE 3-1 Generalized Myasthenia Gravis

Video Display

The patient is a 39-year-old woman who presented in July 1977 with a history of intermittent horizontal diplopia lasting for 2 weeks. Three weeks later, the left upper eyelid started to droop, and, by the end of the day, the eye was closed. She had no ptosis of the right eye (OD) and no generalized fatigue. She consulted an internist and was referred to a neurosurgeon, who noted ptosis OS and weakness of the medial rectus muscle. A computed tomography (CT) brain scan was normal. She was referred for neurological evaluation.

Her past history was negative for previous episodes of fatigue, diplopia or ptosis, nasal speech, or difficulty swallowing.

Analysis of the History

- What are the major presenting symptoms?
- Where are the central nervous system (CNS) lesion(s) likely to be?

CASE 3-1 SYMPTOMS

Symptoms	Location Correlation
Horizontal diplopia	Medial rectus muscle
	Lateral rectus muscle
Progressive ptosis	Levator palpebrae superioris

The analysis guides the clinical examination.

Examination

Ocular Motility/Neurological

- Partial ptosis left eye (OS)
- Lid retraction right eye (OD)
- Enhanced ptosis OD with manual elevation of ptotic lid OS
- Bilateral overaction of the frontalis muscle
- Lid twitch OS
- Fatigable ptosis OS with slight increase on sustained upgaze
- No recovery of ptosis on gentle eye closure
- Impaired ability to bury her eyelashes fully
- Positive lid peek sign
- Mild weakness of medial rectus muscle bilaterally, OS > OD
- Poor convergence
- No nystagmus of the abducting eye
- Normal pupil reflexes
- Weakness of neck flexion
- Motor strength 5/5 throughout
- Normal deep tendon reflexes

What Diagnostic Tests Should Follow?

Tests to confirm a diagnosis of MG are:

- Response to anticholinesterase agents (edrophonium chloride [Tensilon], pyridostigmine bromide [Mestinon], neostigmine)
- Serology (AChR-ab)
- Electrophysiology studies (see later section)
- Chest CT for thymic enlargement/mass

Test Results

Ptosis and neck strength were the selected endpoints for the Tensilon test. An IV dose of 0.2 mL Tensilon produced a positive response with elevation of the ptotic eyelid OS and correction of lid retraction OD. The response lasted 30 seconds and then the left eyelid drooped. A further 0.3 mL of Tensilon resulted in complete recovery of ptosis OS and full neck strength. The remaining 0.5 mL of Tensilon was not given (Figure 3-2A–C).

An objective measure of response is critical to the Tensilon test, and it must be obtained. Positive results are seen in up to 90% of individuals but the Tensilon test should not form the sole basis for diagnosis.

The patient tested positive for antistriatal muscle antibodies, which suggested that she might harbor a thymoma.[25] AChR-ab studies were not done.

A chest x-ray showed a large anterior mediastinal mass. Chest CT and tomograms showed a demarcated, rounded 4 cm mass in the anterior mediastinum directly contiguous and anterior to the inferior portion of the transverse aortic arch. The mass was homogeneous, without evidence of calcification or lobulation. There was no hilar adenopathy (Figure 3-3).

Diagnosis: Generalized Myasthenia Gravis

Treatment

The treatment options for all autoimmune myasthenias are:

- Anticholinesterase agents
- Immunosuppression and immune modulators
- Plasma exchange
- Thymectomy

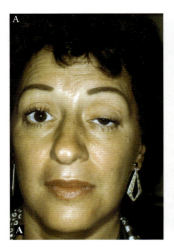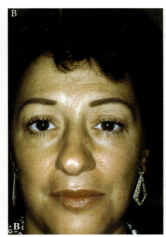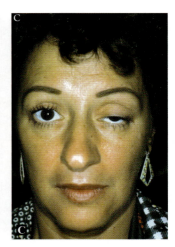

FIGURE 3-2 (A) Patient with myasthenia gravis with partial ptosis of the left eye, lid retraction of the right eye, and bilateral elevation of the eyebrows. (B) Positive Tensilon test with elevation of the ptotic eyelid. Note absent retraction of the right eyelid. (C) Five minutes post Tensilon, return of ptosis left eyelid and retraction of right eyelid.

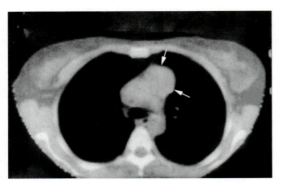

FIGURE 3-3 Chest computed tomogram (CT) shows a large anterior mediastinal mass (*arrows*).

First-line treatment of MG is with anticholinesterase agents, Mestinon, and/or neostigmine. Both drugs increase the half-life of ACh released into the synaptic cleft by inhibiting its hydrolysis by the enzyme AChE and allowing ACh to interact repeatedly with the limited number of AChRs to improve muscle strength.[26,27]

Special Explanatory Note

Corticosteroids are the mainstay of immunosuppressive therapy in MG and induce remission in up to 80% of patients who are given high-dose prednisone therapy (starting at a low dose of 10–20 mg/day and slowly titrating the dose up by 3 mg/day every 5 days to 60 mg/day). Patients usually achieve sustained improvement in 1–3 months.[28] Once the patient is clinically stable, prednisone can be switched to alternate-day therapy and gradually tapered down to a low maintenance dose. When the patient is in remission, steroids can be stopped. Other immunosuppressive drugs include azathioprine,[29] cyclophosphamide,[30] and mycophenolate mofetil.[31]

Plasma exchange aims to remove circulating AChR antibodies and can be effective to treat myasthenic crises; it can be used preoperatively to reduce morbidity, in acute treatment of weak patients, or to gain control of symptoms while immunosuppressants are commenced. Randomized studies are still required to evaluate the efficacy and role of plasma exchange in treatment protocols.[32]

Intravenous immunoglobulin (400 mg/kg/day for 5 days) may be used for some patients who are unable to tolerate or receive plasma exchange.[33,34]

Myasthenic crises are life-threatening episodes of respiratory or bulbar paralysis often provoked by an infection.

Cholinergic crises are caused by excessive anticholinesterase medication leading to a block of neuromuscular transmission that exacerbates weakness associated with cholinergic symptoms (sweating, lacrimation, vomiting, and miosis).

On August 8, 1977, the patient had a thymectomy. The tumor was cystic, overall dimension 11 × 5 × 1 cm, and weighed 45 grams. Pathology revealed a thymolipoma.

On day 1 postsurgery, the patient complained of diplopia in mid-afternoon and marked drooping of her eyelids. The clinical signs on examination are listed in the following chart:

Ocular Motility/Neurological

- Bilateral asymmetrical ptosis, OS > OD
- Bilateral lid twitch
- Palpebral fissure OD 9mm, OS 7 mm
- Increased ptosis bilaterally on prolonged upgaze
- Full vertical gaze
- Bilateral weakness of the medial rectus muscles
- Impaired convergence
- No nystagmus
- No facial weakness
- Bulbar muscles normal
- Neck flexion/mild weakness
- Motor strength 5/5 throughout
- Forced vital capacity normal

Over the next 3 days, she was closely monitored for further signs of GMG. She made an excellent recovery without any medication and was discharged home.

Special Explanatory Note

Thymectomy induces remission in up to 60% of patients with GMG. Clinical improvement is usually delayed at least 6–12 months, but, in some cases, recovery does not occur for several years. The maximal benefit is seen in those patients who undergo thymectomy within 2 years of disease onset.[35–37]

Six weeks later, in September 1977, the patient was readmitted with generalized fatigue, ptosis, diplopia, difficulty chewing, and weakness of the jaw and neck. She had no difficulty swallowing or breathing and no change in the quality of her voice. She was depressed and anxious. The clinical signs at that time are shown in the following chart:

ER Examination

- Bilateral asymmetrical ptosis
- Weakness of the orbicularis oculi and an inability to bury her eyelashes fully
- Increased ptosis on fatigue
- Cogan's lid twitch OS
- Fatigue of horizontal saccades after continuous rapid gaze right and left to the point where the eyes came to a standstill
- Impaired movement of the palate, intact gag reflex, and absent jaw jerk

- Bilateral facial weakness with difficulty pursing her lips and unable to whistle
- Generalized fatigue with inability to sustain the arms elevated for 2 minutes
- Forced vital capacity normal

Treatment

Anticholinesterase inhibitors were prescribed, as was immunosuppression—bearing always in mind that long-term corticosteroid therapy can have serious side effects, with cataracts, diabetes mellitus, hypertension, osteoporosis, weight gain, and psychosis among them.

The patient received Mestinon 60 mg q3h and prednisone 40 mg/day. Twenty-four hours later, there was striking improvement. By day 4, she had fully recovered and was discharged home. Prednisone was tapered and stopped, and Mestinon reduced to 60 mg b.i.d. on follow-up.

Special Explanatory Note

The relationship between MG and thymic pathology, including thymoma, is well known. The thymus gland is thought to be necessary for the deletion of autoreactive T cells and seems to have an important role in the pathogenesis of MG. In early-onset MG patients, the thymus is typically enlarged. In late-onset patients, the thymus is usually atrophic. Approximately 10–15% of MG patients have a thymoma, and 10% of these thymomas are malignant—thus, MG may be considered the most common of the paraneoplastic syndromes in patients with thymoma.[38] Less often recognized extrathymic malignancies and paraneoplastic disorders have also been reported.[39,40]

Neuromuscular transmission failure arises once again in the following case. This time, there is a cautionary flag raised on the use of drugs that may cause transmission to fail.

CASE 3-2 Ocular Myasthenia Gravis

Video Display

The patient is a 46-year-old man with late-onset diabetes and hypertension (Figure 3-4). He presented with a 5-week history of vertical diplopia that began acutely while playing golf. Drooping of the left eyelid developed a few days later and closed the eye. The ptosis completely recovered during sleep, but, immediately on waking in the morning, he had intermittent double vision and within 1 hour drooping of the left eyelid that persisted for the rest of the day. His ophthalmologist referred him for neurological evaluation.

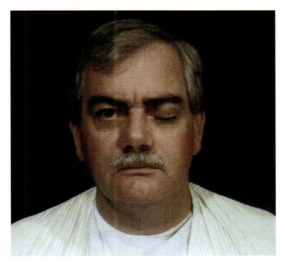

FIGURE 3-4 Patient with unilateral ptosis.

Analysis of the History

- What are the major presenting symptoms?
- Where are the CNS lesion(s) likely to be?

CASE 3-2 SYMPTOMS

Symptoms	Location Correlation
Intermittent diplopia	Extraocular muscles
Unilateral ptosis	Levator palpebrae superioris
Positive sleep test	

The analysis guides the clinical examination.

Ocular Motility

- Complete ptosis of the left (OS) eye
- Mild lid retraction of the right (OD) eyelid
- Unable to bury the eyelashes fully OS
- Overaction of the frontalis muscles
- Full horizontal eye movements
- Normal convergence

Neurological—Selected Signs

- Speech normal
- Tongue moved fully
- Palate and gag reflex normal
- No neck weakness
- Pupils 3 mm OU equally brisk to light and near
- No facial weakness
- Muscle strength 5/5 throughout
- Tendon reflexes symmetric 1+
- Normal gait

Special Explanatory Note

Recovery of ptosis during sleep (the positive sleep test) is reported to have 99% sensitivity and 91% specificity in ptosis due to MG, and the sleep test is an important and safe alternative to tensilon.[41]

Localization and Differential Diagnosis

Myasthenia gravis can mimic a supranuclear, infranuclear, nuclear or ocular motor nerve palsy and all these disorders should be considered in the differential diagnosis of ocular MG. For example, unilateral ptosis due to an oculomotor nerve CN III, palsy sparing the pupil resembles unilateral myasthenic ptosis (compare Case 5-3 Chapter 5 with Case 3-2) A trochlear nerve CN IV; or abducens nerve CN VI palsy are in the differential diagnosis of diplopia, (Chapter 4) Isolated bilateral ptosis due to a nuclear lesion of CN III affecting the central caudal nucleus may be mistaken for ocular MG (Chapter 5). An internuclear opthalmoplegia with weakness of adduction (medial rectus muscle) due to a lesion of the medial longitudinal fasiculus warrants, on occasion, a Tensilon test (Chapter 6).

What Diagnostic Tests Should Follow?

- Ice pack test (bearing in mind that the ice pack test is most likely to give false-negative results in MG patients with complete or nearly complete ptosis).
- Tensilon test
- Chest x-ray
- AChR-ab
- Anti-MuSK-ab

Test Results

The IV Tensilon test was positive, with prompt elevation of the eyelid after 0.3 mL of Tensilon (or 1 mL = 10 mg). The chest x-ray was normal, the AChR-ab negative, and the Anti-MuSK-ab negative.

Diagnosis: Seronegative Ocular Myasthenia Gravis

The diagnosis of MG should be confirmed by at least one of the tests listed below, which also shows their reported sensitivity:[42]

Generalized MG

- Acetylcholine receptor antibodies   80–90%
- MuSK antibodies (in AChR Ab(−) patients)   40–50%
- Repetitive nerve stimulation   75%
- Single fiber electromyography   92–99%

Ocular MG

- Acetylcholine receptor antibodies   40–55%
- MuSK antibodies (in AChR Ab(−) patients)   0 (case reports)
- Repetitive nerve stimulation   50%
- Single fiber electromyography   85–95%

Special Explanatory Note

In MG, the loss of functional AChRs results in a decrement of 10–15% in the compound muscle action potential size on *repetitive nerve stimulation* (RNS), a decrement apparent by the third to fifth stimulus. This decrement may be reversed by exercise or tensilon.[43]

Stimulated single-fiber electromyography (SF-EMG) measures the firing interval of two muscle fibers within the same motor unit. In MG, the firing interval of individual muscle fibers, or *jitter*, is increased, and there may be intermittent blocking of neuromuscular transmission.[44] When the safety margin for transmission is low, these latency variables (jitters) are increased. SF-EMG is positive in 88–99% of all patients with MG.[45,46] This test must be performed by an experienced electrophysiologist (see Case 3-4).

Test Results

The chest CT was normal. The SF-EMG was abnormal, with jitter present in one pair.

Are There Any Hematological Tests Needed?

Because there is an increased prevalence of other autoimmune diseases in these patients, hematological tests must include:

- A complete blood count
- Erythrocyte sedimentation rate
- Antinuclear antibody test
- Thyroid function tests and thyroid antibodies

Test Results

Thyroid function normal was normal, thyroid antibodies were negative, and the hematological tests were all normal.

Treatment

Anticholinesterase inhibitors are the first-line treatment choice. The patient received Mestinon, but failed to respond to the drug, raising the possibility that the Mestinon pills were not absorbed in the stomach. He received instead liquid ambenonium chloride (Mytelase), a cholinesterase inhibitor, at an equivalent neostigmine dose of 60 mg q.i.d. at 8 A.M., 12 P.M., 6 P.M., and 10 P.M. q.d., which resulted in an excellent response and complete recovery. After 3 months, medication was stopped.

In 2003, the patient lacerated his right forearm and was treated at a local hospital with IV antibiotics (drugs unknown) and cephalexin (Keflex) for 1 week. The forearm tendons were then repaired under a local regional anesthetic block. Three days postoperatively, he developed ptosis OD and horizontal diplopia with full eye movements. He had no signs of generalized MG. He was prescribed a short course of Mestinon 60 mg q4h and fully recovered.

Special Explanatory Note

Many drugs have been reported to exacerbate weakness in patients with MG, but not all patients react adversely to the dangerous drugs listed in Table 3-1.[47] Conversely, not all "safe" drugs can be used with impunity in patients with MG. However, *whenever possible,* the drugs listed in Table 3-1 should be avoided, and MG patients should be followed very closely when any new drug is prescribed for them.

TABLE 3-1: Drugs That May Exacerbate Myasthenia Gravis

Antibiotics
Aminoglycosides: e.g., streptomycin, tobramycin, kanamycin
Quinolones: e.g., ciprofloxacin, levofloxacin, ofloxacin, gatifloxacin
Macrolides: e.g., erythromycin, azithromycin,

Nondepolarizing muscle relaxants for surgery
D-Tubocurarine (curare), pancuronium, vecuronium, atracurium
Beta-blocking agents
Propranolol, atenolol, metoprolol

Local anesthetics and related agents
Procaine, Xylocaine in large amounts
Procainamide (for arrhythmias)
Botulinum toxin (Botox exacerbates weakness)

Quinine derivatives
Quinine, quinidine, chloroquine, mefloquine (Lariam)
Magnesium

Modified and reproduced with permission.[47]

A rare subgroup of patients (1–2%) who have low concentrations of AChR-abs may develop MG during penicillamine treatment for rheumatoid arthritis and sometimes for Wilson's disease. Penicillamine-induced MG is indistinguishable from other forms of the disease but typically remits when the drug is stopped.

■ **Clinical Points to Remember About Autoantibodies in Myasthenia Gravis**
- AChR-abs are positive in 85% of patients with GMG.[48–50]
- AChR-abs are positive in 50% of patients with OMG.
- AChR-ab negative does not exclude MG.
- Cases of seronegative GMG are not distinguishable clinically from seropositive cases with AChR-abs.
- Forty percent of AChR-ab seronegative patients with GMG have anti-MuSK antibodies.
- Anti-MuSK antibodies are present in OMG.[51–53]
- Despite the absence of AChR-ab, seronegative MG is an antibody-mediated disease.[54] ■

The leading differential diagnoses of OMG are:

- Mitochondrial cytopathy (chronic progressive external ophthalmoplegia)
- Oculopharyngeal muscular dystrophy
- Thyroid ophthalmopathy

The leading differential diagnoses of GMG are:

- Lambert-Eaton myasthenic syndrome
- Acute Guillain-Barré syndrome
- Fisher syndrome
- Idiopathic myopathies
- Botulism

Two important differential diagnoses for bulbar myasthenia are:

- Amyotrophic lateral sclerosis
- Brainstem stroke

■ **Clinical Points to Remember About Myasthenia Gravis**
- Myasthenia gravis frequently presents with ptosis, diplopia, and painless, fatigable weakness.
- Weakness can be localized for years to the ocular muscles.
- Bulbar weakness causes nasal speech and swallowing difficulties.
- Limb weakness is most pronounced proximally.
- Weakness of neck extension leads to head droop (head ptosis).

- Respiratory muscle weakness can be life-threatening and is best monitored by measurement of forced vital capacity.
- Tendon reflexes are normal.
- A positive anti-AChR-ab test is diagnostic of MG.
- Seronegative MG patients are not distinguishable clinically from AChR-ab positive cases.
- Seronegative MG patients should be tested for anti-MuSK-abs. ■

MuSK Antibody Myasthenic Syndrome

Muscle specific kinase MG (MuSK-MG) was first described by Hoch et al. in 2001.[55] MuSK-MG is immunologically distinct from MG, and the mechanism through which anti-MuSK antibodies (MuSK-abs) cause failure of neuromuscular transmission is not yet clear (Figure 3-5).

Anti-MuSK antibodies have been found in up to 70% of anti-AChR antibody-negative individuals. The disease has a striking prevalence among women, with age of onset ranging from 6 to 68 years and 56% presenting under age 40. The clinical phenotype is characterized by oculobulbar involvement, marked facial weakness, and tongue muscle atrophy, due to significant and persistent bulbar muscle involvement.[56–58]

The case presented here is atypical: the child presented in infancy but remained undiagnosed until she reached the age of 20.

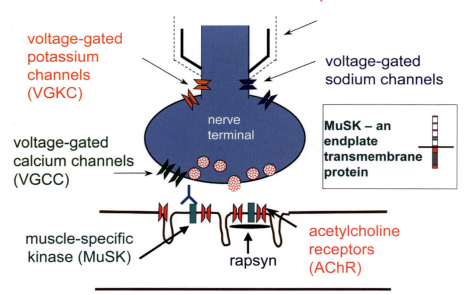

FIGURE 3-5 Neuromuscular junction in MuSK myasthenia gravis.

Courtesy of Professor John Newsom-Davis.

CASE 3-3 MuSK Myasthenia Gravis

Video Display

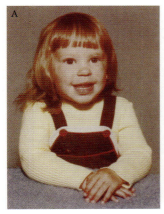 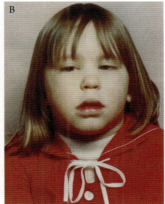 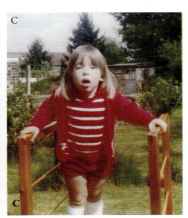

FIGURE 3-6 Facial characteristics associated with myasthenia due to muscle specific kinase antibodies. (A) Before myasthenia diagnosis at age two. (B) At diagnosis and before treatment at age three. (C) Progressive ptosis and facial weakness at age four.

Reproduced with permission.[58]

The patient, a girl aged 3 years, presented with bilateral ptosis and severe facial weakness (Figure 3-6A–C). At the age of 14, a SF-EMG study detected a disorder of neuromuscular transmission, and she was diagnosed with MG. She underwent plasma exchange, which resulted in significant clinical improvement, and she was started on corticosteroid treatment. As soon as her condition stabilized, she was weaned off steroids. At 16, her symptoms returned with bilateral ptosis, weakness of eye closure, profound facial weakness and moderate axial and limb weakness (Figure 3-7).

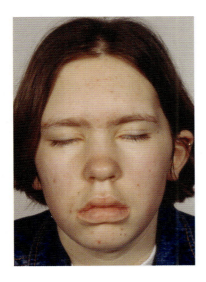

FIGURE 3-7 Patient, age sixteen, with bilateral ptosis, weakness of eye closure, and bilateral facial weakness.

Courtesy of Professor John Newsom-Davis.

Repetitive nerve studies of the right frontalis and orbicularis oculi muscles showed no spontaneous activity, no motor units under voluntary control, and no activity on nerve stimulation. The right orbicularis oris muscle was also studied and showed very few small units (maximum amplitude 50 uV) and a normal profile (duration 5 msec, not polyphasic). Steroids were reintroduced, and she was started on azathioprine as a steroid- sparing immunosuppressive agent. She failed to respond to this drug, and her medication was switched to cyclosporine therapy together with prednisolone. She responded well, and her axial and limb weakness went into remission but her severe facial weakness persisted.

In 2007, at age 20, she relapsed and developed marked nasal speech without dysphagia. A striking clinical finding at that time was severe wasting of the tongue with a triple furrowed appearance[59] (Figure 3-8A).

What Diagnostic Tests Should Follow?

- Brain magnetic resonance imaging (MRI)
- Antibody studies

Test Results

Brain MRI of the facial and tongue muscles (in a similar case) confirmed muscular atrophy, and an abnormally high signal replaced most of the intrinsic tongue musculature (Figure 3-8B–E). Antibody studies showed the patient to be AChR-ab negative and Anti-MuSK-abs positive.

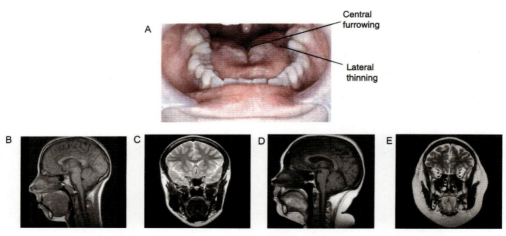

FIGURE 3-8 (A) Photograph demonstrating central tongue wasting (central furrowing) with some lateral thinning, giving a "triple furrowed" tongue in a MuSK antibody–positive patient. (B–C) Magnetic resonance T1 sagittal midline and coronal T2 images of a normal tongue in a healthy individual for comparison. (D–E) Atrophy of the tongue in a MuSK-MG patient with increased T1 and T2 signal in the tongue reflecting fatty replacement.

Modified and reproduced with permission.[59]

Special Explanatory Note

The pattern of muscle involvement, dysarthria (nasal speech), dysphonia, facial weakness, dysphagia (caused by weakness of both tongue and pharyngeal muscles), and fatigable asymmetric ptosis and esotropia, is reported in all cases of MuSK-MG. Involvement of limb muscles is not consistent across cases. Some patients complain only of limb fatigability whereas others have clear-cut weakness present—a feature of this case. Fewer than one in four patients develop facial and pharyngeal weakness with atrophy of the facial muscles and tongue, but it is still not clear why the facial and tongue muscles should be selectively involved.

The clinical phenotype observed in MuSK-MG can vary, and a more limited clinical picture with weakness restricted to neck extensors, shoulder, and respiratory muscles has been reported. Respiratory crises can be remarkably frequent, and, in severely affected patients, periodic exacerbation and respiratory crises require hospitalization, assisted ventilation, and urgent plasma exchange therapy.[60,61]

Newer drugs, such as mycophenolate mofetil, appear to be clinically more effective and may prevent development of muscle wasting.

■ **Clinical Points to Remember About MuSK-MG**

- MuSK-MG presents with predominantly oculobulbar symptoms and facial weakness.
- The age range at onset is from 6 to 68 years. Most patients are young women under 40 years of age.
- Facial muscle atrophy is relatively common in long-standing MuSK-MG.
- There is no substantial thymus pathology.
- Weakness of the limbs may remit with treatment, whereas facial and bulbar weakness persists.
- Patients are seronegative for AChR-abs.
- SF-EMG usually detects a transmission defect in facial muscles but may be normal in limb muscles.
- Plasma exchange is the treatment of choice for exacerbations and respiratory crises.
- Response to treatment with prednisone and azathioprine can be poor, and additional immunosuppressive drugs may be required. ■

Lambert-Eaton Myasthenic Syndrome

The Lambert-Eaton myasthenic syndrome (LEMS) is a relatively rare paraneoplastic disorder of neuromuscular transmission (Figure 3-9).[62]

LEMS is due to an IgG antibody that targets voltage-gated calcium channels (VGCC) at the motor nerve terminal, blocking the calcium influx that normally occurs with nerve depolarization at the motor endplate. This process results in an inadequate presynaptic release of ACh and impaired neuromuscular transmission.[63,64]

Abnormally high titers of VGCC antibodies are found in approximately 90% of patients with LEMS but also in 20–40% of patients with small (oat) cell lung cancer who do not have

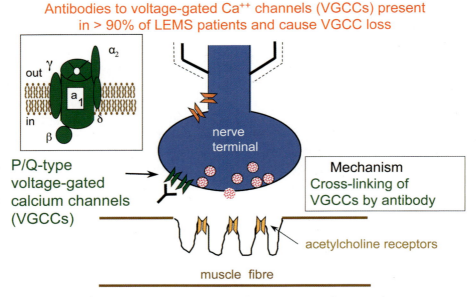

FIGURE 3-9 Neuromuscular junction in Lambert-Eaton myasthenic syndrome.

Courtesy of Professor John Newsom-Davis.

clinical symptoms of LEMS.[65] Thus, a positive VGCC antibody test is not necessarily diagnostic of LEMS. Electromyography (EMG) studies that differentiate between a presynaptic (e.g., LEMS) and a postsynaptic (e.g., MG) neuromuscular transmission disorder are crucial in the diagnosis of LEMS.

The clinical and electrophysiological features of 50 consecutive LEMS cases have been analyzed.[66] Carcinoma was detected in 25, of whom 21 had small-cell lung cancer evident within 2 years of onset of LEMS symptoms, as in the case presented here.

CASE 3-4 Lambert-Eaton Syndrome

No Video Display

The patient is a 67-year-old man who was in good health until March 1998, when he developed increasing muscle weakness and marked generalized fatigue. The muscle weakness affected his legs more than his arms, and he had difficulty getting up from a low chair and climbing stairs. He was unable to run. He was seen by a neurologist at a local hospital and diagnosed with a myopathic disorder. An EMG was done and reported to be normal.

In June 1998, the patient was referred to the neurology clinic with further progression of limb weakness and the onset of a dry mouth.

Analysis of the History

· What are the major presenting symptoms?
· Where are the CNS lesion(s) likely to be?

CASE 3-4 SYMPTOMS

Symptoms	Location Correlation
Generalized fatigue	At this stage idiopathic
Leg weakness	Neuromuscular disorder
Dry mouth	Autonomic nervous system

The analysis guides the clinical examination.

Examination

Ocular Motility/Neurological

· Mild bilateral ptosis
· Normal saccadic and pursuit eye movements
· No facial or bulbar muscle weakness
· Proximal limb weakness
· Symmetrically depressed deep tendon reflexes
· His hand grasp was notably weak when he first grasped the hand of the examiner but by repeatedly grasping it his strength steadily increased (this physiological phenomenon is called post-tetanic facilitation)

Localization and Differential Diagnosis

It is likely that the normal EMG misled the neurologist who originally examined this patient and no RNS studies (which would have been diagnostic for LEMS) were performed.

The patient's symptoms highlight the difference in distribution of muscle weakness between MG and the LEM syndrome.[67] In MG, initial weakness presents with ptosis and involves the extraocular muscles in 90% of cases. In LEMS, proximal muscle weakness in the limbs, especially the legs, is the usual first symptom in more than 95% of cases, mimicking a myopathy. Muscle weakness in MG tends to develop in a craniocaudal direction; in LEMS, it develops in the opposite direction. Oculobulbar weakness in the form of diplopia, ptosis, dysphagia, and dysarthria is relatively uncommon in LEMS and, when present, is usually mild.[68] Autonomic symptoms such as dry mouth (as in this case) and erectile dysfunction in men should prompt clinicians to consider LEMS in the differential diagnosis.

What Additional Tests Should Follow?

· RNS study
· Antibody studies: VGCC, AChR-ab, and anti-Hu
· Search for occult malignancy

Test Results

The RNS showed low-amplitude motor responses and post-tetanic facilitation in all four extremities.

Special Explanatory Note

Normally, increased mobilization of calcium occurs in the nerve terminal following exercise (or electric stimulation of motor nerves), increasing the release of ACh and the amplitude of the muscle action potential—this is post-tetanic facilitation.

The crucial difference between a presynaptic (LEMS) and a postsynaptic (MG) neuromuscular transmission disorder is that brief voluntary exercise (10–15 seconds) or, if necessary, high-frequency repetitive motor nerve stimulation (20–50 Hz), leads to marked facilitation of the muscle action potential (>100%) and increased muscle strength *only in LEMS*. Post-tetanic facilitation is the physiological basis of RNS study[69] and explains postexercise facilitation of the deep tendon reflexes.[70]

Antibody studies showed VGCC antibodies positive. The patient was AChR-ab negative and anti-Hu negative. A chest x-ray/CT scan revealed a 3.5 cm subcarinal mass, clear lungs, and no adenopathy.

After the patient was told the result of his chest x-ray, he admitted that he had been a heavy cigarette smoker. His wife added that he was once "never without one," averaging two packs per day. He stopped smoking 20 years prior to the onset of LEMS.

What Is the Next Step?

A bronchoscopy and needle biopsy were performed. Pathology revealed small (oat) cell lung cancer.

Diagnosis: Lambert-Eaton Myasthenic Syndrome

The patient had paraneoplastic small (oat) cell lung cancer.

Treatment

Treatment of paraneoplastic LEMS must deal with the underlying malignancy. Surgery, chemotherapy, radiation therapy, or a combination are the primary therapies for LEMS associated with cancer of the lung,[71] as well as medication to enhance release of the neurotransmitter ACh.

The drug of choice for the treatment of LEMS is 3,4-diaminopyridine.[72] It acts by blocking potassium channels in the distal motor terminal thus prolonging the VGCC open time and prolonging the motor-nerve action potential, thereby increasing neurotransmitter (ACh) release. It is frequently highly effective in improving muscle strength. This drug was initially approved by the FDA only for compassionate use, and it was unavailable for this patient. When it can be used, the initial dose is 5 mg t.i.d., with a typical maintenance dose of 20 mg t.i.d. Caution is advised because CNS irritability manifested by seizures is a major adverse effect. In addition, immunosuppressive therapy with steroids or azathioprine or immunomodulation with IV immunoglobulin[73] or plasma exchange may be tried.

Surgery was not an option for this patient because his cancer was too extensive. Chemotherapy was started with carboplatin and VP16 for two cycles, plus radiation therapy. Subsequently, the patient received four additional cycles of the same chemotherapy. His last cycle of treatment was on December 17, 1998. He died 3 months later.

> ■ **Clinical Points to Remember About the Lambert-Eaton Myasthenic Syndrome**
> - Increasing fatigue and leg weakness are typically the presenting symptoms.
> - Proximal muscle weakness impairs walking and standing up from a low chair, mimicking a myopathy.
> - Deep tendon reflexes are typically depressed or absent but may be potentiated after 10 seconds of sustained exercise (post-tetanic facilitation).
> - RNS is the electrophysiological study of choice to detect post-tetanic facilitation.
> - Autonomic symptoms, notably a dry mouth, are a guide to diagnosis.
> - High titers of voltage-gated calcium channel antibody against voltage-gated calcium channels are present in 90% of cases with paraneoplastic LEMS.
> - Paraneoplastic LEMS is associated with small (oat) cell lung cancer.
> - The drug of choice is 3, 4-diaminopyridine, which increases the release of the neurotransmitter ACh. ■

BOTULISM

There are many toxic and metabolic disorders of neuromuscular transmission, and botulism is among them. It is caused by the exotoxin of C-botulinum, which acts on the presynaptic region of the NMJ by binding to autonomic and motor nerve terminals, thus reducing the quanta of ACh released at the NMJ. The process resembles the effect of tetanus toxin on spinal interneurons.

In food-borne botulism, the typical initial signs and symptoms of nausea and vomiting, blurred vision, diplopia and associated ptosis, dysarthria, dysphagia, and generalized weakness appear within 12–36 hours of ingestion of tainted food.

The key clinical sign to look for in these cases is nonreactive pupils. This is particularly important because ptosis and extraocular muscle palsies, particularly of the sixth nerve, may at first suggest a diagnosis of MG. Other symptoms of bulbar involvement—nasal quality of the voice, hoarseness, dysarthria, dysphagia, and an inability to phonate—may emerge in quick succession, followed by progressive weakness of muscles of the face, neck, trunk, and limbs and by respiratory insufficiency. Tendon reflexes are lost in cases of severe generalized weakness.

Botulism may also be mistaken for the Guillain Barré syndrome because its onset is rapid, with symmetrical descending paralysis and a mixture of autonomic and parasympathetic dysfunction. Given this, other key botulism markers to watch for are intact sensation and usually normal spinal fluid.

Three types of botulinum toxin (A, B, and E) are indistinguishable by their clinical effects alone, so the patient should receive the trivalent antiserum as soon as the clinical diagnosis is made. Improvement usually begins within a few weeks of onset, first in the eye movements, then in other cranial nerve function. Complete recovery of paralyzed limb and trunk musculature may take months.

MITOCHONDRIAL DISORDERS

Progressive external ophthalmoplegia (PEO) syndrome and Kearns-Sayre syndrome (KSS)[74–76] have an overlapping relationship. These syndromes are the result either of mutations in the mitochondrial genome or of mutations in a few nuclear genes that code for a component of the mitochondrion.[77,78] Mitochondrial transmission of disease occurs in a nonmendelian, mainly maternal pattern, with mitochondrial DNA (mtDNA) inherited exclusively from the maternal lineage. Some families show linkage to chromosome 10q 23, 3-24.3; some families with identical phenotype are linked to chromosome 3p 14/1-21.2; and, in still other families, there is no linkage to either region.

In patients with progressive external ophthalmoplegia, the most commonly found abnormality is a defect that predisposes to multiple mtDNA deletions in three nuclear genes[79]—*ANT1* (adenine nucleotide translocator-1),[80] *TWINKLE* (an adenine nucleotide dependent mtDNA helicase),[81] and *POLG*.[82–84]

Progressive External Ophthalmoplegia

Progressive external ophthalmoplegia is a combination of progressive ptosis and symmetrical external ophthalmoplegia, and it is a common manifestation of mitochondrial disease. Usually, there is no diplopia or strabismus, or at most only transient diplopia, so that the disorder can exist for a long time before it brings the patient to a physician. In clinical practice, nearly all cases of PEO are due to mtDMA deletions, but, in rare cases, the condition can be simulated by a genetically determined muscular dystrophy, including oculopharyngeal dystrophy and a type in which PEO is linked to facioscapulohumeral dystrophy.

The first warning sign of PEO is typically progressive, bilateral ptosis with notably different clinical characteristics from myasthenic ptosis. These differences are shown in Table 3-2.

The appearance of bilateral symmetric ptosis in an 18-year-old girl with PEO is shown in Figure 3-10. As ptosis progresses, the eyelids become abnormally thin due to atrophy of the levator and weakness of the orbicularis oculi muscles, and eyelid closure develops. The combination of weakness of eye closure and eye opening is almost always myopathic. Once begun, PEO progresses relentlessly, impairing conjugate eye movements until the eyes are motionless.

TABLE 3-2: Differentiating Clinical Features in Ptosis Due to Mitochondrial Myopathy and Myasthenia Gravis

Mitochondrial Myopathies		Myasthenia Gravis
Insidious	Onset	Acute
Bilateral (symmetric)	Appearance	Unilateral or bilateral (asymmetric)
No	Ptosis on fatigue	Yes
No	Lid twitch	Yes
No	Recovery with eye closure	Yes
Restricted	Range levator function	Varies
Yes	Weak orbicularis oculi	Yes
Negative	Tensilon test	Positive
Negative	Ice pack test	Positive
Slowly progressive and fixed	Tempo of evolution	Fluctuates ± remission

Kearns-Sayre Syndrome

The Kearns-Sayre syndrome[85] is a progressive, aggressive mitochondrial cytopathy characterized by the combination of:

- Progressive external ophthalmoplegia
- Onset before age 20
- Atypical retinal pigmentosus
- Heart block

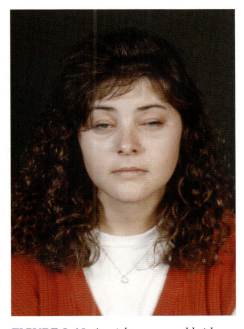

FIGURE 3-10 An eighteen-year-old girl with bilateral asymmetrical ptosis due to progressive external ophthalmoplegia.

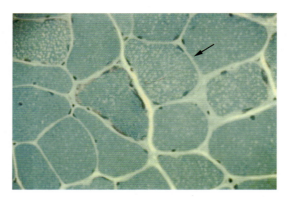

FIGURE 3-11 Skeletal muscle biopsy stained with modified Gomori trichrome stain showing ragged red fibers (*arrow*).

As in PEO, a genetic mutation of mtDNA affects structural genes for the mitochondrial respiratory chain important for energy production throughout the body.[86] The CNS is involved (both muscle and brain) in KSS, as they are in other major CNS syndromes, including mitochondrial encephalomyopathy, lactic acidosis, and stroke-like episodes (MELAS) and myoclonic epilepsy with ragged red fibers (MERRF). In MELAS and MERRF, dysfunction of the CNS dominates the clinical picture.

There is, however, considerable overlap of symptoms and signs among PEO, KSS, MELAS, and MERRF but there is general agreement that cases of PEO, KSS, and mitochondrial myopathy should be considered separately. Their shared feature is the histological abnormality of the muscle mitochondria, which results in *ragged red fibers*, named for the subsarcolemmal and intermyofibrillar collections of membranous (mitochondrial) material in type 1 muscle fibers visualized by the modified Gomori trichrome stain in sections of frozen muscle (Figure 3-11).

The case of KSS presented here illustrates the progressive disabling involvement of multiple organs characteristic of the syndrome.

CASE 3-5 Progressive External Ophthalmoplegia: Kearns-Sayre Syndrome

Video Display

The patient is a 15-year-old boy who presented to an ophthalmologist in 1968 with the insidious onset of slowly progressive asymmetrical ptosis, right eye greater than left (Figure 3-12). No diagnosis was made.

At age 18 he was short in stature (5 ft. 1 in.)

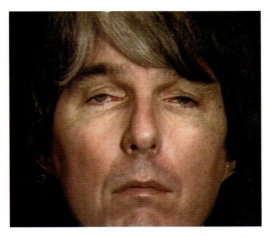

FIGURE 3-12 An eighteen-year-old man with bilateral ptosis and progressive external ophthalmoplegia.

Analysis of the History

- What are the major presenting symptoms?
- Where are the CNS lesion(s) likely to be?

CASE 3-5 SYMPTOMS

Symptoms	Location Correlation
Progressive ptosis	Levator palpebrae superioris
Short stature	Endocrine system

The analysis guides the clinical examination.

Examination

Ocular Motility/Neurological

- Visual acuity 20/20 OU with normal pupils
- Visual fields and fundus examination normal
- Bilateral ptosis
- MRD 2–3 mm with eyebrows immobilized
- Impaired eye movements in all directions of gaze
- Absent Bell's (no deviation of the eyes upward under tight eye closure)
- No bulbar or facial weakness
- Neurological examination normal

Localization and Differential Diagnosis

The differential diagnosis of new onset progressive bilateral ptosis in a young adult includes myasthenia, Musk-MG, botulism, mitochondrial myopathy, myotonic dystrophy and Fisher's syndrome (Case 3-6).

Endocrine dysfunction is common in KSS and, in addition to short stature, other manifestations include hypoparathyroidism, gonadal atrophy, and diabetes mellitus.

What Diagnostic Tests Should Follow?

· Tensilon test
· Chest X-ray

Test Results

The Tensilon test was negative for MG, and the chest x-ray was normal.

Diagnosis: Chronic Progressive External Ophthalmoplegia

Treatment

Ptosis Surgery

Ptosis eventually interferes with vision, and ptosis surgery to raise the eyelids may be necessary. However, these patients also have weakness of the orbicularis oculi affecting eye closure and care must be taken not to overcorrect and impair full eye closure because this leaves the patient at risk of exposure keratopathy.

The patient had bilateral ptosis surgery. Two years later, at age 20, a routine examination of the fundus showed normal optic discs and a mottled salt-and-pepper pigmentary retinal disturbance (Figure 3.13).

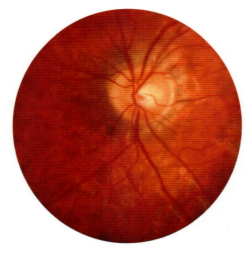

FIGURE 3-13 Fundus photograph of the left eye showing a mottled salt-and-pepper retinal pigmentary disturbance and normal optic disc.

What Other Diagnostic Tests Should Follow?

- Lumbar puncture
- Electrocardiogram (EKG)
- Chest x-ray
- Skeletal muscle biopsy

Test Results

The lumbar puncture showed elevated CSF protein at 120 mg/dL. The EKG showed incomplete right bundle branch block. The chest X-ray revealed cardiomegaly. The skeletal muscle biopsy showed ragged red fibers and a 3.8 kilobase mtDNA deletion.

Diagnosis: Kearns Sayre Syndrome[87,88]

Subsequently, at age 21, audiologic testing revealed bilateral sensory neural hearing loss. Brain MRI showed significant cortical and cerebellar atrophy.[89] At age 24, the patient developed complete heart block and required a pacemaker. Lack of stamina caused him to stop work. (Cardiovascular magnetic resonance imaging can be used to reveal the characteristic pattern of myocardial damage in patients with mitochondrial myopathy.)[90]

Over the next 10 years, advancing multisystem involvement developed, and, by age 50, he was wheelchair bound.

Special Explanatory Note

This patient's extensive multisystem failure (best described as a mitochondrial cytopathy) is characteristic of KSS.[91] Over the 34-year span of his worsening illness, he progressively developed all of KSS's defining disorders:

- PEO
- Atypical pigmentary retinal degeneration
- Heart block and cardiomegaly requiring a pacemaker
- Elevated CSF protein
- Sensory-neural hearing loss
- Ataxia with cerebellar atrophy
- Dysphagia due to pharyngeal dystrophy corrected by cricopharyngeal myotomy
- Blindness
- Proximal myopathy

■ **Clinical Points to Remember About Kearns-Sayre Syndrome**

- Kearns-Sayre syndrome is a mitochondrial cytopathy due to mtDNA deletions.
- Age of onset is usually before 20, with progressive ptosis and external ophthalmoplegia.
- Associated pigmentary retinopathy helps to establish KSS as the diagnosis.
- Skeletal muscle biopsy is positive for ragged red fibers and mtDNA deletions.
- mtDNA deletions affect structural genes for the mitochondrial respiratory chain.
- KSS progressively involves muscle, heart, retina, the endocrine system, the brain, and the liver, resulting in extensive multisystem failure. ■

MUSCULAR DYSTROPHY

Oculopharyngeal Muscular Dystrophy

Oculopharyngeal muscular dystrophy (OPMD) is a rare familial autosomal-dominant myopathy of late life. The syndrome is characterized by dysphagia with ptosis,[92] and it is a variant of restricted cranial myopathy.[93] There is a high incidence of OPMD linked to chromosome 14q11 among the French-Canadian population of the Canadian province of Quebec.[94,95] in whom a GCC repeat expansion has been shown in the PABP2 gene (poly-A binding protein 2).[96]

Oculopharyngeal muscular dystrophy presents with late-onset ptosis, dysarthria, and dysphagia.[97] Ptosis is usually asymmetrical and is followed or accompanied (but seldom preceded) by dysphagia—first for solid food and later for liquids as well. These patients have normal palatal movements and gag reflexes, suggesting that the dysphagia and accompanying regurgitation result from impaired esophageal motility. In a small number of patients, when dysphagia is severe and they are at risk of aspiration pneumonia, cricopharyngeal myotomy has resulted in significant improvement.[98]

■ Clinical Points to Remember About Oculopharyngeal Dystrophy

- Rare autosomal-dominant myopathy linked to chromosome 14q11 in a French-Canadian population.
- GCG repeat expansion in PABP2 gene (poly-A binding protein 2).
- Characterized by late onset (over age 50) ptosis, dysarthria, and dysphagia.
- Simulates OMG and age-related ptosis.
- Dysphagia is progressive, with difficulty swallowing first solid foods and then liquids.
- Risk of choking and aspiration can be prevented by cricopharyngeal myotomy.
- Neurological examination is otherwise normal. ■

A young-onset form of OPMD was reported in two Greek siblings at ages 11 and 14, who presented with bilateral ptosis, upgaze limitation, and skeletal muscle weakness.[99] Muscle biopsy revealed rimmed vacuoles and intranuclear tubulofilamentous inclusions.

The details of Case 1, a 14-year-old boy, are instructive. At age 11, over a period of weeks, he developed nasal speech with nasal regurgitation and bilateral ptosis. The bulbar weakness progressed and, over the next 3 years, he developed leg weakness that left him wheelchair bound. He had increasing ptosis with diplopia, chewing difficulties, and neck weakness, and he developed progressive scoliosis. When examined at age 14, funduscopy showed mild peripheral pigmentation of the retinal epithelium. He had marked bilateral ptosis with external ophthalmoplegia, in particular for upgaze, less so for abduction, and with preserved downgaze. Pupillary reactions were normal. There was bilateral facial weakness and severe wasting weakness of the sternomastoid muscles. Palatal movements were absent, but there was a normal gag reflex. At 16, he required ventilator support at night.

Although the early age of onset, rapid deterioration, and recessive mode of inheritance sets these cases apart from classic late-onset OPMD, all of this disorder's signature symptoms are present (with the notable exception here of the affected extraocular muscles, which, in late-onset OPMD, are usually normal).

Myotonic Dystrophy

Myotonic dystrophy (dystrophia myotonica) is the most common adult form of muscular dystrophy.[100,101] The disease is inherited in an autosomal dominant pattern, and the genetic defect is an expansion of a cytosine, thymine, guanine (CTG) nucleotide repeat residing within the myotonin protein kinase gene on chromosome 19.

In the common early-adult form of the disease, the small muscles of the hand along with the extensor muscles of the forearms are often the first to become atrophied. In other cases, ptosis and thinning of the eyelids and weakness of the facial muscles may be the earliest signs. Atrophy of the masseters leads to narrowing of the lower half of the face, and this, along with the ptosis, frontal baldness, and wrinkled forehead imparts a distinctive physiognomy that, once seen, can be recognized at a glance (the so-called "hatchet face").

Myotonia, characterized by idiomuscular contractions following brief percussion or electrical stimulation of the muscles and delay in relaxation after strong voluntary contraction (for example hand grasp) is diagnostic. Myotonia is not evoked by gentle movements such as eyelid blinks or slow movements of facial expression, but by strong muscle action, hard closure of the eyelids or clenching of the fists, movements that are followed by long delays in relaxation.

ACUTE INFLAMMATORY POLYNEUROPATHY

Guillain Barré and Fisher Syndromes

Acute inflammatory polyneuropathy is generally referred to as the Guillain Barré demyelinative syndrome (GBS).[102,103] This potentially serious condition is the commonest cause of acute or subacute generalized paralysis and, in approximately 60% of cases, it is preceded by a mild respiratory or gastrointestinal infection.

The typical case of GBS is readily identified by the acute onset of paresthesias, slight numbness in the fingers and toes, and weakness that evolves more or less symmetrically over several days to two weeks. Paralysis affects the proximal and distal muscles of the limbs. Typically, the legs are affected first (Landry's ascending paralysis). The weakness can progress to total paralysis and respiratory failure within a few days. Muscle pain is a common symptom, and the cranial muscles may themselves be affected later.

A variant of GBS, first noted by Fisher in 1956[104] and now called *Fisher syndrome*, is characterized by total ophthalmoplegia with ataxia and areflexia in addition to the GBS symptom spectrum. It actually went unrecognized by Fisher until he saw his third case, in which the CSF showed an albuminocytologic dissociation with a total protein of 348 mg/100 mL and no cells. In the first two of Fisher's cases, external ophthalmoplegia was complete, and the eyes were fixed in primary gaze. The third had bilateral sixth-nerve palsy and slight rotary nystagmus; bilateral ptosis developed 2 days later. Fisher was impressed by the presence in his patients of ataxia unaccompanied by sensory loss and "reluctantly interpreted" the clinical signs as manifestations of an unusual and unique disturbance involving the peripheral nervous system.

Other variants of GBS include cervico-brachial-pharyngeal weakness, often with ptosis, bilateral facial or abducens (CN VI) weakness with distal paresthesias, and ophthalmoplegia with GQ_{1b} antibodies. Ptosis with facial weakness is a pattern that overlaps Fisher syndrome in the case presented here.

CASE 3-6 Fisher Syndrome: Facial Diplegia

Video Display

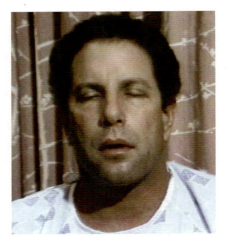

FIGURE 3-14 Patient with bilateral symmetrical ptosis and facial diplegia.

In September 1993, a 47-year-old attorney woke one morning and felt dizzy and unsteady when walking to work (Figure 3-14). The next day, he had horizontal diplopia, slurred speech, and tingling in the right arm and both hands, and was admitted to a local hospital.

His condition deteriorated and, on day 5 of his illness, he had a sensation "like someone had injected my whole mouth with novocaine." On day 10, he was transferred to the Massachusetts General Hospital, at which time he recalled a period of diarrhea 1 week prior to the onset of his symptoms.

Analysis of the History

· What are the major presenting symptoms?
· Where are the CNS lesion(s) likely to be?

CASE 3-6 SYMPTOMS

Symptoms	Location Correlation
Dizziness	Vestibular system
Unsteady gait (ataxia)	Cerebellum
Horizontal diplopia	Lateral rectus/medial rectus muscle
Dysarthria	Facial muscle
Tingling (paresthesia) in the hand	Peripheral sensory system

The analysis guides the clinical examination.

Examination

Neurological

- Speech dysarthric
- Pupils equal sluggishly reacting to light and near
- Bilateral ptosis
- Failed to bury eyelashes on eye closure (weak orbicularis oculi)
- Complete external ophthalmoplegia—eyes fixed in primary gaze with absent convergence
- Bilateral facial weakness, unable to whistle
- Normal tongue and palate movements, gag reflex intact
- Negative Romberg
- Limb and gait ataxia, unable to tandem
- Motor strength 5/5 throughout
- Absent deep tendon reflexes
- Sensory system no abnormality

What Diagnostic Tests Should Follow?

- Stool culture
- Electrophysiological studies
- Antibody studies
- Lumbar puncture

Special Explanatory Note

A stool culture for *Campylobacter jejuni* is important. It is particularly worth noting that *C. jejuni* may be the responsible trigger in GBS and Fisher syndrome because anti-GQ_1b antibodies bind to surface epitopes on this organism, and its lipopolysaccharide fraction may molecularly mimic the ganglioside.[105]

Electrophysiological nerve conduction studies are a dependable diagnostic indicator of GBS. They will show reduction in amplitude of the compound muscle action potential, slow conduction velocity, conduction block in motor nerves, prolonged distal latencies (reflecting distal conduction block), and prolonged or absent F responses (indicating involvement of proximal segments of the nerves and roots)—all reflecting focal demyelination. The H-reflex is delayed or absent, confirmed by loss of ankle jerks.

A number of autoantibodies directed at components of nerve ganglioside are inconsistently present in GBS. The most important is the anti-GQ_1b IgG antibody,[106] which is found in almost all cases with ophthalmoplegia.[107]

Test Results

Stool cultures were positive for *C. jejuni*. Electrodiagnostic studies showed normal nerve conduction velocity and normal F waves. The anti-GQ_1b IgG antibody was positive.

A lumbar puncture at the local hospital showed albuminocytologic dissociation with an elevation of the CSF protein to 102 mg/mL and no cells.

Albuminocytologic dissociation refers to an elevation of CSF protein, and the CSF is acellular. In GBS and Fisher syndrome, the CSF protein is usually normal during the first few days of symptoms, but then begins to rise, reaching a peak in 4–6 weeks and persisting at a variably elevated level for many weeks. The increase in CSF protein reflects the widespread inflammatory disease of the nerve roots but has no prognostic significance.

Treatment

Plasma exchange[108,109] is the treatment of choice for GBS and Fisher syndrome. The patient received a total of six sessions of plasma exchange and ciprofloxacin 500 mg. p.o., b.i.d. His condition slowly improved. First, he regained a few degrees of eye movement—an ability to just open his eyes although still with marked bilateral ptosis—and improvement in facial diplegia although still unable to smile or whistle.

At 4 months, ptosis and ophthalmoplegia had resolved completely. He had mild residual facial weakness at that time but his speech was 90% back to normal. He had 5/5 muscle strength throughout with no ataxia.

It is worth noting that intravenous immunoglobulin (IG) 0.4g/kg/day for 5 consecutive days is as effective as plasma exchange, is easier to administer, and safer because there is no need for large IV access.

■ **Clinical Points to Remember About Fisher Syndrome**

- Fisher syndrome is an idiopathic acute inflammatory demyelinative polyneuropathy—a variant of GBS.
- The diagnostic triad is external ophthalmoplegia (or abducens (CN IV) nerve palsy) ataxia and areflexia.
- Facial diplegia is commonly associated.
- Stool cultures are typically positive for *C. jejuni*.
- Anti-GQ_{1b} antibody is invariably present in ophthalmoplegia cases.
- Cerebrospinal fluid shows albuminocytologic dissociation a few days after the onset of the disorder.
- Nerve conduction studies show reduced amplitude of the compound muscle action potential, slow conduction velocity, conduction block in motor nerves, prolonged or absent F responses, and a delayed or absent H reflex.
- Patients respond slowly to plasma exchange and IV immunoglobulin. ■

Special Explanatory Note

A number of autoantibodies directed at components of nerve ganglioside are detectable in patients with GBS. Where ophthalmoplegia is a feature of the GBS case, as it is in Fisher Syndrome, anti-GQ_1b is uniformly present. In approximately one-third of patients with a predominantly motor presentation and axonal damage, antibodies to the GM_1 ganglioside are present, and they appear to be triggered largely by *C. jejuni* infections. Notably, infection with the same bacteria also triggers an acute demyelinative form of GBS.

SELECTED REFERENCES

1. Gorelick PB, Rosenberg M, Pagano RJ. Enhanced ptosis in myasthenia gravis. *Arch Neurol.* 1981;38:531.
2. Lepore FE. Unilateral ptosis and Hering's law. *Neurology.* 1988;38:319–322.
3. Cogan DG. Myasthenia gravis: a review of the disease and a description of lid twitch as a characteristic sign. *Arch Ophthalmol.* 1965;74:217–221.
4. Osher RH, Griggs RC. Orbicularis fatigue: the 'peek' sign of myasthenia gravis. *Arch Ophthalmol.* 1979;97:677–679.
5. Gay AJ, Salmon ML, Windsor CE. Hering's law, the levators, and their relationship in disease states. *Arch Ophthalmol.* 1967;77:157–160.
6. Schechter RJ. Ptosis with contralateral lid retraction due to excessive innervation of the levator palpebrae superioris. *Ann Ophthalmol.* 1978;10:1324–1328.
7. Kansu T, Subutay N. Lid retraction in myasthenia gravis. *J Clin Neuro-ophthalmol.* 1987;7:145–150.
8. Marino M, Barabesino G, Pinchera A, Manetti L, Ricciardi R, Rossi B, Muratorio A, Braverman LE, Mariotti S, Chiovato L. Increased frequency of euthyroid ophthalmopathy in patients with Graves' disease associated with myasthenia gravis. *Thyroid.* 2000;10(9):799–802.
9. Toth C, McDonald D, Oger J, Brownell K. Acetylcholine receptor antibodies in myasthenia gravis are associated with greater risk of diabetes and thyroid disease. *Acta Neurol Scand.* 2006;114:124–132.
10. Golnik KC, Pena R, Lee AG, Eggenberger ER. An ice test for the diagnosis of myasthenia gravis. *Ophthalmology.* 1999;106:1282–1286.
11. Movaghar M, Slavin ML. Effect of local heat versus ice on blepharoptosis resulting from ocular myasthenia. *Ophthalmology.* 2000;107:2209–2214.
12. Kubis KC, Danesh-Meyer HV, Savino PJ, Sergott RC. The ice test versus the rest test in myasthenia gravis. *Ophthalmology.* 2000;107:1995–1998.
13. Daroff RB. The office Tensilon test for ocular myasthenia gravis. *Arch Neurol.* 1986; 43:843–844.
14. Ing EB, Ing SY, Ing T, Ramocki JA. The complication rate of edrophonium testing for suspected myasthenia gravis. *Can J Ophthalmol.* 2000;35:141–145.
15. Seybold ME. The office Tensilon test for ocular myasthenia gravis. *Arch Neurol.* 1986;43:842–843.
16. Leigh RJ, Zee DS. *The Neurology of Eye Movements.* 4th ed. New York: Oxford University Press; 2006.
17. Engel AG. The neuromuscular junction. In: Engel AG, Franzini-Armstrong C, eds. *Myology: Basic and Clinical.* 2nd ed. New York: McGraw-Hill; 1994: 261–302.
18. Luchanok U, Kaminski HJ. Ocular myasthenia: diagnostic and treatment recommendations and the evidence base. *Curr Opin Neurol.* 2008;21:8–15.
19. Kupersmith MJ, Latkany R, Homel P. Development of generalized disease at 2 years in patients with ocular myasthenia gravis. *Arch Neurol.* 2003;60:243–248.
20. Kusner LL, Puwanant A, KIaminski HJ. Ocular myasthenia: diagnosis, treatment, and pathogenesis. *Neurologist.* 2006;12:3231–239.
21. Vincent A, Clover L, Buckley C, Evans J, Rothwell PM and the UK Myasthenia Gravis Survey. Evidence of under-diagnosis of myasthenia gravis in older people. *J Neurol Neurosurg Psychiat.* 2003;74(8):1105–1108.
22. Kupersmith MJ, Ying G. Ocular motor dysfunction and ptosis in ocular myasthenia gravis: effects of treatment. *Br J Ophthalmol.* 2005;890:1330–1334.
23. Vincent A, Lang B, Kleopa KA. Autoimmune channelopathies and related neurological disorders. *Neuron.* 2006;52:123–138.

24. Kanazawa M, Shimohata T, Tanaka K, Nishizawa M. Clinical features of patients with myasthenia gravis associated with autoimmune diseases. *Eur J Neurol.* 2007;142:1403–1404.

25. Aarli JA, Skeie GO, Mygland A, Gilhus NE. Muscle striation antibodies in myasthenia gravis. Diagnostic and functional significance. *Ann NY Acad Sci.* 1998;841:505–515.

26. Drachman DB. Therapy of myasthenia gravis. *Handb Clin Neurol.* Elsevier Amsterdam. 2008;91:253–272.

27. Skeie GO, Apostolski S, Evoli A, Gilhus NE, Hart IK, Harms L, Hilton-Jones D, Melms A, Verschuuren J. Guidelines for treatment of autoimmune neuromuscular transmission disorders. *Eur J Neurol.* 2010;17:893–902.

28. Miano MA, Bosley TM, Heiman-Patterson TD, Reed J, Sergott RC, Savino PJ, Schatz NJ. Factors influencing outcome of prednisone dose reduction in myasthenia gravis. *Neurology.* 1991;41(6):919–921.

29. Palace J, Newsom-Davis J. A randomized double-blind study of prednisolone alone or with azathioprine in myasthenia gravis. *Neurology.* 1998;50:1778–1783.

30. Drachman DB, Adams RN, Hu R, Jones RJ, Brodsky RA. Rebooting the immune system with high dose cyclophosphamide for treatment of refractory myasthenia gravis. *Ann NY Acad Sci.* 2008;1132:305–314.

31. Phan SJ, Sanders DB, Siddiqi ZA. Mycophenolate mofetil in myasthenia gravis: The unanswered question. *Expert Opin Pharmacother.* 2008;9(14):2545–2551.

32. Gajdos P, Chevret S, Clair B, Tranchant C, Chastang C. Clinical trial of plasma exchange and high-dose intravenous immunoglobulin in myasthenia gravis. Myasthenia Gravis Clinical Study Group. *Ann Neurol.* 1997;41:789–796.

33. Achiron A, Barak YH, Miron S, Sarova-Pinhas I. Immunoglobulin treatment in refractory myasthenia gravis. *Muscle Nerve.* 2000;23(4):551–555.

34. Zinman L, Ng E, Bril V. IV immunoglobulin in patients with myasthenia gravis: A randomized controlled trial. *Neurology.* 2007;68:837–841.

35. Lanska DJ. Indications for thymectomy in myasthenia gravis. *Neurology.* 1990; 40:1828–1829.

36. Gronseth GS, Barohn RJ. Practice parameter: thymectomy for autoimmune gravis (an evidence-based review). *Neurology.* 2000;55:7–15.

37. Hankins JR, Mayer RF, Satterfield JR, Turney SZ, Attar S, Sequeira AJ, Thompson BW, McLaughlin JS. Thymectomy for myasthenia gravis: 14-year experience. *Ann Surg.* 1985;201(5):618–625.

38. Siao P, Zukerberg LR. Case records of the Massachusetts General Hospital. Weekly clinicopathological exercises. Case 15–2000. A 69-year-old man with myasthenia gravis and a mediastinal mass. *N Engl J Med.* 2000;342(20):1508–1514.

39. Tormoehlen LM, Pascuzzi RM. Thymoma, myasthenia gravis, and other paraneoplastic syndromes. *Hematol Oncol Clin North Am.* 2008;22(3):509–526.

40. Tanakaya K, Konaga E, Takeuchi H, Yasui Y, Takeda A, Yunoki Y, Murakami I. Colon carcinoma after thymectomy for myasthenia gravis: report of a case. *Surg Today.* 2002;32(10):896–898.

41. Odel JG, Winterkorn JM, Behrens MM. The sleep test for myasthenia gravis. A safe alternative to Tensilon. *J Clin Neuro-ophthalmol.* 1991;11:288–292.

42. Benatar M. A systematic review of diagnostic studies in myasthenia gravis. *Neuromuscul Disord.* 2006;16:459–467.

43. Costa J, Evangelista T, Conceicao I, Carvalho M. Repetitive nerve stimulation in myasthenia gravis—relative sensitivity of different muscles. *Clin Neurophysiol.* 2004;115:2776–2782.

44. Lange DJ. Electrophysiologic testing of neuromuscular transmission. *Neurology.* 1997;48(suppl):S46–S51.

45. Padua L, Stalberg E, LoMonaco M, Evoli A, Batocchi A, Tonali PA. SFEMG in ocular myasthenia gravis diagnosis. *Clin Neurophysiol.* 2000;111:1203–1207.

46. Valls-Canals J, Povedano M, Montero J, Pradas J. Stimulated single-fiber EMG of the frontalis and orbicularis oculi muscles in ocular myasthenia gravis. *Muscle Nerve.* 2003;28:501–503.

47. Drachman DB. Myasthenia gravis and other diseases of the neuromuscular junction. In: Longo DL, Fauci AS, Kasper DL, Hauser SL, Jameson JL, Loscalzo J, eds. *Harrison's Principles of Internal Medicine.* 18th eds. McGraw Hill; New York 2012;2: Ch 386;3480–3486.

48. Lindstrom JM, Seybold ME, Lennon VA, Whittingham S, Dyane DD. Antibody to acetylcholine receptor in myasthenia gravis: Prevalence, clinical correlates and diagnostic value. *Neurology.* 1976;26:1054–1059.

49. Vincent A, Newsom-Davis J. Acetylcholine receptor antibody as a diagnostic test for myasthenia gravis: results in 153 validated cases and 2967 diagnostic assays. *J Neurol Neurosurg Psychiat.* 1985;48:1246–1252.

50. Vincent A, Bowen J, Newsom-Davis J, McConville J. Seronegative generalized myasthenia gravis: clinical features, antibodies, and their targets. *The Lancet Neurol.* 2003;2:99–105.

51. Bennett DLH, Millis KR, Riordan-Eva P, Barnes PRJ, Rose MR. Anti-MuSK antibodies in a case of ocular myasthenia gravis. *J Neurol Neurosurg Psychiat.* 2006;77:564–565.

52. Caress JB, Hunt CH, Batish SD. Anti-MuSK myasthenia gravis presenting with purely ocular findings. *Arch Neurol.* 2005;62:1002–1003.

53. Hanisch F, Eger K, Zierz S. MuSK-antibody positive pure ocular myasthenia gravis. *J Neurol.* 2006;253:659–660.

54. Vincent A, Li Z, Hart A, Barrett-Jolley R, Yamamoto T, Burges J. Wray D, Byrne N, Molenaar P, Newsom-Davis J. Seronegative myasthenia gravis: Evidence for plasma factor(s) interfering with acetylcholine receptor function. *Ann NY Acad Sci.* 1993;681:529–538.

55. Hoch W, McConville J, Helms S, Newsom-Davis J, Melms A, Vincent A. Auto-antibodies to the receptor tyrosine kinase MuSK in patients with myasthenia gravis without acetylcholine receptor antibodies. *Nat Med.* 2001;7(3):365–368.

56. Evoli A, Tonali PA, Padua L, Monaco ML, Scuderi F, Batocchi AP, Marino M, Bartoccioni E. Clinical correlates with anti-MuSK antibodies in generalized seronegative myasthenia gravis. *Brain.* 2003;126:2304–2311.

57. Oh SJ. Muscle-specific receptor tyrosine kinase antibody positive myasthenia gravis current status. *J Clin Neurol.* 2009;5:53–64.

58. Parr J, Jayawant S, Buckley C, Vincent A. Childhood auto-immune myasthenia. In: Dale RC, Vincent A, eds. *Inflammatory and Autoimmune Disorders of the Nervous System in Children.* McKeith Press; 2010:388–405.

59. Farrugia ME, Robson MD, Clover L, Anslow P, Newsom-Davis J, Kennett R, Hilton-Jones D, Matthews PM, Vincent A. MRI and clinical studies of facial and bulbar muscle involvement in MuSK antibody-associated myasthenia gravis. *Brain.* 2006;129:1481–1492.

60. Guptill JT, Sanders DB. Update on MuSK antibody positive myasthenia gravis. *Curr Opin Neurol.* 2010;23:530–535.

61. Guptill JT, Sanders DB, Evoli A. Anti-MuSK antibody myasthenia gravis: Clinical findings and response to treatment in two large cohorts. *Muscle Nerve.* 2011; 44:36–40.

62. Lambert EH, Eaton LM, Rooke ED. Defect of neuromuscular conduction associated with malignant neoplasms. *Am J Physiol.* 1956;187:612–613.

63. Fukunaga H, Engel AG, Lang B, Newsom-Davis J, Vincent A. Passive transfer of Lambert-Eaton myasthenic syndrome with IgG from man to mouse depletes the presynaptic membrane active zones. *Proc Natl Acad Sci USA.* 1983;80:7636–7640.

64. Lambert EH, Lennon VA. Selected IgG rapidly induces Lambert-Eaton myasthenic syndrome in mice: complement independence and EMG abnormalities. *Muscle Nerve.* 1988;11:1133–1145.

65. Lennon VA, Kryzer TJ, Griesmann GE, O'Suilleabhain PE, Windebank AJ, Woppmann A, Miljanich GP, Lambert EH. Calcium-channel antibodies in the Lambert-Eaton syndrome and other paraneoplastic syndromes. *N Engl J Med.* 1995;332:1467–1474.

66. O'Neill JH, Murray NMF, Newsom-Davis J. The Lambert-Eaton myasthenic syndrome. A review of 50 cases. *Brain.* 1988;111(3):577–596.

67. Wirtz PW, Sotodeh M, Nijnuis M, Van Doorn PA, Van Engelen BG, Hintzen RQ, De Kort PL, Kuks JB, Twijnstra A, De Visser M, Visser LH, Wokke JH, Wintzen AR, Verschuuren JJ. Difference in distribution of muscle weakness between myasthenia gravis and the Lambert-Eaton myasthenic syndrome. *J Neurol Neurosurg Psychiat.* 2002;73(6):766–768.

68. Burns TM, Russell JA, LaChance DH, Jones HR. Oculobulbar involvement is typical with Lambert-Eaton myasthenic syndrome. *Ann Neurol.* 2003;53:270–273.

69. Tim RW, Sanders DB. Repetitive nerve stimulation studies in the Lambert-Eaton myasthenic syndrome. *Muscle Nerve.* 1994;17:995–1001.

70. Odabasi Z, Demirci M, Kim DS, Lee DK, Ryan HF, Claussen GC, Tseng A, Oh SJ. Postexercise facilitation of reflexes is not common in Lambert-Eaton myasthenic syndrome. *Neurology.* 2002;59(7):1085–1087.

71. Chalk CH, Murray NME, Newsom-Davis J, O'Neill JH, Spiro SG. Response of the Lambert-Eaton myasthenic syndrome to treatment of associated small-cell lung carcinoma. *Neurology.* 1990;40:1552–1556.

72. Sanders DB, Massey JM, Sanders LL, Edwards LJ. A randomized trial of 3,4-diaminopyridine in Lambert-Eaton myasthenic syndrome. *Neurology.* 2000; 43:603–607.

73. Rich MM, Teener JW, Bird SJ. Treatment of Lambert-Eaton syndrome with intravenous immunoglobulin. *Muscle Nerv.* 1997;20:614–615.

74. Holt IJ, Harding AE, Morgan-Hughes JA. Deletions of muscle mitochondrial DNA in patients with mitochondrial myopathies. *Nature.* 1988;331:717–719.

75. Zeviani M, Moraes CT, DiMauro S, Nakase H, Bonilla E, Schon EA, Rowland LP. Deletions of mitochondrial DNA in Kearns-Sayre syndrome. *Neurology.* 1988; 38:1339–1346.

76. Moraes CT, DiMauro S, Zeviani M, Lombes A, Shanske S, Miranda AF, Nakase H, Bonilla E, Werneck LC, Servidei S, Nonaka I, Koga Y, Spiro AJ, Brownell AKW, Schmidt B, Schotland DL, Zupanc M, DeVivo DC, Schon EA, Rowland LP. Mitochondrial DNA deletions in progressive external ophthalmoplegia and Kearns-Sayre syndrome. *N Engl J Med.* 1989;320:1293–1299.

77. Newman NJ. Mitochondrial disease and the eye. *Ophthalmol Clin North Am.* 1992; 5:405–424.

78. Mitsumoto H, Aprille JR, Wray SH, Nemni R, Bradley WG. Progressive external ophthalmoplegia (PEO): clinical, morphologic and biochemical studies. *Neurology.* 1983;33(4):452–461.

79. Hirano M. DiMauro S. Ant1, Twinkle, POLG, and TP. New genes open our eyes to ophthalmoplegia. *Neurology.* 2001;57:2163–2165.

80. Kaukonen J, Juselius JK, Tiranti V, Kyttala A, Zeviani M, Comi GP, Keranen S, Peltonen L, Suomalainen A. Role of adenine nucleotide translocator 1 in mtDNA maintenance. *Science.* 2000;289:782–785.

81. Spelbrink JN, Li FY, Tiranti V, Nikali K, Yuan QP, Tariq M, Wanrooij S, Garrido N, Comi G, Morandi L, Santoro L, Toscano A, Fabrizo G-M, Somer H, Croxen R, Beeson D, Poulton J, Suomalainen A, Jacobs HT, Zeviani M, Larsson C. Human mitochondrial DNA deletions associated with mutations in the gene encoding Twinkle, a phage T7 gene 4-like protein localized in mitochondria. *Nat Genet.* 2001;28:223–231.

82. Van Goethen G, Dermaut B, Lofgren A, Martin JJ, Van Broeckhoven C. Mutation of POLG is associated with progressive external ophthalmoplegia characterized by mtDNA deletions. *Nat Genet.* 2001;28:211–212.

83. Agostino A, Valletta L, Chinnery PF, Ferrari G, Carrara F, Taylor RW, Schaefer AM, Turnbull DM, Tiranti V, Zeviani M. Mutations of ANT1, Twinkle, and POLG1 in sporadic progressive external ophthalmoplegia (PEO). *Neurology.* 2003; 60:1354–1356.

84. Hudson G, Deschauer M, Taylor RW, Hanna MG, Fialho D, Schaefer AM, He L-P, Blakely E, Turnbull DM, Chinnery PF. POLG1, C10ORF2, and ANT1 mutations are uncommon in sporadic progressive external ophthalmoplegia with multiple mitochondrial DNA deletions. *Neurology.* 2006;66:1439–1441.

85. Kearns TP, Sayre GP. Retinitis pigmentosa, external ophthalmoplegia and complete heart block: unusual syndrome with histological study in one of two cases. *AMA Arch Ophthalmol.* 1958;60(2):280–289.

86. Van Goethen G, Martin JJ, Van Broeckhoven C. Progressive external ophthalmoplegia characterized by multiple deletions of mitochondrial DNA: unraveling the pathogenesis of human mitochondrial DNA instability and the initiation of a genetic classification. *Neuromolecular Med.* 2003;3(3):129–146. Review.

87. Kosmorsky G, Johns DR. Neuro-ophthalmologic manifestations of mitochondrial DNA disorders: chronic progressive external ophthalmoplegia, Kearns-Sayre syndrome, and Leber's hereditary optic neuropathy. *Neurol Clin.* 1991;9(1):147–161.

88. Zeviani M, Moraes CT, DiMauro S, Nakase H, Bonilla E, Schon EA, Rowland LP. Deletions of mitochondrial DNA in Kearns-Sayre syndrome. *Neurology.* 1988; 38:1339–1346.

89. Wray SH, Provenzale JM, John DR, Thulborn KR. MR of the brain in mitochondrial myopathy. *Am J Neuroradiol.* 1995;16(5):1167–1173.

90. Yilmaz A, Gdynia HJ, Ponfick M, Rosch S, Lindner A, Ludolph AC, Sechtem U. Cardiovascular magnetic resonance imaging (CMR) reveals characteristic pattern of myocardial damage in patients with mitochondrial myopathy. *Clin Res Cardiol.* 2012;10(4):255–261.

91. Evans OB, Parker CC, Haas RH, Naidu S, Moser HW, Bock HGO. *Inborn Errors of Metabolism of the Nervous System.* In: Bradley WG, Daroff RB, Fenichel GM, Marsden CD, eds. *Neurology in Clinical Practice.* Vol II. 3rd ed. Butterworth Henemann; Boston 2000;68:1595–1662.

92. Taylor EW. Progressive vagus-glossopharyngeus paralysis with ptosis. A contribution to the group of family diseases. *J Nerv Ment Dis.* 1915;42:129–139.

93. Victor M, Hayes R, Adams RD. Oculopharyngeal muscular dystrophy. A familial disease of late life characterized by dysphagia and progressive ptosis of the eyelids. *N Engl J Med.* 1962;267:1267–1272.

94. Barbeau A. The syndrome of hereditary late onset ptosis and dysphagia in French Canada. In: Kuhn W, ed. *Symposium über progressive Muskeldystrophie, Myotonie, Myasthenie, 1965.* Berlin: Springer-Verlag; 1966:102–109.

95. Barbeau A. Oculopharyngeal muscular dystrophy in French Canada. In: Brunette JK, Barbeau A, eds. *Progress in Neuro-ophthalmology.* Amsterdam: Excerpta Medica; 1969. Vol 2, Int Congress Ser 5:176.

96. Stajch JM, Gilchrist JM, Lennon F, Lee A, Yamaoia L, Helms B, Gaskell PC, Donald L, Roses AD, Vance JM, Pericak-Vance MA. Confirmation of linkage of oculopharyngeal muscular dystrophy to chromosome 14q11.2-q13. *Ann Neurol.* 1996;40:801–804.

97. Neetens A, Martin JJ, Brais B, Wein B, Dreuw B, Tijssen CC, Ceuterick C. Oculopharyngeal muscular dystrophy (OPMD). *Neuro-ophthalmology.* 1997; 17(4):189–200.

98. Hardiman O, Halperin JJ, Farrell MA, Shapiro BE, Wray SH, Brown RH. Neuropathic findings in oculopharyngeal muscular dystrophy. A report of seven cases and a review of the literature. *Arch Neurol.* 1993;50:481–488.

99. Rose MR, Landon DN, Papadimitriou A, Morgan-Hughes JA. A rapidly progressive adolescent-onset oculopharyngeal somatic syndrome with rimmed vacuoles in two siblings. *Ann Neurol.* 1997;41:25–31.

100. Batten FE, Gibb HP. Myotonia atrophica. *Brain.* 1909;32:187–205.

101. Brook JD, McCurrach ME, Harley HG, Buckler AJ, Church D, Aburatai H, Hunter K, Stanton VP, Thirion JP, Hudson T. Molecular basis of myotonic dystrophy: expansion of a trinucleotide (CTG) repeat at the 3N end of a transcript encoding a protein kinase family member. *Cell.* 1992;69:385–395.

102. Guillain G, Barre JA, Strohl A. Le reflexe medico-plantaire: Etude de ses caracteres graphiques et de son temps perdu. *Bulletins et memoires de la Societe desMedecins des Hopitaux de Paris.* 1916;40:1459–1462.

103. Guillain G, Barre JA, Strohl A. Sur un syndrome de radiculonevrite avec hyperalbuminose du liquid cephalo-rachidien sans reaction cellulaire. Remarques sur les caracteres cliniques et graphiques des reflexes tendineux. *Bulletins et memoires de la Societe desMedecins des Hopitaux de Paris.* 1916;40:1462–1470.

104. Fisher M. An unusual variant of acute idiopathic polyneuritis (syndrome of ophthalmoplegia, ataxia and areflexia. *N Engl J Med.* 1956;255:57–65.

105. Sheikh KA, Nachamkin I, Ho TW, Willison HJ, Veitch J, Ung H, Nicholson M, Li CY, Wu HS, Shen BQ, Cornblath DR, Asbury AK, McKhann GM, Griffin JW. Campylobacter jejuni lipopolysaccharides in Guillain-Barre syndrome. Molecular mimicry and host susceptibility. *Neurology.* 1998;51:371–378.

106. Willison HJ, Plomp JJ. Anti-ganglioside antibodies and the presynaptic motor nerve terminal. *Ann NY Acad Sci.* 2008;1132:114–123.

107. Yuki N, Sato S, Tsuji S, Ohsawa T, Miyatake T. Frequent presence of anti-GQ$_{1b}$ antibody in Fisher's syndrome. *Neurology.* 1993;43:414–417.

108. McKhann GM, Griffin JW, Cornblath DR, Mellits ED, Fisher RS, Quaskey SA and the Guillain-Barre Syndrome Study Group. Plasmapheresis and Guillain-Barre syndrome: Analysis of prognostic factors and the effect of plasmapheresis. *Ann Neurol.* 1988;23:347–353.

109. van Door PA, Ruts L, Jacobs BC. Clinical features, pathogenesis, and treatment of Guillain-Barre syndrome. *Lancet Neurol.* 2008;7:939–950.

| 4 |

THE EXTRAOCULAR MUSCLES
AND DIPLOPIA

THE EXTRAOCULAR MUSCLES

There are six extraocular muscles for each eye. The *lateral rectus, medial rectus, superior rectus,* and *inferior rectus* muscles are, respectively, responsible for moving the eye outward (abduct), inward (adduct), superiorly (up), and inferiorly (down). Depending on eye position, the rectus muscles can also produce torsional eye movements.

The two oblique muscles, the *superior oblique* and *inferior oblique,* are responsible for vertical and torsional eye movements.

The four rectus muscles originate in a common tendinous ring at the apex of the orbit and insert into the sclera of the eyeball.

The superior oblique muscle originates on the sphenoid bone in the posterior medial orbit and passes anteriorly through a fibrous pulley (the trochlear) on the medial superior orbital rim to insert on the superior surface of the eye to produce *intorsion*, which moves the upper pole of the eye inward. The inferior oblique originates along the anterior medial orbital wall, attaches to the inferior bony orbit, and inserts on the inferior surface of the eye to produce *extorsion,* which moves the upper pole of the eye outward.

The oculomotor (III), trochlear (IV), and abducens (VI) cranial nerves (CN) enter the orbit through the superior orbital fissure. The trochlear nerve supplies the superior oblique, the abducens nerve supplies the lateral rectus, and the oculomotor nerve supplies the remaining four extraocular muscles (as well as the levator palpebrae and iris sphincter muscles) (Figure 4-1).[1,2]

Each extraocular muscle has a specific action, shown with their innervation by CN III, IV, and VI in Table 4-1.

The *oculomotor nuclei* (CN III) innervate three of the extraocular muscles and the inferior oblique that lie near the midline in the upper midbrain at the level of the superior colliculus ventral to the periaqueductal gray matter (Table 4-2).

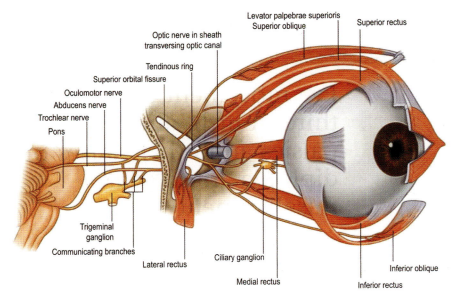

FIGURE 4-1 Innervation of the extraocular muscles. The oculomotor (III), trochlear (IV), and abducens (VI) nerves enter the orbit through the superior orbital fissure.

Reproduced with permission.[2]

The *trochlear nuclei* that innervate the superior oblique muscle lie in the lower midbrain at the level of the inferior colliculus.

The *abducens nuclei* that innervate the lateral rectus muscle lie on the floor of the fourth ventricle in the mid- to lower pons.

Cranial nerves III (oculomotor) and VI (abducens) exit the brainstem ventrally; CN IV (trochlear) exits the brain dorsally. In their intact state, these muscles and the cranial nerves that innervate them are responsible for every movement of the eyes signaled by the cortex.

TABLE 4-1: Actions and Innervation of the Extraocular Muscles

Muscle	Main Actions	Innervation
Lateral rectus	Abduction	Abducens nerve (CN VI) (outward) movement of the eye
Medial rectus	Adduction	Oculomotor nerve (CN III) (inward) movement
Superior rectus	Elevation, intorsion	Oculomotor nerve (CN III) and adduction; intorsion increases with adduction
Inferior rectus	Depression, extorsion	Oculomotor nerve (CN III) and adduction; extorsion increases with adduction
Inferior oblique	Elevation, extorsion	Oculomotor nerve (CN III) and abduction; extorsion increases with abduction
Superior oblique	Depression, intorsion	Trochlear nerve (CN IV) and abduction; intorsion increases with abduction

Reproduced with permission.[2]

TABLE 4-2: Subnuclei of the Oculomotor Nucleus (CN III) and the Muscles Innervated

Subnucleus	Muscles Innervated	Side Innervated
Dorsal	Inferior rectus	Ipsilateral
Intermediate	Inferior oblique	Ipsilateral
Ventral	Medial rectus	Ipsilateral
Edinger-Westphal	Pupillary constrictors	Bilateral (parasympathetic) lens ciliary muscles
Central caudal	Levator palpebrae superior	Bilateral
Medial	Superior rectus	Contralateral

Reproduced with permission.[2]

DIPLOPIA

Diplopia or double vision is the commonest subjective complaint associated with a lesion affecting the extraocular muscles, their neuromuscular junctions, the ocular motor nuclei or nerve, or supranuclear projections in the brainstem that maintain alignment of the eyes.[3]

Seeing double is due both to lack of visual fusion and misalignment of the visual axes of the eyes (the line connecting the fovea with the fixation point). This causes the image of an object to fall on noncorresponding areas of the two retinas, and, because each retina has corresponding areas in the cerebral cortex that interpret each image represented as a single perception in the same location in visual space, when images fall on noncorresponding areas, they are interpreted as an object seen in two different locations in space (Figure 4-2).[4]

Diplopia is a frightening symptom for patients to encounter, and it carries a broad differential diagnosis of ocular disorders and myopathic or neurologic conditions affecting ocular alignment. This makes it particularly important to have a clear understanding of the anatomic and physiological mechanisms that may be responsible for patients seeing double—or complaining simply of "blurred" or "fuzzy vision." If blurred vision is corrected with one eye covered, the patient is experiencing diplopia, and it is important, always, to consider diplopia in evaluating vague symptoms like "fuzziness."

There are two principal types of diplopia, *monocular* and *binocular,* and a history focused on this distinction is critical for narrowing evaluation further.[5] In monocular diplopia, only the affected eye will see double so that covering each eye in turn will reveal the affected eye. In contrast, in binocular diplopia from ocular misalignment, diplopia disappears with either eye closed and returns with both eyes viewing. However, there are conditions that can produce bilateral monocular diplopia, for example, a cataract in one eye and a lesion of the cornea in the other.

Once the type of diplopia has been determined, the history needs to focus on the involved eye in patients with monocular diplopia, on the brainstem/cranial nerves in patients with binocular diplopia, and on the cerebral cortex in patients with polyopia.

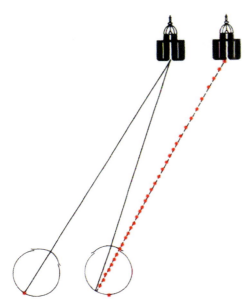

FIGURE 4-2 Disparate retinal images. The image of a distant object lies on the fovea of the left eye but, because of an esotropia in the right eye (due to a right lateral rectus weakness, for instance) the image lies medial to the fovea. Each retinal element corresponds to a specific subjective visual direction. Consequently, the subject localizes the same object in two different directions and experiences diplopia. The broken line indicates the perceived direction of the false image.

Reproduced with permission.[4]

Monocular Diplopia

Monocular diplopia is usually caused by an ocular disorder. With rare exceptions, *unilateral* or *bilateral* monocular diplopia is due to a refractive error caused by uncorrected astigmatism (e.g., keratoconus), corneal disease, cataract, or macular disease, but it can also be due to incorrectly prescribed glasses. Patients with any of these conditions nearly always describe seeing a fainter, slightly displaced superimposed image called "ghosting." If looking through a pinhole eliminates ghosting, then the diplopia is likely to be caused by a refractive abnormality (or early cataract). If refraction with a rigid contact lens improves diplopia, then the cause is likely to be an irregular corneal surface. Treatment of monocular diplopia is specific to the etiology. It may require refraction, rigid contact lens use, cataract extraction, or laser keratectomy.

Patients with monocular diplopia due to macular disease frequently describe a break, bend, or distortion of the viewing edge leading to a double or distorted image that is not improved by looking through a pinhole. Macular disease can be detected by a neurologist using an Amsler grid, which is a grid pattern of small boxes with a central fixation point. The patient is asked to view the grid wearing his near correction glasses and then to say whether all the lines are straight or whether any lines are missing, bent, or blurry. Macular disease typically produces a curvature distortion of the lines in the grid pattern (*metamorphopsia*). Macular disease can also lead to significant image distortion or difference in image size when one eye is compared with the other (*aniseikonia*). The discrepancy of image size and shape prevents fusion of images despite normal visual alignment and results in diplopia. Common macular causes of monocular diplopia are epiretinal membranes or retinal or choroidal folds.

Monocular double vision may be nonorganic or "functional." When patients tell you that they see two distinct images, and gross abnormality of the eye (e.g., lens subluxation) is ruled out, a psychogenic cause should be considered. Patients with functional diplopia may even complain of triple or quadruple vision.

Binocular Diplopia

Binocular diplopia is usually caused by strabismus, which can be a *comitant* or *incomitant* misalignment of the visual axes.[6] *Comitant deviation* describes an ocular misalignment that is independent of the direction of gaze. That is to say, it *does not change* in different positions of gaze with either eye fixating. Comitant misalignments are typically the nonparalytic strabismus most frequently observed in cross-eyed children. When a previously asymptomatic comitant misalignment becomes "symptomatic," it is said to "break down." The breakdown can be as subtle as a slip perhaps from a *phoria* (the relative deviation of the visual axes during monocular viewing of a single target) to a *tropia* (the relative deviation of the visual axes during binocular viewing of a single target). In some patients, the slip can go back and forth between phoria and tropia, particularly as the patient becomes fatigued.

Incomitant deviation describes an ocular misalignment that varies with the direction of gaze and changes according to which eye is fixating. Most incomitant misalignments are paralytic or mechanical in origin and are most frequently seen in incomitant deviations. (CN III, IV, and VI palsies), orbital restriction muscle paralysis, (tumors, thyroid exophthalmos), myasthenia gravis (MG), and inflammatory orbital myositis.

The term *primary deviation* is used to describe the deviation of the paretic eye while the normal eye is fixing. The deviation of the normal eye while the paretic eye is fixating is *secondary deviation,* which is larger than primary deviation in comitant strabismus (Figure 4-3).

Table 4-3 shows a comparison between nonparalytic and paralytic ocular misalignment.

THE DIPLOPIA HISTORY

Although it may seem daunting at first to determine which extraocular muscle is responsible for a patient seeing double, an accurate diagnosis can be achieved with a careful history and a clinical examination based on a clear understanding of the anatomy and physiology involved.

The onset of diplopia is usually acute, and it often brings a patient to the emergency room. There are important questions the examiner must ask—in particular, whether the diplopia is monocular or binocular, its onset, and duration. The patient's answers help establish the tempo of evolution, severity, and pathogenesis of the underlying condition.

- Does your double vision go away when you cover either eye? (A "yes" confirms binocular diplopia.)
- How did your double vision start? Acutely or gradually?
- How long have you had double vision?

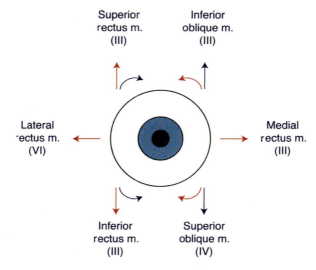

FIGURE 4-3 Diagram of right eye (examiner's view showing direction of primary (red) and secondary (blue) actions of the six extraocular muscles (m) and the ocular motor nerve (III, IV, or VI) which innervates each.

Reproduced with permission.[1]

- Is this the first time it has occurred?
- Is double vision present all the time?
- Has it increased in severity, or improved, or has it fluctuated since it started?
- Is it worse at the end of the day when you are tired?
- Is it better after a good night's sleep?

If *binocular diplopia* is confirmed, the most important question to ask is whether the images are *horizontally*, *vertically*, or *obliquely* displaced. Patients are often doubtful about their answer to this

---

TABLE 4-3: Non-Paralytic versus Paralytic Ocular Misalignment

Feature	Non-Paralytic (Comitant Misalignment)— Does not Vary with Gaze Position	Paralytic (Incomitant Misalignment)— Varies with Gaze Position
Age of onset	Childhood	Any age
Diplopia	Rare	Frequent
Amblyopia	Common	Infrequent
Comitance	Typical	Rare
Full eye movements	Yes	No
Other neurological finding	Rare	Common

Reproduced with permission.[3]

question, and, in such cases, I ask them to tell me what they see when they look across the room—at distance, then at near, then to both sides of the room, then up and down. I ask them to show me *with their hands* the position of the images (a good technique to detect obliquely tilted images in CN IV palsy) and then I ask:

- Are the images separated side-by-side or one on top of the other?
- Is the diplopia (separation of the image) greater at distance (typical of a sixth-nerve palsy)? Or at near (typical of a medial rectus palsy)?
- Is the diplopia greater looking right, left, up, or down?
- Is there any corrective head position that makes the diplopia better (typical of a fourth-nerve palsy)?
- If the diplopia is intermittent, can you see the image split apart into two, and can you refocus the images into a single image by blinking or closing your eyes (suggestive of a decompensated phoria)?
- How long does the double vision last, seconds or minutes?

Associated Symptoms

The history should conclude with a symptomatic inquiry for associated neurological symptoms: for example, eye (periorbital) pain suggests a diabetic mononeuropathy, monocular visual loss suggests an orbital apex syndrome, dizziness (vertigo) suggests a vestibular disorder, drooping of the eyelids (ptosis) supports a CN III palsy or MG, and headache suggests raised intracranial pressure.

A significant past history of strabismus as a child, treatment with prism glasses or ocular surgery, previous episodes of diplopia, head or eye trauma, vascular risk factors (hypertension, hyperlipidemia, diabetes mellitus), the patient's medications, and use of alcohol and/or drugs are all important to the history.

HORIZONTAL DIPLOPIA OR SEEING DOUBLE SIDE-BY-SIDE

Horizontal displacement of the image tells the examiner that the medial or lateral recti are involved, and, if the diplopia is worse with either near or far fixation, this narrows causation further: if worse with near vision, muscles of convergence are impaired, which implicates at least one of the medial recti.

Determining which direction of gaze makes the diplopia worse identifies which eye is responsible since the *images are most widely separated when looking in the direction of the paretic muscle*. For example, when a patient complains that his horizontal diplopia is worse at distance (suggesting a differential diagnosis of a sixth-nerve palsy vs. divergence insufficiency) but also worsens looking to the right (suggesting weakness of the left medial rectus or the right lateral rectus muscle), the right lateral rectus muscle is the cause because the diplopia is worse at distance. However, if the patient says his horizontal diplopia is worse at near (suggesting medial rectus muscle weakness), and it also worsens looking to the left (suggesting weakness of the right medial rectus and left lateral rectus), the right medial rectus muscle is the cause because the diplopia is worse at near.

Isolated weakness of the medial or lateral rectus muscles (isolated medial or lateral rectus paresis) deserves special attention.

Isolated weakness of the medial rectus muscle results in horizontal diplopia and an outward deviation of the eye (exotropia) because the medial rectus no longer opposes the action of the lateral rectus muscle. The causes of apparently isolated medial rectus paresis include a fascicular third-nerve palsy, MG, orbital myositis, and orbital disease—for example, restriction of movement due to the orbitopathy of Graves disease or entrapment of the medial rectus (limiting full abduction) due to fracture of the floor of the orbit.

Isolated weakness of the lateral rectus muscle (isolated lateral rectus paresis) is a common presentation and is most often due to a lesion of CN VI. It results in horizontal diplopia and inward deviation of the eye (esotropia) due to the unopposed action of the medial rectus muscle. The causes of isolated lateral rectus paresis also include MG, orbital myositis, muscle trauma, and orbital disease, in addition to an extensive list of central nervous system (CNS) disorders affecting CN VI (Chapter 5).

Lesions of the CNS involving the CN III oculomotor nucleus also affect the medial rectus, but not in isolation since the motor neurons controlling the medial rectus muscle lie in three separate locations within the oculomotor nucleus complex.

A lesion affecting the medial longitudinal fasciculus results in impairment of adduction on the side of the paretic medial rectus muscle and is associated with abducting nystagmus of the opposite eye, the principal manifestation of *internuclear ophthalmoplegia*. The medial longitudinal fasciculus contains axons from the vestibular nuclei that carry signals for the vertical vestibular ocular reflex (VOR), smooth pursuit, gaze-holding, and otolith-ocular reflexes (Chapter 6). This accounts for the presence of a skew deviation in association with an internuclear ophthalmoplegia.[7]

The differential diagnosis of horizontal diplopia should always include supranuclear paresis of convergence (*convergence insufficiency*) and paresis of divergence (*divergence insufficiency*), which can be mimicked by bilateral CN VI palsies.

VERTICAL DIPLOPIA OR SEEING DOUBLE ONE IMAGE ON TOP OF THE OTHER

There are twice as many extraocular muscles involved in vertical eye movements as in horizontal eye movements, and, not surprisingly, the range of movement disorders is correspondingly greater. In horizontal movements, the lateral/medial recti have only primary actions, whereas the muscles controlling vertical gaze have primary, secondary, and tertiary actions. When the images are vertically displaced and move farther apart looking up, then the inferior oblique and/or superior rectus muscles may be weak. When the images move farther apart looking down, then the superior oblique or the inferior rectus muscles may be weak.[8] *Images are most widely separated when looking in the direction of action of the paretic muscle* (Figure 4-4).[9]

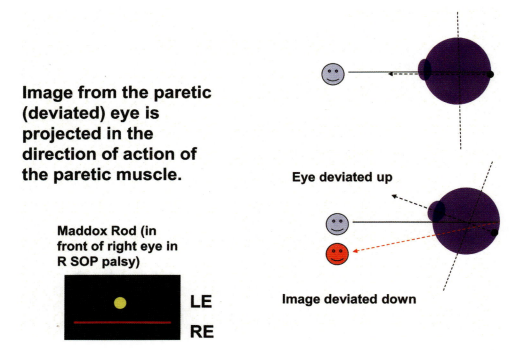

FIGURE 4-4 Evaluation of vertical deviation: Subjective testing of diplopia.

Reproduced with permission.[9]

Vertical diplopia is an important symptom of *restrictive orbital processes* such as thyroid-associated orbitopathy, which is often accompanied by forward displacement of the globe (*exophthalmos*), or with periorbital swelling. Mechanical limitation of motion occurs with entrapment of the extraocular muscles following traumatic fracture of the floor of the orbit or with a spontaneous fracture due to bone loss associated with sinus disease. The ipsilateral eye may be *enophthalmic* (backward displacement) and smaller in appearance.

The Forced Duction Test

Patients suspected of having mechanical limitation of motion due to an entrapment syndrome should be referred to an ophthalmologist for *forced duction testing*, which employs passive movement of the eye to distinguish limited movement caused by paresis of a muscle from that caused by mechanical restriction of its antagonist. The test requires anesthetizing the eyeball with a topical anesthetic and grasping the conjunctiva with fine-toothed forceps near the limbus on the non-limited side opposite to the direction in which the eye is to be moved. The patient is asked to looktoward the side of limited motion and an attempt is made by the examiner to move (with gentle force) the eye in that direction. If there is no resistance, the test is negative. If resistance is encountered, the test is positive and mechanical restriction is the cause of the motility defect.

Mechanical limitation can also be inferred if intraocular pressure increases substantially when the patient attempts to look in the direction of the gaze limitation.

The Palpebral-Oculogyric Reflex: Bell's Reflex

In cases of vertical diplopia with limited upgaze, the *palpebral-oculogyric reflex* (Bell's phenomenon or reflex) is helpful in differentiating a supranuclear (premotor) lesion from a nuclear or infranuclear lesion. Bell's reflex is the normal upward and outward rotation of the globe elicited during forceful eye closure, for example, squeezing the eyes shut as if there is soap in them. A normal Bell's reflex in cases of vertical diplopia with limited upgaze indicates a supranuclear lesion with intact nuclear and infranuclear oculomotor nerve function for upgaze. An absent Bell's reflex is characteristic of inferior entrapment syndromes, age-related double elevator palsy, and CN III palsy due to paresis of the superior rectus and inferior oblique muscles, but it must be kept in mind that Bell's reflex is absent in 50% of the normal population.

Skew Deviation Versus Trochlear Nerve Palsy

In cases of vertical diplopia with vertical misalignment and hypertropia, differentiating skew deviation from paresis of the superior oblique muscle can sometimes be difficult. This can happen because skew deviation closely mimics a palsy of the CN IV trochlear nerve,[10,11] the nerve innervating the superior oblique.

Skew deviation is a vertical misalignment caused by a supranuclear lesion that asymmetrically disrupts the utriculo-ocular pathway, causing an imbalance of vestibular tone in the roll plane.[12–16] The utricle mediates the static ocular counter-roll reflex, which generates partially compensatory torsional eye movements during static head roll.[17–19]

Skew deviation is often associated with other neurological signs. When accompanied by ocular torsion and head tilt, it forms a symptom triad called the *ocular tilt reaction*. In the ocular tilt reaction, the pathologic head tilt is *ipsilateral* to the hypotropic eye, reflecting the underlying pathological mechanism, and ocular torsion is such that the upper poles of both eyes rotate in the same direction as that of the head tilt (i.e., the hypotropic eye is extorted and the hypertropic eye is intorted).

In contrast, and worth remembering, the head tilt in trochlear nerve palsy is *contralateral* and is a compensatory mechanism to minimize the amount of hypertropia.

The Upright-Supine Test

In skew deviation, abnormal torsion and vertical misalignment are *head position-dependent*.[20] Normally, with the head upright, the utricles lie in an earth-horizontal plane. When the head changes from an upright to a supine position, the orientation of the utricles changes to an earth-vertical plane. This new orientation in the supine position leads to a reduction of vertical misalignment in skew deviation.

The underlying pathophysiology of skew deviation is the rationale for the upright-supine test,[21–22] which is positive for skew when the vertical deviation decreases by at least 50% from the upright to the supine position. This test supplements the classic Park's three-step test[23] in differentiating skew from trochlear nerve palsy.

Fundus Examination

A skew deviation versus a trochlear nerve palsy can also be differentiated by fundus examination and by the patient's perspective viewing a horizontal line. In skew deviation, the fundus is intorted in the hypertropic eye (Figure 4-5A).[24] In trochlear nerve superior oblique palsy, the fundus is extorted in the hypertropic eye (Figure 4-5B).

The patient's perspective viewing a horizontal line also helps differentiate a skew deviation from a trochlear superior oblique palsy: with a skew deviation, the patient sees two oblique parallel lines (Figure 4-5C); with a trochlear superior oblique palsy, the patient sees two lines that converge toward the side of the palsy (Figure 4-5D).

The absence of extorsion of the fundus in the supine position is consistent with abnormal torsion of the eye in skew deviation—it either decreases substantially or disappears completely in the supine position (with the head in neutral position).

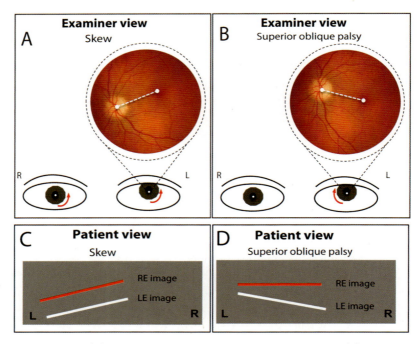

FIGURE 4-5 (A) Skew: intorsion of the fundus in the hypertropic eye. (B) Superior oblique palsy: extorsion of the fundus in the hypertropic eye. (C–D) Shows patient's perspective viewing of a horizontal line. (C) Skew: Lines are oblique and parallel. (D) Superior oblique palsy: Lines converge toward the side of a left fourth-nerve palsy.

Reproduced with permission.[24]

TABLE 4-4: Clinical Characteristics of Trochlear Nerve Palsy vs. Skew Deviation

Trochlear Nerve Palsy	Skew Deviation
Hypertropia in primary position	Hypertropia in primary position
Incomitant, hypertropia worse on gaze to opposite side acutely, may become comitant with time	Incomitant, comitant, or alternating
Hypertropia worse on ipsilateral head tilt	Hypertropia may or may not change with head tilt
Compensatory head tilt contralateral to the hypertropic eye	Pathologic head tilt contralateral to the hypertropic eye
Extorsion of the hypertropic eye	Intorsion of the hypertropic eye (extorsion of the hypotropic eye)
Usually no other neurologic signs (unless caused by trauma or lesions in brainstem)	Usually has other neurologic signs (e.g., gaze-evoked nystagmus, gaze palsy, dysarthria, ataxia, hemiplegia)

Reproduced with permission.[21]

Table 4-4 provides an anatomic recap of the clinical characteristics of a trochlear nerve palsy with paresis of the superior oblique muscle versus skew deviation.

EPISODIC DIPLOPIA

Episodic diplopia—horizontal, vertical, and/or oblique, lasting seconds or minutes only—occurs either spontaneously or in ocular neuromyotonia after sustained eccentric gaze. The episodes may occur infrequently or many times in a single day, and the patient can usually tell which eye is involved.

Ocular Neuromyotonia

Ocular neuromyotonia is a rare disorder in which sustained contractions of the extraocular muscles are due to repetitive firing in the peripheral ocular motor nerves. For example, diplopia occurring after downward gaze sustained for 10–20 seconds with gaze then returned to central position is usually followed by a refractory period with normal baseline ocular motility between attacks. Patients with ocular myotonia have often had prior radiation to the sella or parasellar region, months or even years before the onset of diplopia. In most cases, a single nerve is involved (CN III in 55% of cases).[25–27] A neurovascular compressive syndrome may be causal in idiopathic cases.[28] Treatment with carbamazepine may abolish symptoms.

The pathogenesis of ocular neuromyotonia is thought to be related to unstable axonal membranes, ephaptic neural transmission following peripheral nerve injury, or changes in neural activity following denervation. Most patients with ocular neuromyotonia benefit from membrane-stabilizing agents such as carbamazepine.[29]

CEREBRAL CAUSES OF MULTIPLE IMAGES

Polyopia (perseveration of a visual image in space) is a rare symptom, and its mechanism is unknown. It is reported with a maximum of four multiple images in two cases with occipital lobe trauma and visual field defects, in one patient with diffuse cerebral dysfunction due to encephalitis, and in another patient with a defect in visual fixation of unknown etiology. Polyopia may occur as a toxic side effect of methylenedioxymethamphetamine (Ecstasy).[30,31]

Palinopsia (visual preservation) is a similar illusory visual phenomenon, defined as the persistence or recurrence of visual images after the stimulus object has been removed.[32,33]

In the immediate persistent type of palinopsia, the persistent image is usually superimposed upon the scene in view. This happened to one of my patients who was watching the news over dinner—on looking away from the television, she saw the face of the anchor superimposed on her dinner plate for several minutes before the image faded. This type of palinopsia has some similarity to the normal experience of an afterimage observed after prolonged viewing of a bright object. In other cases of palinopsia, the image may be multiplied across otherwise intact visual fields. Some patients may experience a delayed type of palinopsia in which the image of a previously seen object reappears after an interval of minutes to hours, sometimes reappearing for days or even weeks. These patients may also experience both the immediate and delayed forms of palinopsia.

The most common cause of palinopsia is a parieto-occipital vascular lesion with incomplete homonymous hemianopia.[34] Palinopsia may also occur as a toxic side effect of lysergic acid diethylamide[35] and, more rarely, after certain prescription medication(s) such as Klonopin, interleukin 2, and trazodone.[36] Palinopsia associated with psychiatric conditions, for example schizophrenia, should only be considered illness-related in the absence of drugs or cerebral disease.[37]

THE DIPLOPIA EXAMINATION

A complete ophthalmological assessment should be made in patients presenting with monocular diplopia. *Binocular diplopia requires the cause of misalignment of the visual axes to be determined.*

Head Position

The diplopia examination should begin the moment the patient enters the room. The first really important observation is the position and/or the movement of the patient's head. Does it change in any way? Keep in mind that *changes in head posture serve to minimize or eliminate diplopia by positioning the eyes away from the movement field of a paretic muscle.* The head is usually turned or tilted to the position where action of the paretic muscle is least required (i.e., toward the side of the paretic muscle). A patient with a right sixth-nerve palsy, for example, may habitually turn her head to the right so that her eyes are deviated to the left in the orbit while she views objects straight ahead.

Similarly, patients with vertical extraocular muscle paresis may carry their head flexed or extended. A patient with a right fourth-nerve palsy and paresis of the superior oblique muscle may slightly flex his head down and turn his face to the left, away from the paretic eye—these compensatory movements position the eyes out of the field of the right superior oblique muscle. This patient may also tilt his head toward the side opposite the paretic muscle (i.e., to the left) to lessen the torsion required of the paretic right superior oblique muscle. This position permits fusion of the images. In contrast, the patient with monocular paralysis of elevation will tend to keep the head elevated and positioned in the direction of the paretic eye movement.

Some patients adopt a head posture that actually increases the distance between the two images, allowing one of the images to be more easily ignored. One way to determine whether an abnormal head posture is related to diplopia is to cover one eye. If the abnormal head posture disappears on covering one eye, then it is likely to be associated with diplopia.

Ocular Alignment

Paresis of the ocular muscles causing specific misalignments of the eyes are the markers telling the examiner which cranial nerves are involved. For example, an exotropia—outward deviation of the eye—is due to paresis of the medial rectus muscle, which is innervated by CN III, the oculomotor nerve.

The lateral rectus muscle innervated by CN VI, the abducens nerve, is involved in an esotropia, an inward deviation of the eye. Paresis of the superior oblique muscle, which is innervated by CN IV, the trochlear nerve, gives rise to hypertropia and vertical deviation of the eyes in primary gaze.

Unquestionably, the examination to assess ocular alignment is important for localizing the eye signs—and it must include objective tests that do not rely on the patient's description of image separation.

- Use the corneal reflection test (or the Krimsky test) to detect subtle degrees of misalignment.
- Use the cover-uncover test over one eye to detect a tropia.
- Use the alternate cover test to detect a phoria.
- Use the red glass or the Maddox rod test to more clearly distinguish the image the patient sees.

The *corneal reflection test* is often overlooked by neurologists as a way of assessing ocular alignment, but it is very useful. It involves simply asking the patient to look at a bright light held in front of the face. At a distance of approximately 33 cm, the reflected light spot should fall near the center of the pupil. Eccentric location of a reflected light spot indicates misalignment of the eye, with 1 mm of deviation from center corresponding to 7 degrees of ocular deviation.

The ophthalmologist's *Krimsky test* includes placing a prism over the nonfixating deviated eye and increasing or decreasing the strength of the prism (measured in diopters) until the reflected light spot is in the center of both pupils.[38,39] The light's reflection in the center of the pupil indicates alignment of the visual axes, quantified by the amount of prism required to neutralize the deviation.

The *cover-uncover test* is more sensitive than the Krimsky test for detecting tropias (misalignment with both eyes viewing). Tropias are abnormal. Both eyes could be tested in sequence, and the same observations made. The test confirms which is the deviated eye by looking for the movement of redress (the corrective movement) when the cover is removed from the eye.

- If the uncovered eye moves to take up fixation, it can be assumed that, under binocular viewing conditions, the eye was not aligned with fixation and a manifest deviation was present (a tropia).
- Inward movement of the uncovered eye indicates an exotropia.

- Outward movement of the uncovered eye indicates an esotropia.
- A vertical movement down indicates a hypertropia.
- A vertical movement up indicates a hypotropia.

The examiner should determine whether the tropia is *comitant* or *incomitant* by seeing if the magnitude of the deviation of the eye varies or remains the same in the eight cardinal positions of gaze (horizontal and oblique; hyperdeviation up, hypodeviation down).

If there is a vertical deviation of the eyes, the eye with a hyperdeviation is conventionally referred to as *hypertropic*. For example, a hyperdeviation of the right eye is a *right hypertropia*.

Cover testing for ocular misalignment is straightforward. In Figure 4-6 the patient is fixing with the nonparetic right eye. Upon occlusion of the right eye, the misaligned left eye is forced to fixate.

- *Esotropic* eyes move laterally to fixate
- *Exotropic* eyes move medially to fixate
- *Hypertropic* eyes move downward to fixate

Thus, the ocular deviations can be determined by the direction of the fixation movements.[1]

The *alternate cover test* is a test for phorias (misalignment with one eye viewing). Look for the movement of redress (the corrective movement) when the cover is switched to the other eye. Horizontal phorias, usually exophoria, may be present in normal subjects viewing a near target. Vertical phorias tend to be abnormal.

The *red glass test* helps to more clearly distinguish the image seen by each eye. The red glass is always placed in front of the patient's right eye, and the patient fixes on a single light as the object of regard. First and always, the patient should be asked if he sees one or two lights. If the eyes are misaligned, the patient sees two lights (red and white). He should identify the colors of the two images and say whether the red light is to the right or to the left of the white light, or above or below.

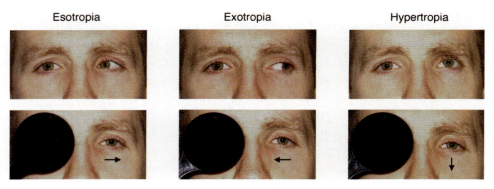

FIGURE 4-6 Cover testing for ocular misalignment. In each case, the patient is fixing with the nonparetic right eye. On occlusion of the right eye, the misaligned left eye is forced to fixate.
- *Esotropic* eyes move laterally to fixate.
- *Exotropic* eyes move medially to fixate.
- *Hypertropic* eyes move downward to fixate.
Thus, the ocular deviations can be determined by direction of the fixation movements.

Reproduced with permission.[1]

If the right eye is *exotropic* due to paresis of the medial rectus muscle (innervated by the oculomotor nerve [CN III]), the patient will see the red light to the left of the white light. This is *crossed diplopia* (Figure 4-7A–B).

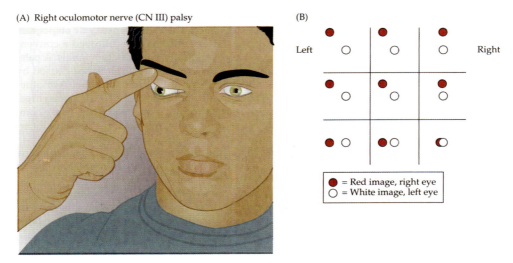

FIGURE 4-7 Oculomotor nerve (CN III) palsy. (A) Appearance of the eyes in the presence of a right oculomotor nerve palsy. (B) Red glass testing with a right oculomotor nerve palsy. A red glass was placed over the right eye, and results are drawn as seen from the patient's perspective.

Reproduced with permission.[2]

If the patient has an *esotropia* due to paresis of the lateral rectus muscle (innervated by the abducens nerve [CN VI]), the patient will see the red light to the right of the white light. This is *uncrossed diplopia* (Figure 4-8A–B).

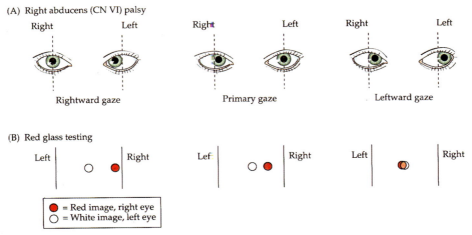

FIGURE 4-8 Abducens nerve (CN VI) palsy. (A) Appearance of the eyes in three different positions of gaze, in the presence of a right abducens nerve palsy. (B) Red glass testing in the same three positions of gaze, with a right abducens nerve palsy. A red glass was placed over the right eye, and results are drawn as seen from the patient's perspective.

Reproduced with permission.[2]

If an eye is *hypertropic* due to a vertical deviation of the eyes caused by paresis of the superior oblique muscle (innervated by the trochlear nerve (CN IV)) the patient will see the red light from the hypertropic eye below the white light from the contralateral eye (Figure 4-9A–C).

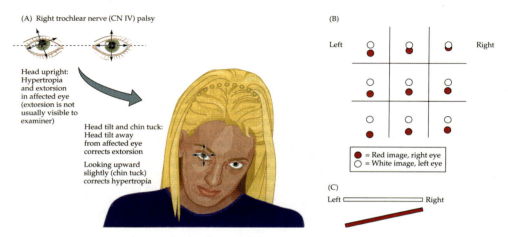

FIGURE 4-9 Trochlear nerve (CN IV) palsy. (A) Appearance of the eyes in the presence of a right trochlear nerve palsy. Hypertropia can be compensated for by tucking the chin and looking up slightly. Extorsion can be compensated for by tilting the head away from the affected eye. (B) Red glass testing with a right trochlear nerve palsy. A red glass was placed over the right eye, and results are drawn as seen from the patient's perspective. (C) Position of a horizontal red line with a red glass over the right eye.

Reproduced with permission.[2]

Once a patient indicates that there is clear separation of images when he is fixating on the light held straight ahead, the examiner can determine the point of maximum vertical separation of the images by having the patient look at the light held in the other diagnostic positions of gaze.

The *Maddox rod test* is a variation of the red glass test except that the patient sees a red line rather than a red dot (Figure 4-10). A Maddox rod is a series of parallel cylinders that convert the image of a single light into a line. The rod can be oriented to make the line vertical or horizontal. By convention, the rod is placed over the right eye and the patient is asked to fixate on a white light either at distance or near. The relationship of the red line to the white light seen from the left eye, whether it is to the left or to the right, above or below, characterizes the type of ocular misalignment.

Ductions and Versions

Ductions during monocular viewing test the movement of each eye (ocular motility) while the other eye is covered. All the extraocular muscles contribute to alignment of the visual axes in all

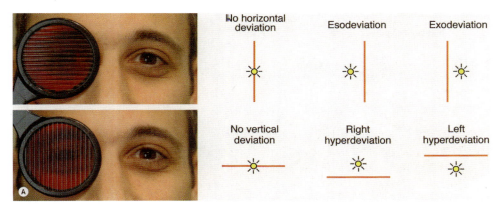

FIGURE 4-10 Maddox rod testing for ocular misalignment drawn from the patient's perspective. A binocular patient's right eye sees a red line, while the uncovered left eye sees the white light. *Top row*: To evaluate horizontal ocular deviations, the bars on the Maddox rod are aligned horizontally, so the patient sees a vertical red line with the right eye. If there is no horizontal deviation, the patient perceives the red line passing through the white light (depicted in yellow for illustrative purposes). If the eyes are esodeviated, the red line, whose image would abnormally fall on the nasal retina, appears to the right of the white light ("uncrossed diplopia"). Exodeviated eyes would result in the red line appearing to the left of the light ("crossed diplopia") because the red image would abnormally fall on the temporal retina. *Bottom row*: (A) to evaluate vertical deviations, the bars are oriented vertically, so the patient will see a horizontal red line with the right eye. The red line passes through the white light when there is no vertical deviation, whereas a red line perceived below the light implies a right hyperdeviation, and a white light perceived below the red line indicates a left hyperdeviation (i.e., the lower image corresponds to the hyperdeviated eye).

Reproduced with permission.[1]

positions of gaze, and limited duction will indicate paralysis of a muscle or restriction of its antagonist. To test this, the patient is asked to look fully in nine diagnostic positions of gaze: straight ahead, right, left, up, down, up and to the right, up and to the left, down and to the right, down and to the left.

Ductions are always full in nonparalytic strabismus, and testing ductions answers the question of whether an esotropia is a nonparetic strabismus (with full range of movement with monocular viewing) or a paretic strabismus.

Versions refer to the range of ocular motion during binocular viewing. Testing versions in the nine cardinal diagnostic positions of gaze further refines diagnosis. Eye movements in seven of the nine diagnostic positions are shown in Figure 4-11.[40]

Conventionally, diagnostic eye positions are recorded in an H fashion from the patient's perspective.[41] This method helps identify the paretic muscle more clearly because each position of gaze corresponds with the main action of a particular extraocular muscle.

In the absence of visible restriction of eye movements by ocular muscle weakness, diplopia should be further tested by occluding each eye in turn. The rule in these cases is that *the outer image comes from the paretic eye.* For example, if the patient reports diplopia in the left field of

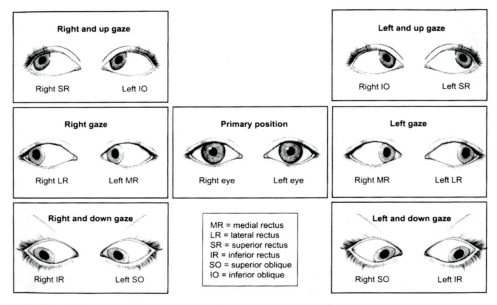

FIGURE 4-11 Eye movements in seven diagnostic positions of gaze.

Reproduced with permission.[40]

gaze, and the outer image disappears with the right eye covered, the patient has a right medial rectus palsy.

DIPLOPIA WITH FULL EYE MOVEMENTS

A phoria is a latent visual axis deviation held in check by fusion—that is to say, a misalignment of the eyes that occurs only when binocularity is interrupted. Patients with a phoria usually complain of intermittent transient diplopia or difficulty focusing for seconds only, and many patients close their eyes or blink to refix the single image when they see an image break apart, for example, while watching TV. Patients who can do this have a phoria until proven otherwise. They retain full eye movements.

Decompensated Phoria

The case presented here of an elderly man with transient diplopia strikes a cautionary note. It illustrates the care with which a diagnosis of an episodic (decompensated) phoria should be approached.

CASE 4-1 Episodic Diplopia: Ocular Myasthenia Gravis

Video Display

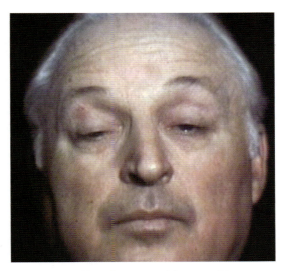

FIGURE 4-12 Sixty-five-year-old man with episodic diplopia and bilateral ptosis.

In 1974, a 65-year-old physician in good health and on no medication presented with intermittent horizontal double vision that troubled him when driving toward the end of the day (Figure 4-12). He consulted an ophthalmologist who found that he had full eye movements and bilateral ptosis. A diagnosis of age-related ptosis and a decompensated phoria was made. He was prescribed prism glasses but frequently needed to renew them and get a stronger prism correction. Ultimately, over 4 months, he had five pairs of prism glasses prescribed. The patient referred himself for evaluation.

The diplopia history revealed that he had:

- Intermittent horizontal diplopia at distance and near lasting seconds only.
- A single image with one eye covered.
- Difficulty driving at the end of the day because the cars in front of him appeared to be double.
- Occasional episodes of blurred vision reading.
- He frequently saw TV images split horizontally into two images side by side. By closing his eyes for a second or two, he could refocus a single image.
- Intermittent drooping of his eyelids particularly at the end of the day.
- If he gently closed his eyes when he brought his car to a stop at traffic lights, his eyelids opened more fully.
- No past history of diplopia, ptosis, or muscle fatigue.

Analysis of the History

· What are the major presenting symptoms?
· Where are the CNS lesion(s) likely to be?

CASE 4-1 SYMPTOMS

Symptoms	Location Correlation
Ptosis	Levator palpebrae superioris
Episodic diplopia	Extraocular muscles

The analysis guides the clinical examination.

Examination

Eyelid Examination

· Bilateral ptosis with almost complete closure of his eyes
· Slight increase in ptosis on fatigue
· Overaction of the orbicularis oculi
· Positive lid twitch
· Transient recovery of ptosis on gentle eye closure
· Impaired ability to bury his eyelashes fully

Ocular Motility

· No head turn or tilt
· Eye movements full in all positions of gaze
· Normal horizontal and vertical saccades
· Normal smooth pursuit
· Impaired convergence
· Normal oculocephalic reflex
· Normal Bell's reflex—eyes deviated up under closed lids
· Corneal reflex test—subtle horizontal misalignment
· Alternate cover testing showed an exophoria

Localization and Differential Diagnosis

Multiple pairs of prism glasses over a short period of time suggest a decompensated phoria since the ability to hold fusion relaxes with age and fatigue. However, diplopia driving home at night is suggestive of MG.

What Diagnostic Test Should Follow?

- Tensilon test
- Chest scan
- Antibody studies

Test Results

The patient received a test dose of 0.2 mL edrophonium chloride (Tensilon) without any side effects, followed by a dose of 0.3 mL, resulting in prompt elevation of the eyelids. A full dose of 1 mL (10 mg) of Tensilon was not given. The chest CT was normal. A test for acetylcholine receptor antibody (AChR) was negative.

Diagnosis: Ocular Myasthenia Gravis

Treatment*

- Anticholinesterase inhibitor
- Immunosuppression

Treatment was started with pyridostigmine (Mestinon) 60 mg q4h and prednisone 20 mg/day, which resulted in complete resolution of the diplopia and less marked ptosis.

The patient was followed for 4 years with no sign of generalized MG—he remained seronegative for AChR antibody.

Special Explanatory Note

A decompensated phoria is the commonest cause of postoperative diplopia in the recovery room and a very common side effect of drugs such as anticonvulsants, antidepressants, antipsychotics, sleeping pills, antihistamines, and alcohol. Serial upgrades of prism glasses due to an increasing horizontal deviation and convergence insufficiency is a key sign of a progressive motility disorder consistent with ocular MG.

Loss of Binocular Fusion

A further and particularly rare variant of diplopia with full eye movements but loss of binocular fusion may occur in patients with pituitary tumors, chiasmal compression, and complete or almost complete bitemporal hemianopia (a visual field defect with bilateral blindness in the temporal half-field). Kirkham reported this phenomenon in a woman whose symptoms emerged when precision visual tasks demanded near fixation to undertake—for example, cutting her fingernails pruning roses and reading. When reading she noted gaps appearing in the lines of print or in individual words. Occasionally, the page appeared to split into two parts and separate vertically, making it impossible to scan the page. Changing the position of her head had no effect. She also noted intermittent distortion of other objects, splitting and separation vertically of shelves, cars, people's faces, and bodies.[42] Kirkham's patient had two visual perception disorders previously seen in association with bitemporal hemianopia.[43] The first consisted of difficulties with depth perception, referred to as "chiasmatic postfixational blindness." The second consisted of horizontal or vertical separation of images (occurring in the absence of a muscle paresis) resulting in nonparetic diplopia.

Chiasmatic postfixational blindness describes symptoms of impaired depth perception, caused by a blind area beyond the fixation point, present in patients with bitemporal hemianopia. An image of an object posterior to fixation falls on the blind nasal retina (temporal half field), and objects in the central field of vision disappear (Figure 4-13). Patients with postfixation blindness have difficulty with precision tasks that demand close up central vision, for example threading a needle, and may complain of difficulty focusing and judging distance.

Horizontal or vertical separation of images occurring in the absence of a muscle palsy is called the *hemifield slide phenomenon*. Because of the overlap of the receptive fields of retinal ganglion cells in the vertical median strip, normal visual fields appear uniform and without interruption in the midline, but if the physiological linkage between the two hemifields is lacking, patients with bitemporal hemianopia experience field instability, with binocular vision possible only when the eyes are still, not when the eyes are moving. This is referred to as a motor imbalance, and it makes maintaining the two hemifields in juxtaposition to each other difficult, allowing a preexisting or intermittent *exotropia* (XT), a preexisting or intermittent *esotropia* (ET), or a hyperdeviation to produce startling results in which objects appear to overlap (XT), separate horizontally (ET), or diverge vertically (Figure 4-14). These symptoms occur intermittently.

Nonparetic diplopia has also been reported in patients who have an alternating superior altitudinal field defect in one eye and an inferior altitudinal field defect in the other (referred to as *heteronymous altitudinal field defects*). These cases illustrate nonparetic diplopia may be due to generalized loss of fusion rather than to the particular topography of the visual field defect.[44]

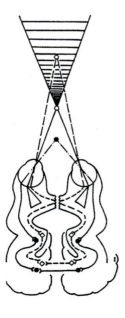

FIGURE 4-13 Chiasmatic postfixational blindness: The shaded area represents the blind area beyond the fixation point, which is present in patients with a bitemporal hemianopia.

Reproduced with permission.[42]

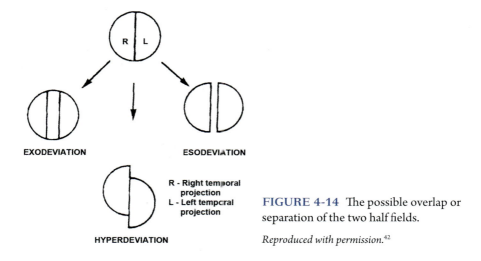

EXODEVIATION

ESODEVIATION

R - Right temporal
projection
L - Left temporal
projection

HYPERDEVIATION

FIGURE 4-14 The possible overlap or separation of the two half fields.

Reproduced with permission.[42]

DIPLOPIA WITH PARETIC EYE MOVEMENTS

The presence of an obvious ocular misalignment in primary gaze with deviation of one or both eyes is an important clinical clue in patients with diplopia. The deviation may be an esotropia (inward deviation), an exotropia (outward deviation), or a hypertropia (upward deviation). Table 4-5 summarizes the range of causes that can give rise to significant ocular misalignment.

TABLE 4-5: Ocular Deviation in Primary Gaze Diagnostic Indicators

Esotropia (inward)
Nonparalytic strabismus
Sixth-nerve palsy
Lateral rectus weakness
Divergence insufficiency
Medial rectus (entrapment)
Myasthenia gravis

Exotropia (outward)
Nonparalytic strabismus
Third-nerve palsy
Unilateral wall-eyed internuclear ophthalmoplegia
Paralytic pontine exotropia
Convergence insufficiency
Myasthenia gravis

Hypertropia (upward)
Fourth-nerve palsy
Skew deviation
Monocular paresis of downgaze
Fracture of the floor of the orbit with muscle entrapment
Myasthenia gravis

Evaluating Esotropia

An esotropia raises the immediate question: is the deviation due to a nonparalytic strabismus or to a paralytic disorder? The case presented here illustrates the diagnostic work up.

CASE 4-2 Evaluating An Esotropia: Abducens Nerve Palsy

Video Display

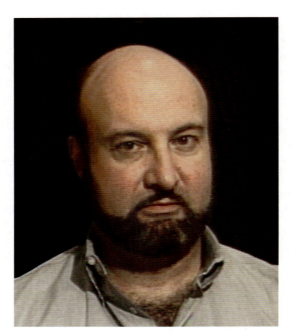

FIGURE 4-15 Patient with a right head turn and a left esotropia.

The patient is a 45-year-old pharmaceutical executive who presented in October 1990 with acute diplopia (Figure 4-15). Nine days prior to admission, he flew back to Boston from San Francisco after a hectic business trip feeling jet lagged and fatigued. Four days later, he made a day trip to New York. On the following morning, a Saturday, he awoke with a severe generalized headache that persisted for 2 days. On Monday, he was well enough to go to work, but, on Tuesday, he had headache, left sided retro-orbital pain, and double vision with objects side-by-side. He came to the emergency room.

A diplopia history revealed:

- Horizontal diplopia at distance, not at near.
- The images were horizontal side-by-side and became farther apart on gaze left.
- A single image with one eye covered.

- When driving, the cars in front of him appeared to be "double."
- Turning his head to the right and keeping his eyes straight enabled him to see a single image.
- No pain on eye movement (to suggest an orbit process).
- Past history significant for a transient episode of horizontal diplopia, without drooping of the eyelids, 18 months prior to this attack. At that time, he did not seek medical advice and could not recall if one eye was deviated or not.
- Family history positive for diabetes in both grandparents.

Analysis of the History

- What are the major presenting symptoms?
- Where are the CNS lesion(s) likely to be?

CASE 4-2 SYMPTOMS

Symptoms	Location Correlation
Headache	Intracranial
Retro-orbital pain	Orbit
Horizontal diplopia	Lateral rectus muscle
	Medial rectus muscle

The analysis guides the clinical examination.

Examination

Ocular Motility

- Head turn to the right to place his eyes in primary gaze
- No ptosis
- Esotropia left eye (OS) with right eye (OD) fixating
- Left lateral rectus muscle paresis
- Limited range of abduction OS monocular viewing
- Full horizontal gaze to the right
- Full adduction OD
- Normal convergence
- Full vertical gaze
- Normal pupillary and corneal reflexes
- No nystagmus
- No exophthalmos, ocular pulsation, or ocular bruit
- Lower cranial nerves intact

There were no other focal findings on neuro-ophthalmological and neurological examination.

Localization and Differential Diagnosis

Microinfarction of the abducens nerve is the commonest cause of a painful sixth-nerve palsy in patients with diabetes mellitus and/or systemic vascular disease (hypertension, hyperlipidemia). In this patient, a nondiabetic without risk factors for ischemia, it is essential to rule out a compressive lesion.

What Diagnostic Tests Should Follow?

· Chest x-ray
· Brain computed tomography (CT)

Test Results

Chest x-ray normal. The brain CT (1990) showed complete opacification and mucosal thickening of the left mastoid sinus, no evidence of a cavernous sinus lesion or bony destructive process.

Diagnosis: Unilateral Mastoiditis with Petrous Apicitis

Prognosis

The diplopia resolved spontaneously over a period of 4 weeks. Three years later, in February 1993, a few days after a severe upper respiratory infection complicated by sinusitis and headache, he again developed horizontal double vision and inward deviation of his left eye (esotropia).

A brain CT (1993) with and without contrast, with coronal images through the petrous bones, cavernous sinus, and orbit showed the left petrous apex was completely opacified without evidence of bone destruction or definite bone expansion. Opacification of several inferior and posterior mastoid air cells was also noted on the left. The right petrous apex was well pneumatized.

Treatment

The patient was seen in consultation by an otolaryngologist and received a 2-week course of intravenous antibiotics. He made a complete recovery.

Special Explanatory Note

When petrous apicitis is associated with the clinical triad of otorrhea, retro-orbital pain, and a sixth-nerve palsy, it is referred to as *Gradenigo's syndrome* (although in Gradenigo's original report of 57 cases, fewer than half presented with the classic triad).[45,46]

Computed tomography is considered the imaging study of choice in these cases because it provides detailed imaging of bone, and most apex lesions show up as erosion of bone plus opacification of the air cells of the petrous apex.[47] Failure to make the diagnosis of petrous apicitis may lead to serious morbidity and mortality. Intravenous antibiotics are recommended for at least 2–3 weeks.

Evaluating Exotropia

The presence of an exotropia in primary gaze raises the same question as an esotropia: is the deviation due to a nonparalytic strabismus or to a paralytic disorder? The case presented here illustrates the same step-by-step approach to the diagnosis.

CASE 4-3 Evaluating An Extropia: Fascicular Oculomotor Nerve Palsy

Video Display

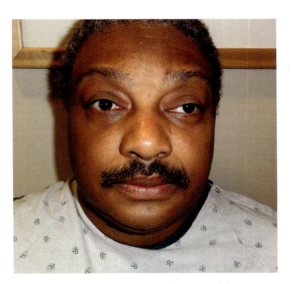

FIGURE 4-16 Fifty-one-year-old man with diplopia at near and exotropia.

The patient is a 51-year-old man with multiple vascular risk factors (hypertension, hyperlipidemia) and a history of inconsistent medicine compliance (Figure 4-16). He presented with a 1-day history of acute onset of blurry vision at 7:30 A.M. while working at his desk, and he noted for the first time intermittent double vision. He had no associated symptoms, in particular no headache or dizziness.

He went to the ER at the Massachusetts Eye and Ear Infirmary and was found to have high blood pressure 198/97, pulse 70 regular, and was referred to the Massachusetts General Hospital (MGH) for admission. In the MGH ER, he complained that his "eyes were not coordinated."

His history was negative for transient ischemic attacks or cardiovascular disease.

A diplopia history revealed:

- Diplopia only for reading and at near.
- When he closed each eye individually, his vision was "near normal."

- Images were side-by-side and further apart when he looked to the right.
- No eye pain or pain on eye movement.
- No history of strabismus as a child or the need to wear prism glasses.
- He was on no medication and denied substance abuse.

Analysis of the History

- What are the major presenting symptoms?
- Where are the CNS lesion(s) likely to be?

CASE 4-3 SYMPTOMS

Symptoms	Location Correlation
Multiple vascular risk factors	
Diplopia at near	Medial rectus muscle
Partial ptosis	Levator palpebrae superioris

The analysis guides the clinical examination.

Examination

Ocular Motility

- No head turn
- Slight ptosis left eye (OS)
- Exotropia left eye (OS) with the right eye (OD) fixating
- Left medial rectus paresis
- Slow adducting saccades OS
- Limited range of adduction OS with monocular viewing
- Full horizontal conjugate gaze to the left
- Full horizontal gaze to the right (OD) with no abducting nystagmus
- Convergence impaired OS, the eye moved down and out attempting to converge
- Convergence normal OD
- Normal pupillary and corneal reflexes

The ocular motility signs are illustrated in Figure 4-17A–D.

There were no other findings on neurological examination.

Within 24 hours, ptosis OS progressed, almost closing the exotropic left eye (Figure 4-17). Weakness of upgaze OS was noted at this time.

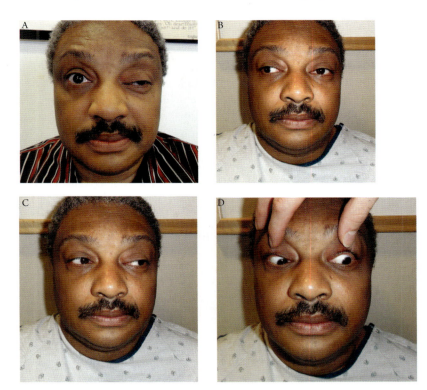

FIGURE 4-17 (A) Marked ptosis of the left eye, lid retraction of the right eye. (B) Paresis of adduction of the left eye looking to the right. (C) Full eye movements looking to the left. (D) Monocular impairment of convergence of the left eye, which deviates down and out.

Localization and Differential Diagnosis

Given the major symptoms and signs—diplopia at near and paresis of the medial rectus muscle—the differential diagnoses to consider are:

- Ocular myasthenic paresis, especially with the development of ptosis.
- Internuclear ophthalmoplegia (INO), characterized by weakness of adduction of the left eye; but, in the absence of nystagmus in the abducting eye, an INO is ruled out.
- A partial progressive CN III palsy sparing the pupil (a leading contender).
- A partial fascicular CN III palsy (a rare disorder).

What Diagnostic Tests Should Follow?

- Tensilon test
- Brain magnetic resonance imaging (MRI)
- Brain magnetic resonance angiography (MRA)

Test Results

The Tensilon test was negative after a full intravenous dose (10 mg) of Tensilon. Brain MRI showed a left paramedian midbrain infarct (DWI bright ADC dark) ventral to the Sylvian aqueduct in the region of the medial longitudinal fasciculus (MLF) and the oculomotor nucleus complex and several old lacuna infarcts in the thalamus, putamen, and left paramedian pontine tegmentum just above the level of the sixth-nerve nucleus.

Fluid attenuated (FLAIR) images showed nonspecific bihemispheric diffuse white matter foci consistent with microvascular disease.

Brain MR angiogram showed moderate narrowing of the right vertebral artery origin and mild narrowing of the proximal segment of the right posterior cerebral artery.

Diagnosis: Unilateral Midbrain Infarct

The diagnosis included partial left fascicular third-nerve palsy affecting fascicles to the medial rectus, superior rectus and the levator palpebrae superioris muscles.

Treatment

Blood pressure control is essential in this patient.

Prognosis

The patient was discharged home on antihypertension medication. He was followed for 2 months, by which time his eye movements had completely recovered.

Special Explanatory Note

Partial isolated fascicular oculomotor nerve palsies are rare and, in some patients, may be misdiagnosed as an ischemic partial CN III nerve palsy.

Magnetic resonance imaging is invaluable in differentiating the two disorders. In this case, it clearly showed the topographical location of an infarct involving the left oculomotor nucleus complex in the midbrain.

Evaluating Hypertropia

The presence of a hypertropia raises the question: is it due to a trochlear nerve palsy with paresis of the superior oblique muscle or to a skew deviation/ocular tilt reaction? (see Chapter 8).

CASE 4-4 Evaluating A Hypertropia: Post-Traumatic Trochlear Nerve Palsy

Video Display

The patient is a 32-year-old left-handed athletic chemistry teacher who presented with intermittent vertical double vision when reading late in the evening (Figure 4-18). The

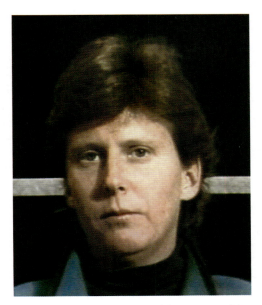

FIGURE 4-18 Thirty-two-year-old woman with diplopia and a right head tilt.

images were one on top of the other, and, on occasion, one image was slightly slanted. She had no diplopia with one eye covered.

She consulted an ophthalmologist who documented a 2 diopter esotropia and hypotropia and prescribed prism reading glasses, which helped. She consulted a neurologist at the same time because her vision lost focus when she turned her head from side to side quickly. The neurologist noted only a "lag of abduction" of the right eye and obtained a brain MRI with gadolinium, a blood study for AChR antibody, and thyroid tests, all of which were normal.

In December 1992, she referred herself for a second opinion. At that time, she said that she could correct her diplopia by changing the position of her head or by covering one eye. Her history was negative for strabismus as a child, prism glasses, head or eye trauma and transient ptosis or fatigue.

Analysis of the History

· What are the major presenting symptoms?
· Where are the CNS lesion(s) likely to be?

CASE 4-4 SYMPTOMS

Symptoms	Location Correlation
Vertical diplopia corrected by head tilt	Trochlear nerve palsy

The analysis guides the clinical examination.
Diplopia history:

- A single image with one eye covered
- Vertical separation of the images greatest in downgaze and to the opposite side
- Tilting her head to the right corrected the diplopia.
- When the patient viewed a horizontal bar, the two images were slanted with respect to each other, with the apparent intersection of the lines pointing toward the right (the side of the fourth-nerve palsy). This feature helps to distinguish trochlear nerve palsy from skew deviation, in which the two lines appear parallel.

Ocular Motility

- Right head tilt
- Hypertropia of the right eye (OD)
- Paralysis of the right superior oblique muscle with absent depression and intorsion
- Overaction of the right inferior oblique muscle looking to the left with upward deviation of the eye in adduction
- Normal cranial nerves CN III, V, and VI

The neurological examination was normal.

Localization and differential diagnosis

Patients who present with a chief complaint of vertical diplopia usually have a palsy of the trochlear nerve or skew deviation but consideration should also be given to the syndrome of overaction of the inferior oblique. In the absence of a history of head trauma, MRI with and without gadolinium, may show relevant brianstem lesions, infiltrative or inflammatory processes involving the long course of the fourth nerve. When imaging the head and orbit show no abnormality and test results for diabetes and myasthenia are negative, then the outcome is usually favourable. Rarely, movements of the superior oblique tendon are restricted in the trochlea by tendosynovitis, adhesions, tumor, metastases or trauma resulting in impaired elevation of the adducted eye—an acquired Brown's syndrome. Occasionally, in some patiens, when they attempt to look up there is initally restriction and limited elevation but after an audible click, the eye does eventually elevate. This orbital disorder is the superior oblique click-syndrome.

What Diagnostic Tests Should Follow?

- Parks-Bielschowsky Three-Step Test

Steps to follow are:

Step 1. Determine which eye is hypertropic in primary position (four possible muscles).

Example: If there is a right hypertropia in primary position, then the depressors of the right eye (inferior rectus [IR] and superior oblique [SO]) or the elevators of the left eye (superior rectus [SR]) and inferior oblique [IO]) are weak (these muscles are outlined in red in Figure 4-19).

Step 2. Determine whether the hypertropia increases on right or left gaze (two possible muscles).

- The vertical rectus muscles (SR and IR) have their greatest vertical action when the eye is *abducted.*
- The oblique muscles (SO and IO) have their greatest vertical action when the eye is *adducted.*
- Example: If a right hypertropia increases on left gaze, then the oblique muscles of the right eye (SO and IO) or the vertical rectus muscles of the left eye (SR and IR) are involved (outlined in blue in Figure 4-19).

Step 3. Determine whether the hypertropia increases on right or left head tilt.

- During right head tilt, the right eye intorts (SO and SR) and left eye extorts (IO and IR).
- During left head tilt, the right eye extorts (IO and IR) and left eye intorts (SO and SR).
- Example: If a right hypertropia increases on right head tilt, then the intortors of the right eye (SO and SR) or the extorters of the left eye (IO and IR) are involved (outlined in green in the Figure 4-19).

Because the right superior oblique is outlined in all three test steps, the diagnosis is a right fourth-nerve palsy.

Three-step test confirmed a right superior oblique palsy.

Test Results

Three-step test confirmed a right superior oblique palsy.

The cover/uncover test revealed:

- Hypertropia OD primary gaze
- Hypertropia most marked with right head tilt
- Hypertropia diminished, almost absent with left head tilt
- Hypertropia almost fully corrected with prism glasses at distance

The three-step test confirmed a right superior oblique palsy.

Example: Right fourth nerve palsy

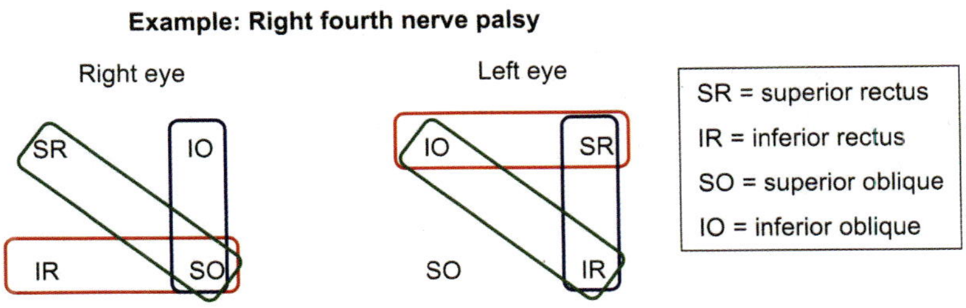

FIGURE 4-19 The Parks-Bielschowsky three-step test.

Reproduced with permission.[40]

What Additional Tests Are Needed?

· Neuroimaging of the orbit and brain
· Review of old photographs if possible to determine the duration of the head tilt

Test Results

A CT of the orbits with bone windows was normal. A review of old soccer team photographs established a 14-year duration of the right head tilt, and a history of trauma not previously volunteered by the patient was elicited. In 1978, she was hit by a lacrosse ball and sustained a black eye and swelling of the right side of her face. She was startled by the blow but not knocked out. The injury took several days for her to recover but, during that time, she did not recall having double vision.

Special Explanatory Note

As already noted, old photographs are well worth asking for. A review of this patient's soccer photograph indicated the presence of a head tilt in 1980 (Figure 4-20).

The head tilt was a clue with a question: could her present condition be a decompensated *congenital* CN IV palsy presenting in adult life with the onset of presbyopia? If this were the case, the congenital nature of the lesion would be confirmed by evidence of chronicity; that is, overaction of the ipsilateral inferior oblique muscle and a large vertical fusional amplitude (the ability to fuse vertically separated images in spite of increasing strengths of vertical prism placed over the affected eye).

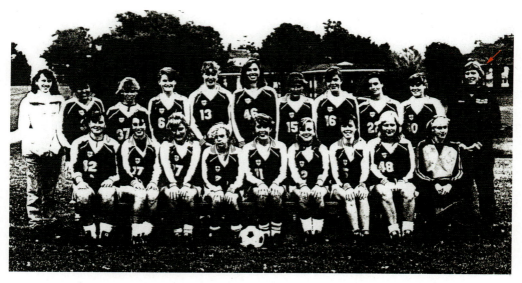

FIGURE 4-20 A soccer team photograph taken 14 years before the onset of vertical diplopia. The patient is standing in the second row on the right (*arrow*). Her head tilts to the right.

In patients with an acquired fourth-nerve palsy, this ability is absent and they must, as in this case, use prism glasses to correct their double vision.

Cautionary note: This patient tilted her head to the right, *ipsilateral* to the right CN IV palsy, which increased the separation of the images and allowed one image to be suppressed.

Diagnosis: Post-Traumatic Fourth-Nerve Palsy

Treatment

- Strabismus surgery
- Botulinum toxin injection
- Prism glasses

Trauma is one of the most common causes of acquired CN IV palsies.[48–51] Strabismus surgery is elected by some patients because of increasing double vision or an inability to carry on normal activities (e.g., in the case of a dentist). However, the initial impact of an acute superior oblique palsy on an active patient's life can also be relieved by a single injection of botulinum toxin type A (Botox) into the ipsilateral inferior oblique muscle.

The patient declined strabismus surgery and elected to wear prism glasses. Botox therapy was not available at the time.

Worth noting: this case of a post-traumatic long-standing CN IV palsy is really a blueprint for clinically evaluating vertical diplopia and hypertropia. The cost implications of getting the diagnosis right are significant.

SELECTED REFERENCES

1. Liu GT, Volpe NJ, Galetta SL, eds. *Neuro-ophthalmology: Diagnosis and Management.* 2nd ed. Philadelphia: Saunders/Elsevier; 2010.
2. Blumenfeld H. *Neuroanatomy through clinical cases.* 2nd ed. Sunderland, MA: Sinauer Associates; 2010.
3. Sharpe JA. Analysis of diplopia. *Med Clin N Am.* 1986;35:5002–5026.
4. Leigh RJ, Zee DS. *The Neurology of Eye Movements.* 4th ed. New York: Oxford University Press; 2006.
5. Danchaivijitr C, Kennard C. Diplopia and eye movement disorders. *J Neurol Neurosurg Psychiat.*2004;75(suppl IV):iv24–iv31.
6. Brazis PW, Lee AG. Acquired binocular horizontal diplopia. *Mayo Clin Proc.* 1999; 74(9):907–916.
7. Zwergal A, Cnyrim C, Arbusow V, Glaser M, Fesl G, Brandt T, Strupp M. Unilateral INO is associated with ocular tilt reaction in pontomesencephalic lesions: INO plus. *Neurology.* 2008;71(8):590–593.
8. Brazis PW, Lee AG. Binocular vertical diplopia. *Mayo Clin Proc.* 1998;73(1):55–66.
9. Leigh RJ, Zee DS. With permission 2013.
10. Donahue SP, Lavin PJ, Hamed LM. Tonic ocular tilt reaction simulating a superior oblique palsy: Diagnostic confusion with the 3-step test. *Arch Ophthalmol.* 1999; 117:347–352.
11. Keane JR. Ocular skew deviation: analysis of 100 cases. *Arch Neurol.* 1975;32:185–190.
12. Brandt T, Dieterich M. Skew deviation with ocular torsion: a vestibular brainstem sign of topographic diagnostic value. *Ann Neurol.* 1993;33:528–534.

13. Brodsky MC, Donahue SP, Vaphiades M, Brandt T. Skew deviation revisited. *Surv Ophthalmol.* 2006;*51*:105–128.

14. Wong AMF, Sharpe JA. Cerebellar skew deviation and the torsional vestibulo-ocular reflex. *Neurology.* 2005;*65*:412–419.

15. Westheimer G, Blair SM. The ocular tilt reaction—a brainstem oculomotor routine. *Invest Ophthalmol.* 1975;*14*:833–839.

16. Dieterich M, Brandt T. Ocular torsion and tilt of subjective visual vertical are sensitive brainstem signs. *Ann Neurol.* 1993;*33*:292–299.

17. Collewijn H, Van der Steen J, Ferman L, Jansen TC. Human ocular counterroll: assessment of static and dynamic properties from electromagnetic scleral coil recordings. *Exp Brain Res.* 1985;*59*:185–196.

18. Hamasaki I, Hasebe S, Ohtsuki H. Static ocular counterroll: video-based analysis after minimizing the false-torsion factors. *Jpn J Ophthalmol.* 2005;*49*:497–504.

19. Goltz HC, Mirabella G, Leung JC, Blakeman AW, Colpa L, Abuhaleeqa K, Wong AMF. Effects of age, viewing distance and target complexity on static ocular counterroll. *Vision Res.* 2009;*49*(14):1848–1852.

20. Parulekar MV, Dai S, Buncic JR, Wong AMF. Head position-dependent changes in ocular torsion and vertical misalignment in skew deviation. *Arch Ophthalmol.* 2008;*126*(7):899–905.

21. Wong AMF. Understanding skew deviation and a new clinical test to differentiate it from trochlear nerve palsy. *J AAPOS.* 2010;*14*:61–67.

22. Wong AMF, Colpa L, Chandrakumar M. Ability of an upright-supine test to differentiate skew deviation from other vertical strabismus causes. *Arch Ophthalmol.* 2011;*129*(12):1570–1575.

23. Parks MM. Isolated cyclovertical muscle palsy. *Arch Ophthalmol.* 1958;*60*:1027–1035.

24. Kheradmand A, Bronstein A, Zee DS. Clinical bedside examination. Chapter 12. In: Bronstein A, ed. *Oxford Textbook of Vertigo and Imbalance.* New York: Oxford University Press, 2013.

25. Lessell S, Lessell I, Rizzo JF. Ocular neuromyotonia after radiation therapy. *Am J Ophthalmol.* 1986;*102*:766–770.

26. Purvin VA. Ocular motor complications of radiation therapy. *North America Neuro-ophthalmology Society Annual Meeting Syllabus.*2010;317–323.

27. Shults WT, Hoyt WF, Behrens M, MacLean J, Saul RF, Corbett JJ. Ocular neuromyotonia: a clinical description of six patients. *Arch Ophthalmol.* 1986;*104*:1028–1034.

28. Tilikete C, Vial C, Niederlaender M, Bonnier PL, Vighetto A. Idiopathic ocular neuromyotonia: a neurovascular compression syndrome? *J Neurol Neurosurg Psychiat.* 2000;*69*:642–644.

29. Frohman EM, Zee DS. Ocular neuromyotonia: clinical features, physiological mechanisms, and response to therapy. *Ann Neurol.* 1995;*37*:620–626.

30. Bender M. Polyopia and monocular diplopia of cerebral origin. *Arch Neurol.* 1945;*54*:323–338.

31. Lopez JR, Adomato BT, Hoyt WF. "Entomopia": a remarkable case of cerebral olyopia. *Neurology.* 1993;*43*:2145–2146.

32. Bender MB, Feldman M, Sobin AJ. Palinopsia. *Brain.* 1968;*91*:321–328.

33. Meadows JUC, Munro SSF. Palinopsia. *J Neurol Neurosurg Psychiat.* 1977;*40*:5–8.

34. Michel EM, Troost BT. Palinopsia: cerebral localization with computed tomography. *Neurology.* 1980;*30*:887–889.

35. Kawasaki A, Purvin V. Persistent palinopsia following ingestion of lysergic acid diethylamide (LSD). *Arch Ophthalmol.* 1996;*114*:47–50.

36. Hughes MS, Lessell S. Trazodone-induced palinopsia. *Arch Ophthalmol.* 1990;*108*:399–400.

37. Pomeranz HD, Lessell S. Palinopsia and polyopia in the absence of drugs or cerebral disease. *Neurology.* 2000;*54*:855–859.

38. Choi R, Kushner BJ. The accuracy of experienced strabismologists using the Hirschberg and Krimsky tests. *Ophthalmology.* 1998;*105*:1301–1306.

39. Miller NR, Newman NJ, Biousse V, Kerrison JB, eds. *Walsh & Hoyt's Clinical Neuro-Ophthalmology THE ESSENTIALS.* 2nd ed. Philadelphia: Lippincott, Williams & Wilkins; 2008. Section 111;Ch 16:331–343.

40. Wong AMF. *Eye Movement Disorders.* New York: Oxford University Press; 2008.

41. Bardram MT. Oculomotor pareses and nonparetic diplopia in pituitary adenomata. *Acta Ophthalmol (Copenhagen).* 1949;*27*(2):225–258.

42. Kirkham TH. The ocular symptomatology of pituitary tumours. *Proc R Soc Med.* 1972;*65*:517–518.

43. Nachtigaller H, Hoyt WF. Visual perception disorders in bi-temporal hemianopsia and displacement of the visual axes. *Klinische Monatsblatter fur Augenheilkunde.* 1970;156:821–836.

44. Borchert MS, Lessell S, Hoyt WF. Hemifield slide diplopia from altitudinal visual field defects. *J Neuro-ophthalmol.* 1996;16:107–109.

45. Gradenigo G. Ueber Die Paralyse Des Nervus Abducens Bei Otitis. *Arch Ohrenheilkunde.* 1907;74:149–187.

46. Sherman SC, Buchanan A. Gradenigo Syndrome: A case report and review of a rare complication of otitis media. *J Emerg Med.* 2004;27:253–256.

47. Damrose EJ, Petrus LV, Ishiyama A. Radiology forum: quiz case 2. Diagnosis: petrous apicitis with secondary abducens nerve palsy. *Arch Otolaryngol Head Neck Surg.* 2001;127:715–717.

48. Rush JA, Younger BR, Paralysis of cranial nerves III, IV, and VI. *Arch Ophthalmol.* 1981;99:76–79.

49. von Noorden GK, Murray E, Wong SY. Superior oblique paralysis: a review of 270 cases. *Arch Ophthalmol.* 1986;104:1771–1776.

50. Mansour AM, Reinecke RD. Central trochlear palsy. *Surv Ophthalmol.* 1986;30:279–297.

51. Keane JR. Fourth nerve palsy: historical review and study of 215 inpatients. *Neurology.* 1993;43:2439–2443.

| 5 |
CRANIAL NERVES THREE, FOUR, SIX, AND THEIR SYNDROMES

THE OCULOMOTOR NERVE

Cranial nerve three (CN III) is the oculomotor nerve. It innervates the extraocular muscles; the superior, inferior, and medial rectus (MR) muscles; both levator palpebrae superioris muscles; and the pupillary constrictor muscle and ciliary body. By any measure, it is an important nerve, and, when damaged or injured, the consequences are invariably serious.

The Oculomotor Nucleus Complex

The oculomotor nucleus complex lies in the midbrain at the level of the superior colliculus and red nucleus (Figure 5-1). It extends rostrocaudally close to the midline for about 8 mm, ventral and dorsal to the Sylvian aqueduct, separated by the periaqueductal gray, and dorsal to the two medial longitudinal fascicule. The nucleus consists of four lateral paired subnuclei which innervate the superior, inferior, and MR muscles, as well as the inferior oblique muscles.[1]

A single midline subnucleus, the central caudal nucleus (CCN), innervates both levator palpebrae superioris muscles. It is important to note that the superior rectus subnuclei allow axons from one superior rectus subnucleus to cross within the nucleus and pass through the contralateral superior rectus subnucleus (without synapse) to innervate the contralateral superior rectus muscle.[2,3]

The MR motor neuron subgroups lie in three distinct clusters of subnuclei—areas A, B, and C (Figure 5-2). The A-group extends into the medial longitudinal fasciculi (MLF).[4,5]

The difference in function of the A, B, and C subgroups is still unclear. The C group is known to project to nontwitch fibers in the medial and inferior rectus muscles, and neurons from midline area S project to nontwitch fibers in the inferior oblique and superior rectus muscle. These fibers

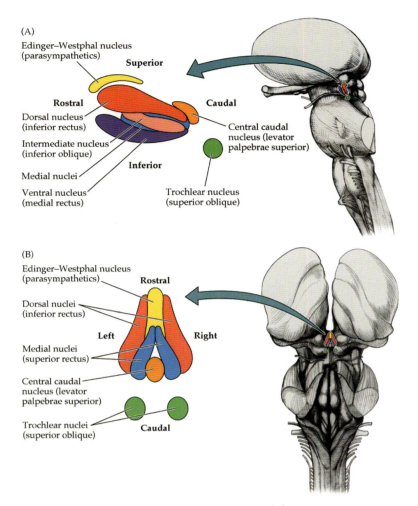

(A)

Edinger–Westphal nucleus (parasympathetics)

Superior

Rostral

Caudal

Dorsal nucleus (inferior rectus)

Central caudal nucleus (levator palpebrae superior)

Intermediate nucleus (inferior oblique)

Medial nuclei

Inferior

Ventral nucleus (medial rectus)

Trochlear nucleus (superior oblique)

(B)

Edinger–Westphal nucleus (parasympathetics)

Rostral

Dorsal nuclei (inferior rectus)

Left

Right

Medial nuclei (superior rectus)

Central caudal nucleus (levator palpebrae superior)

Trochlear nuclei (superior oblique)

Caudal

FIGURE 5-1 The oculomotor nucleus complex. (A) Left lateral view. (B) Dorsal view. The trochlear nuclei are also shown.

Reproduced with permission.[3]

are thought to be particularly capable of the sustained contraction needed for convergence and gaze holding. Neurons from areas A, B, and C all receive inputs from the contralateral abducens nucleus via the MLF.

The parasympathetic nuclei that lie in the Edinger-Westphal nucleus (EWN) (shown in yellow in Figure 5-1A–B) form a V-shape as they curve over the dorsal rostral aspect of the nucleus and connect across the midline. These nuclei supply preganglionic parasympathetic innervation to the ciliary ganglion, and they control pupillary constriction and accommodation. Bilateral dilated pupils unreactive to light and near can be expected with lesions affecting the EWN.

OCULOMOTOR NUCLEUS

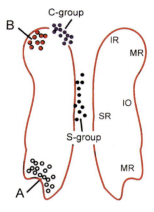

FIGURE 5-2 Schema of the anatomy of the three groups of medial rectus motoneurons, A, B, and C identified by injecting isotope into the medial rectus muscle. IR, inferior rectus; MR, medial rectus; SR, superior rectus; IO, inferior oblique.

Reproduced with permission.[5]

■ **Clinical Points to Remember About Lesions of the Oculomotor Nucleus Complex**

- A unilateral lesion of the oculomotor nucleus complex can affect all or nearly all of the ocular muscles, causing bilateral signs:
  - Bilateral asymmetrical ptosis
  - Ipsilateral cranial nerve (CN) III palsy with contralateral superior rectus palsy
  - Ipsilateral internal ophthalmoplegia[6]
- A lesion selectively affecting the CCN innervating the levator muscles causes bilateral ptosis only—the eye movements are relatively spared.[7,8]
- A lesion selectively sparing the CCN causes bilateral CN III palsy with or without internal ophthalmoplegia.[9]

This case presented with bilateral ptosis.

CASE 5-1 Bilateral Ptosis: Nuclear Oculomotor Nerve Palsy

Video Display

The patient is a 52-year-old man with hypertension and hyperlipidemia who awoke one morning unable to open his eyes (Figure 5-3). When he tried to walk, he had to tilt his head backward and look down. He was admitted as an emergency to the Massachusetts General Hospital.

CASE 5-1 SYMPTOMS

Symptoms	Location Correlation
Bilateral ptosis	Levator palpebrae superioris
	CN III central caudal nucleus

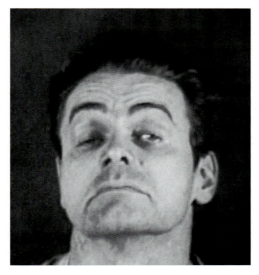

FIGURE 5-3 Fifty-two-year-old man with bilateral ptosis and exotropia of the left eye. Note his backward head tilt.

Examination in the ER

Neuro-ophthalmological

- BP 210/92, pulse regular
- Head tilt backward
- Bilateral asymmetrical ptosis, greater in the right eye (OD)
- Overaction of the frontalis muscles
- Pupils equal, constricting equally briskly to light and near

Ocular Motility of the Left Eye (OS)

- Exotropia (unopposed action of the lateral rectus)
- Paralysis of all extraocular muscles innervated by CN III
- Convergence absent
- Cranial nerves four (CN IV), five (CN V), and six (CN VI) normal

Ocular Motility of the Right Eye (OD)

- Central in primary gaze
- Paresis of superior rectus muscle (paresis of elevation)
- All the other extraocular muscles innervated by CN III normal
- Cranial nerves four (CN IV), five (CN V), and six (CN VI) normal

The neurological examination was normal.

Localization and Differential Diagnosis

The differential diagnosis of apoplectic bilateral ptosis is:

- Midbrain infarction or hemorrhage.
- Metastatic disease.

Bilateral asymmetrical ptosis, unilateral oculomotor nerve (CN III) palsy OS, and contralateral paresis of the superior rectus muscle OD are diagnostic of a left oculomotor nuclear palsy sparing the pupils. The etiology of a focal midbrain lesion in a patient with severe hypertension is likely to be an infarction.

What Diagnostic Tests Should Follow?

- Brain magnetic resonance imaging (MRI) with attention to the midbrain.
- Holter monitor to rule out atrial fibrillation.

Test Results

A computed tomogram (CT) of the brain was normal (MRI was not available). Readings from the Holter monitor were also normal.

Diagnosis: Left Oculomotor Nuclear Palsy

A diagnosis of midbrain infarction was made.

Treatment

Medication to treat hypertension and hyperlipidemia was prescribed. The patient was followed by his primary care doctor. He fully recovered in 10 weeks.

Special Explanatory Note

The EWN and parasympathetic pupillary fibers were spared in this case, consistent with infarction of the caudal segment of the oculomotor nucleus complex affecting the motor neurons for the levator palpebrae superioris in the CCN.

A similar case came to autopsy in 1974. The patient was a 72-year-old hypertensive woman who presented with bilateral ptosis and a right (ipsilateral) partial CN III palsy, which fully recovered. She died of a myocardial infarct 3 years later. The sole abnormality in the brainstem at autopsy was a triangular-shaped cavitary infarct, principally involving the right side of the midbrain tegmentum, with the apex extending across the midline just ventral to the cerebral aqueduct (Figure 5-4). The rostrocaudal extent of the lesion measured only 3 mm. The location of the midline infarct coincided precisely with the caudal end of the third-nerve nuclear complex in the area of the CCN. thus affecting the excitatory burst neurons that activate the levator palpebrae superioris muscle in both eyes.[10]

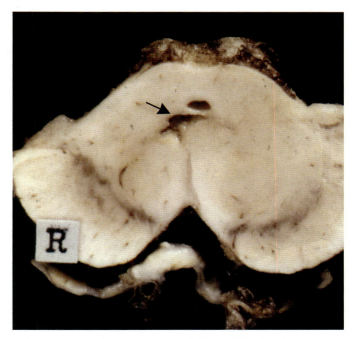

FIGURE 5-4 Gross appearance of the midbrain shows a triangular-shaped cavitary infarct (*arrow*) in the right tegmentum with the apex extending across the midline ventral to the cerebral aqueduct.

Reproduced with permission.[10]

There have since been numerous single case reports with clinicopathological and/or neuroimaging correlation of focal vascular or mass lesions affecting selected regions of the oculomotor nucleus.[11] Table 5-1 provides a modified list of Daroff's clinical rules to allow precise localization of signs of oculomotor nuclear lesions.[12,13]

The Oculomotor Fasciculus

The fascicular portion of the third nerve consists of axons from all the subnuclei of the extraocular muscles, and from the EWN and the CCN. After leaving the nucleus, the fascicles sweep ventrally and laterally and diverge widely to pass through the MLF, the tegmentum, the red nucleus, and the substantia nigra, and then converge to exit the brainstem medial to the cerebral peduncles. To illustrate this, Castro et al.[14] proposed a two-dimensional model in which the fibers for the inferior oblique (IO), superior rectus (SR), MR, levator palpebrae (LP) and inferior rectus (IR) muscles lie in the tegmentum from lateral to medial (Figure 5-5).

The span of the divergent axons (approximately 3 mm in the sagittal plane and 6 mm in the actual transverse plane) is wide enough to explain selective involvement of individual axons in isolated extraocular muscle palsies.[15–17]

TABLE 5-1: Signs Identifying Oculomotor Nuclear Lesions

Nuclear Lesions

Unilateral third-nerve palsy with contralateral superior rectus paresis and bilateral partial ptosis

Bilateral third-nerve palsy with spared levator function and presence or absence of internal ophthalmoplegia

Possible Nuclear Lesions

Bilateral total third-nerve palsy

Bilateral ptosis

An isolated weakness of a single muscle (inferior rectus, inferior oblique) but not the levator, superior rectus, or medial rectus muscle

Unlikely Nuclear Lesions

Unilateral third-nerve palsy, with or without internal ophthalmoplegia, accompanied by normal contralateral superior rectus function

Unilateral internal ophthalmoplegia

Unilateral ptosis

Isolated unilateral or bilateral medial rectus weakness

Reproduced with permission.[13]

This model adds further clarity to the brain MRI of a 26-year-old woman recently hospitalized with multiple strokes causing a left hemiplegia and a right CN III fascicular lesion characterized by partial ptosis and paresis of the superior rectus muscle. Brain MRI showed a small infarct in the right ventral midbrain tegmentum affecting CN III fascicles, a left parieto-occipital infarct, and multiple other small infarctions (Figure 5-6A–B). The infarcts were attributed to vasculitis due to the use of ecstasy (3,4-methylene-dioxy-N-methylamphetamine).[18]

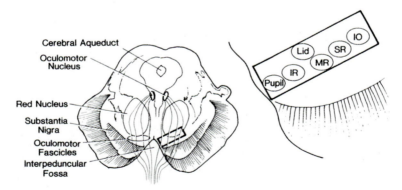

FIGURE 5-5 Schematic diagram of the midbrain at the level of the superior colliculus. The oculomotor fascicular fiber course is adopted from histologic sections. The proposed model of the oculomotor fascicular organization in the ventral midbrain tegmentum from lateral to medial is as follows: inferior oblique (IO), fascicles; superior rectus (SR) fascicles; medial rectus (MR) fascicles; levator palpebrae (lid) fascicles; inferior rectus (IR) fascicles; and most medially, the pupillary fibers.

Reproduced with permission.[14]

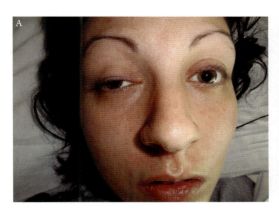
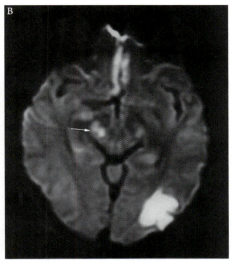

FIGURE 5-6 (A) Patient with partial right ptosis and paresis of the superior rectus muscle. (B) Magnetic resonance imaging, axial DWI through the level of the midbrain, shows infarcts in the right cerebral peduncle (*arrow*) affecting the oculomotor fascicles, left parieto-occipital lobe, and multiple other infarctions.

■ **Clinical Points to Remember About Lesions of the Oculomotor Fasciculus**

- A lesion affecting all the fascicles causes an isolated CN III palsy with or without involvement of the pupil.[19]
- Infarction involving the lateral portion of the fasciculus can cause isolated monocular elevation paresis, suggesting that the fibers intended to innervate the SR and IO, the elevator muscles of the eye are in the lateral portion.[20,21]
- Lesions of the oculomotor fascicles can mimic an isolated peripheral oculomotor nerve palsy affecting the superior or inferior division of CN III.
- Fascicular lesions (like nuclear lesions) may be ischemic, hemorrhagic, compressive, infiltrative, traumatic, and, in rare cases, inflammatory.[22]   ■

The neurologic signs in oculomotor fascicular syndromes have been recognized for more than a century, and they permit precise topographical lesion localization:

- *Weber's syndrome* is an ipsilateral CN III palsy with contralateral hemiplegia due to a lesion of the cerebral peduncle.[22]
- *Nothnagel's syndrome* is an ipsilateral CN III palsy with ipsilateral cerebellar ataxia due to a lesion in the area of the superior cerebellar peduncle.
- *Benedikt's syndrome,* which was first described and named by Charcot in 1893, is an ipsilateral CN III palsy with contralateral hemitremor (or chorea) due to a more extensive lesion affecting the cerebral peduncle, adjacent red nucleus, and substantia nigra.

Claude's syndrome is an ipsilateral CN III palsy with contralateral cerebellar ataxia due to simultaneous involvement of the cerebellar efferent fibers to the thalamus (the dentatorubrothalamic pathway from the superior cerebellar peduncle).[23,24] Claude published his "Syndrome pédunculaire de la région du noyau rouge" in 1912.[25,26]

The Oculomotor Nerve

The oculomotor nerve (CN III) exits the brainstem ventrally and emerges from a sulcus on the medial aspect of the cerebral peduncle and passes forwards and laterally to skirt the lateral margin of the posterior clinoid process. The nerve then courses along the roof of the cavernous sinus before entering the lateral wall. Between the brain stem and the posterior clinoid process the nerve crosses the subarachnoid space in the interval bounded by the margin of the tentorial notch laterally, the dorsum sellae anteriorly, and the brain stem posteriorly. This interval is called the tentorial gap.

As the nerve crosses the tentorial gap it has certain important vascular and cerebral relations. Superior relations are the posterior communicating and posterior cerebral arteries. The superior cerebrebellar artery runs beneath the nerve as it travels laterally to pass beneath the tentorium. It should be emphasised that a portion of the uncal region of the temporal lobe is, in the majority of cases, a normal content of the tentorial gap and a customary superior relation of the third nerve.

Within the cavernous sinus, the nerve runs along the lateral wall together with the trochlear nerve (CN IV), and the ophthalmic (VI) and maxillary (V2) divisions of the trigeminal nerve (CN V). As CN III leaves the cavernous sinus, it divides into a superior and an inferior division, which pass through the superior orbital fissure (SOF) to enter the orbit within the annulus of Zinn.

Acquired syndromes of the oculomotor nerve are common. They are caused by nearly every pathological process affecting the CNS. A complete third-nerve lesion will paralyze all of the extraocular muscles, leaving intact only the LR (innervated by the abducens nerve [CN VI]) and the SO muscle (innervated by the trochlear nerve [CN IV]). Complete ptosis results from paralysis of the levator (Figure 5-7A) and because of the unopposed action of the LR muscle the eye rests in a down-and-out (exotropic) position (Figure 5-7B). Because of the unopposed action of the LR muscle, the eye comes to lie in a down-and-out (exotropic) position at rest (Figure 5-7B). When assessing SO function in patients with an oculomotor nerve palsy, the ability of the SO to intort the eye is particularly important. In such cases, the absence of intorsion when the patient attempts to depress the eye while it is abducted indicates lack of SO function as well.

A CN III palsy with headache is an emergency, as seen in Case 5-2 presented here.

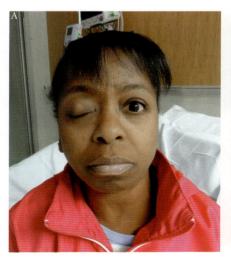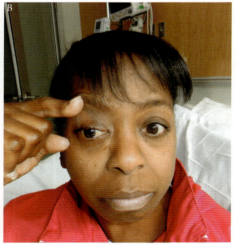

FIGURE 5-7 Complete right oculomotor nerve palsy. (A) Unilateral ptosis. (B) The eye is down and out—exotropia—and the pupil dilated and fixed.

CASE 5-2 Oculomotor Nerve Palsy: Syphilitic Meningitis

No Video Display

The patient is a 50-year-old man with type 2 diabetes who presented in September 1996. Five months prior to admission (PTA), he had flu-like symptoms with mild fever, frequent chills, drenching night sweats, sinus congestion, and diffuse myalgia in the chest, abdomen, legs, and the soles of the feet which resolved over 2 weeks. He lost 20 pounds in weight over 3 months. His physician diagnosed a viral syndrome.

Three days PTA, he woke with ptosis of the right eye, and, when he held the eyelid up, he had double vision, worse on gaze left. He also experienced decreased auditory acuity, right ear worse than left, and gait instability due to impaired balance. He tended to lean to one side or the other.

He was admitted to a local hospital. He denied vertigo, tinnitus, and ear ache. He had begun to experience difficulties with short-term memory and word-finding. For several weeks, he had also suffered from a dull bifrontal throbbing headache that intensified 3 days PTA. The headache woke him from sleep. He denied photophobia, phonophobia, or stiff neck. A brain scan was normal. A lumbar puncture was attempted unsuccessfully. He was transferred to the Massachusetts General Hospital.

Past history was negative for trauma, previous ptosis, diplopia, and drug or alcohol abuse. He worked as a consultant and traveled frequently in the United States but not abroad. He walked his dog in the woods in the summer.

Analysis of the History

· What are the major presenting symptoms?
· Where are the CNS lesion(s) likely to be?

CASE 5-2 SYMPTOMS

Symptoms	Location Correlation
Febrile Headache	Intracranial
Ptosis and double vision	Oculomotor nerve (CN III)
Decreased hearing	Auditory nerve (CN VIII)

The analysis guides the clinical examination.

Examination

Neurological

- Temperature 100.3°F, pulse regular, BP 150/80
- No neck stiffness, lymphadenopathy, or skin rash
- Oriented ×3, impaired short-term memory, 0/3 at 3 minutes
- Speech—mild word finding difficulty
- Complete right (OD) third-nerve palsy sparing the pupil
- Cranial nerves IV, V, VI normal
- Cranial nerve VIII bilateral deafness
- Right pronator drift and slowness of dexterous hand/finger movements
- Reflexes 2+ bilaterally, plantar responses equivocal
- No finger/nose or heel/shin ataxia
- Gait ataxia, unable to tandem walk
- Sensory system normal

Localization and Differential Diagnosis

An inflammatory/infectious meningeal process is the major consideration in a patient with fever, headache, and a CN III palsy. The differential diagnosis includes aseptic (i.e., bacterial cultures negative) meningitis due to viral disease and bacterial meningitis including Lyme disease (*Borrelia burgdorferi*).

What Diagnostic Tests Should Follow?

- Blood culture ×3
- AIDS/HIV tests
- Spinal tap/examination and culture of the cerebrospinal fluid (CSF)
- Audiogram

Special Explanatory Note

Acquired immunodeficiency syndrome (AIDS) is a viral disease associated with a retrovirus, human immunodeficiency virus (HIV). HIV infection is characterized by an acquired depression of all cell-mediated immunity, manifested by CD4+/CD8+ lymphocytosis as a result of reduction in CD4+ cells. The failure of immune function explains the development of a wide range of opportunistic infections and unusual neoplasms. All organ systems and the CNS are vulnerable, with the CNS susceptible not only to disease due to immunosuppression but to the AIDS virus infection per se.[27]

Test Results

Blood cultures ×3 negative

- HIV antibody nonreactive
- Serum immunoglobulin (Ig)G 20, IgA 490 (both elevated), IgM 52

- Fluorescent treponemal antibody absorption (FTA-ABS) test reactive 1 to 120
- CSF increased cells, white blood cells (WBCs) 755/cubic mm, 20% polys, 56% lymphs
- Elevated protein 142 mg/dL (range 40–200 mg/dL)
- Increased gammaglobulin IgA 72.9, IgG 23.2 (both elevated), no banding
- Positive serologic reagin tests—Venereal Disease Research Laboratory (VDRL) slide test reactive at 1 to 2 dilution
- Rapid plasma reagin (RPR) test reactive at 1 to 64 dilution
- Normal glucose content 64 mg/dL
- Cultures and cytology for acute bacterial or chronic fungal meningitis, tuberculosis, Lyme disease, or lymphomatous meningitis were negative
- Audiogram revealed moderate to severe bilateral sensory neural hearing loss

Special Explanatory Note

The serological diagnosis of syphilis depends on the presence of one of two types of antibodies—nonspecific or nontreponemal (reagin) antibodies and specific treponemal antibodies. The common test for reagin is the VDRL slide test. If the VDRL is positive in the CSF, it is diagnostic of neurosyphilis. Serum reactivity alone demonstrates exposure to the organism in the past but does not identify the presence of neurosyphilis. The FTA–ABS test for antibodies directed specifically against treponemal antigens is the test in common use. This patient is seropositive for syphilis and confirmed for CNS neurosyphilis (the VDRL test was positive in the CSF).

What Neuroimaging Studies Should Follow?

- Brain MRI
- Magnetic resonance angiography (MRA)

Brain MRI was normal. The brain MRA showed irregularity of the horizontal (A1) segment of the anterior cerebral artery involving the origin of the recurrent artery of Heubner, which appeared occluded. There was slight beading of the basilar artery and the posterior cerebral arteries, right more than left.

Diagnosis: Meningeal and Meningovascular Syphilis, Oculomotor Nerve Palsy Sparing the Pupil and Bilateral Sensory Neural Deafness

Treatment

The patient was treated with crystalline penicillin G intravenously 4 million units q4h for 14 days. The third-nerve palsy completely recovered in 2 months. The patient returned to his normal baseline and energy level. He was left with slight impairment of short-term memory and bilateral deafness.

The thought sequence in this patient's diagnostic workup was important. The comparative rarity of fever with third-nerve involvement and headache and the potential for infection associated with frequent travel were a combination of interest. The febrile CN III palsy suggested the serology and CSF studies, which led to the diagnosis and treatment of neurosyphilis—a now uncommon disease and easily overlooked.

SYNDROMES OF THE SUBARACHNOID SPACE

Isolated involvement of CN III in the subarachnoid space posterior to the cavernous sinus can be located anywhere between the ventral surface of the midbrain, where the nerve exits, and the posterior clinoid process, where the nerve enters the cavernous sinus. The paresis may be total (complete) or partial. A total CN III palsy is characterized by ptosis, paralysis of all the extraocular muscles innervated by the third nerve, a dilated nonreactive pupil (iridoplegia), and paralysis of accommodation (cycloplegia). Partial (incomplete) CN III palsies may spare the pupil or have partial motility defects. The terms "total" and "partial" refer only to the extent to which the eyelid and the individual CN III innervated extraocular muscles are involved.

Uncal Herniation

Transtentorial herniation of the uncus (the undersurface of the temporal lobe) forced downwards into the tentorial gap and through the tentorial notch due to raised intracranial pressure leads to compression of the oculomotor nerve (CN III) stupor, coma and death. Acute compression of the pupillo-constrictor fibres in the upper sector of the third nerve[28] is particularly marked on the ipsilateral side of the lesion and the first indication that impaired consciousness is due to uncal herniation is given by the pupil. The pupillary changes develop in the following order: First, the pupil on the affected side constricts: this phase is very brief. Thus, unless the patient is examined in the early stages and at very short intervals, the constriction phase is missed. Secondly, the pupil on the affected side slowly dilates, becomes unresponsive to light and fixed in full dilation (a so-called "blown pupil"). Minutes to several hours (8 to 13) may elapse before full dilation occurs. Third, ultimately, pupil changes begin to appear in the contralateral pupil sometimes before the terminal stage is reached on the ipsilateral side. There is an initial constriction which may persist for several minutes (10 to 55) followed by dilation so that several hours after the onset of uncal herniation both pupils are fully dilated and fixed[29] (In rare cases of uncal herniation, the opposite pupil may be the first to dilate[30] but its initial enlargement may also be a false localizing sign in intraparenchymal frontal hemorrhage).[31] With further progression, paresis of the extraocular muscles and a complete CN III palsy and ipsilateral hemiplegia develop (Kernohan's notch syndrome).[32] With still further progression, loss of corneal reflexes, posturing, and respiratory arrest occur.

A *cautionary clinical note:* neurologists sometimes use the acronym "PERRLA" in the chart to document that "pupils are equal, round, and reactive to light and accommodation." Acronyms are easier to write if one is in a rush, but they often fail to reflect exactly what was tested.[33] A more descriptive sentence is preferable: for example, "pupils: equal and equally brisk constricting to light. Near response could not be tested due to the patient's obtunded state." Transient fluctuation in pupillary diameter is normal and is termed *hippus.* A useful scale for pupil reactivity is: 3+ normal brisk reaction; 2+ slightly sluggish; and 1+ sluggish.

Aneurysmal Compression of the Oculomotor Nerve

With pupil involvement (dilated pupil sluggish to ligh and near or fixed dilated pupil)

- *A painful oculomotor nerve palsy involving the pupil is due to compression by an intracranial aneurysm until proved otherwise.* These patients require urgent admission.
- A common location for an aneurysm is at the junction of the internal carotid artery (ICA) and the posterior communicating artery (PoCA). More than 90% of these patients show symptoms of a CN III palsy prior to rupture and subarachnoid hemorrhage,[34] but sudden severe pain in or around the eye, which may be due to hemorrhage enlarging the aneurysmal sac to which the CN III nerve is attached, is often the presenting symptom, and pain may occur several hours before signs of CN III palsy appear. Aneurysmal compression often involves the pupil well in advance of complete CN III palsy.

With pupil sparing:

- Pupil sparing can occur with aneurysmal compression of CN III.[35] In one retrospective study of 84 patients with posterior communicating aneurysms, seven initially had normal pupils (representing 8% of the total and 14% of those with CN III palsies).[36] In four of the seven patients, pupil involvement developed within 5 days, and in one patient pupil involvement developed in 4 months.
- This suggests that pupil sparing may occur more often than previously thought in patients with posterior communicating aneurysms with CN III involvement.

Oculomotor syndromes due to compression by an aneurysm are:

- Painful CN III palsy involving the pupil
- Painful CN III palsy sparing the pupil
- Progressive CN III palsy sparing the pupil
- Isolated ptosis[37]
- Ptosis and mydriasis[38]
- Pupillary light-near dissociation[39]
- Transient CN III palsy[40,41]
- Pupil sparing CN III palsy with aberrant regeneration[42]
- Dorsal midbrain syndrome (from giant basilar aneurysm in the posterior fossa)[43]

Patients with painful CN III palsies should be closely observed for at least a week for the development of pupil involvement and/or studied noninvasively with MRA or CT angiography (CTA), the neuroimaging studies of choice for painful CN III palsy with and without sparing of the pupils. *When headache is an associated symptom, a spinal tap to rule out subarachnoid hemorrhage is mandatory.* Depending on the results of noninvasive neuroimaging, a conventional three-vessel angiogram may be appropriate in patients with pupil involvement. Posterior communicating artery aneurysms tend to project posterolaterally to compress CN III as it travels toward the cavernous sinus. Conventional angiography in a young woman with a painful CN III palsy involving the pupil illustrates this; see Figure 5-8A–C.

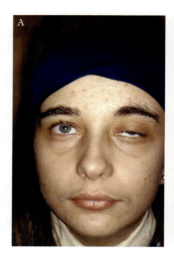
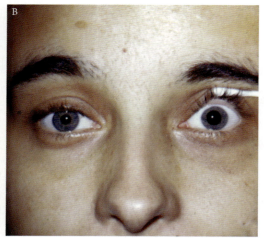

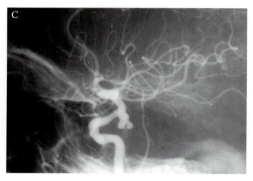

FIGURE 5-8 (A) Twenty-six-year-old woman with partial ptosis of the left eye due to a painful CN III palsy involving the pupil. (B) The pupil is dilated and fixed. (C) Left internal carotid arteriogram shows a lobulated aneurysm at the junction of the internal carotid and posterior communicating artery.

The aneurysm was successfully surgically clipped. Clipping versus interventional coil embolization are equally effective.[44] Advanced age, diabetes, delayed interventions, and complete CN III palsy at presentation are indicators of a poor prognosis for recovery.

Microinfarction with Pupil Sparing

Microinfarction is the most frequent cause of a pupil-sparing oculomotor nerve palsy.[45] In most instances, the patient has diabetes mellitus or hypertension, atherosclerosis, and hyperlipidemia.[46] Typically, severe eye pain or retro-orbital pain precedes the onset of ptosis and diplopia by 1–4 days and usually stops when paralysis of the third nerve is complete.

There is general agreement that a normal pupil in most cases excludes an aneurysm as the cause of a CN III palsy; however, the diagnostic approach in cases with pupil sparing is unsettled,[47] and the best approach to diagnosing an isolated painful oculomotor palsy is to obtain noninvasive angiography (MRA or CTA) in all patients with or without pupil sparing.

The case presented here reflects this approach.

CASE 5-3 Diabetic Oculomotor Nerve Palsy: Sparing The Pupil

Video Display

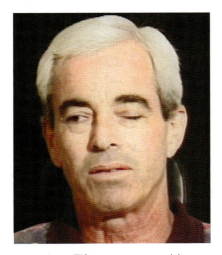

FIGURE 5-9 Fifty-seven-year-old diabetic man with a left third-nerve palsy sparing the pupil.

The patient is a 57-year-old man who carried a diagnosis of atrial fibrillation, coronary artery disease post coronary artery bypass graft, and diabetes mellitus (Figure 5-9).

Four days PTA, he developed bifrontal headache and retro-orbital eye pain accompanied by double vision looking down. He reported that the double vision involved "diagonal images" and was worse on looking to the left. He had no nausea, vomiting, or eye pain.

One day PTA he developed ptosis of the left eye. He was seen in the Massachusetts General Hospital ER and admitted as an emergency. His history was notable for:

- *Coronary artery disease with multivessel coronary artery bypass grafts in 1991.*
- *Diabetes mellitus (insulin controlled).*
- *Hypercholesterolemia.*
- *Atrial fibrillation (he was not on anticoagulation).*
- *Heavy cigarette smoking in the past.*

Analysis of the History

- What are the major presenting symptoms?
- Where are the CNS lesion(s) likely to be?

CASE 5-3 SYMPTOMS

Symptoms	Location Correlation
Headache	
Retro-orbital eye pain	Trigeminal nerve, first division
Diplopia	Oculomotor nerve
Ptosis	Levator palpebrae superioris CN III

The analysis guides the clinical examination.

Examination

Neuro-ophthalmological

- Visual acuity 20/20 OU
- Normal fields and fundus examination
- Pupils equal, reacting equally briskly to light and near

Ocular Motility Signs Confined to the Left Eye (OS)

- Ptosis OS
- Complete CN III palsy OS
- Cranial nerve IV and VI normal
- Corneal reflex normal
- No proptosis or ocular pulsation

Cardiovascular

- Blood pressure 120/70
- Pulse: atrial fibrillation
- Temporal artery pulses normal and nontender
- No carotid or ocular bruits

The neurological examination was normal.

Localization and Differential Diagnosis

The combination of symptoms and signs—atrial fibrillation, coronary artery disease, diabetes mellitus, headache, retro-orbital eye pain, and a progressive CN III palsy over 4 days, sparing the pupil—is consistent with microinfarction of the oculomotor nerve.

The important differential diagnosis of a painful CN III palsy sparing the pupil must, in a patient with headache, include a ruptured intracranial aneurysm and subarachnoid hemorrhage.

Cautionary note: dilation of the pupil with a topical mydriatic (for example, tropicamide ophthalmic solution USP, 1%) in a patient with a painful and/or progressive pupil-sparing. CN III palsy should never be performed The examiner must always be able to serially monitor pupil size and response to light and near because dilation of the pupil (mydriasis) may be delayed for days in aneurysmal compression of the oculomotor nerve.

What Diagnostic Tests Should Follow?

- Hematological tests
- Spinal tap to rule out xanthochromia (yellowish discoloration of the CSF indicative of blood)
- Brain MRI
- Brain MRA or CTA

Test Results

Results of the hematological tests:

- Complete blood count normal
- Blood sugar elevated 180 mg/100 mL
- Erythrocyte sedimentation rate normal
- C-reactive protein and fibrinogen normal
- Blood lipids normal

The CSF analysis showed no xanthochromia, protein 39 mg/mL, and sugar 77 mg/dL; no cells. The brain MRI and MRA were both normal.

On day 2, six days after the onset of symptoms, the patient became pain free. The pupil remained normal.

Diagnosis: Microinfarction of the Oculomotor Nerve

Treatment

Treatment of a patient with a "medical" CN III palsy, consists of controlling all stroke risk factors, hypertension, diabetes, and hyperlipidemia. The CN III palsy recovered completely in 16 weeks. He was referred to a cardiologist for evaluation of atrial fibrillation and Coumadin therapy.

Special Explanatory Note

Pupil sparing in diabetic ophthalmoplegia must never divert attention from the potential severity of the condition. Two autopsy cases of diabetic ophthalmoplegia localized the lesion to the intracavernous segment of CN III, with histological features of an ischemic neuropathy resembling those noted in peripheral ischemic mononeuropathy multiplex associated with diabetes mellitus.[48,49] In these two autopsy cases, a meticulous search for occluded arteries was fruitless but hyalinization of interneural arterioles was apparent. In an additional case, the ischemic lesion localized to the subarachnoid portion of the nerve.[50]

Localization in the intracavernous segment of CN III suggests the possibility of watershed ischemia because the infarct is positioned between the territories of the carotid branches, usually the tentorial branch of the meningohypophyseal trunk in the cavernous sinus, and recurrent collaterals—or twigs—of the posterior cerebral artery, the PoCA, or the basilar artery posteriorly. In all three autopsy cases the central core of the nerve was most severely involved, sparing the peripherally located pupillary fibers and thus explaining the preservation of the pupillary reaction.

■ **Clinical Points to Remember About Microinfarction of CN III with Pupil Sparing**

- An acute CN III ophthalmoplegia may be the initial manifestation of diabetes mellitus.
- Eye pain typically stops when diabetic ophthalmoplegia is complete.
- Persistent eye pain or headache in a pupil-sparing CN III can occur in aneurysmal compression and calls for a CTA to rule out an aneurysm and a spinal tap to rule out a subarachnoid hemorrhage.
- Microinfarction of CN III in a diabetic patient recovers, on average, in 12–16 weeks. ■

Ophthalmoplegic Migraine

Ophthalmoplegic migraine has its onset in childhood, usually in children with a family history of migraine.[51–53] A CN III palsy may occur at the time of headache or as it abates. As a rule, the palsy recovers completely within a month although occasionally it may become permanent. Recurrent painless oculomotor palsies in children are considered a variant of ophthalmoplegic migraine.[54] In some cases, MRI may demonstrate thickening and enhancement of a portion of the cisternal third nerve that can mimic a mass lesion (schwannoma). The differential diagnosis includes ischemia, inflammation, or demyelination.

SYNDROMES OF THE CAVERNOUS SINUS

A complete cavernous sinus syndrome is characterized by involvement of unilateral CN III (with and without pupil involvement), CN IV, and CN VI accompanied by facial sensory loss involving CN V (VI first division and VII) and by a Horner's syndrome due to involvement of the sympathetic nerve supply to the eye. Although headache is not thought to be a symptom of a cavernous sinus syndrome, pituitary apoplexy is a memorable and important exception to this traditional rule.

Pituitary Apoplexy

Pituitary apoplexy causing a CN III palsy sparing the pupil is a syndrome of the cavernous sinus. Its key symptoms—sudden severe headache and somnolence—were the initial symptoms in the brief but remarkable case presented here.

The patient was a 65-year-old man who presented with severe headache, somnolence, bilateral CN III palsies sparing the pupils, and a left CN VI palsy (Figure 5-10A–B). He was suspected to have had a subarachnoid hemorrhage. A spinal tap in the ER showed more than 300 red blood cells and xanthochromia. Brain MRI showed a large pituitary tumor extending bilaterally into the cavernous sinus. An immediate transsphenoidal resection of the tumor (a chromophobe adenoma with hemorrhage) and massive corticosteroid replacement therapy resulted in a rapid and complete recovery.

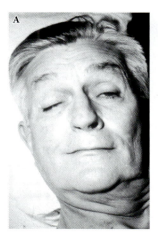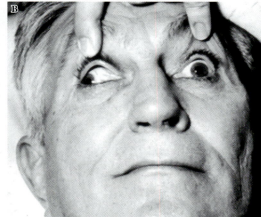

FIGURE 5-10 Pituitary apoplexy. (A) Acute bilateral asymmetric ptosis due to bilateral third-nerve palsies. (B) Marked exotropia in the right eye due to the unopposed action of the lateral rectus muscles. The left eye is straight in primary gaze due to an associated left abducens nerve palsy.

Pituitary apoplexy is life-threatening.[55] Its signs—sudden severe headache, somnolence, ophthalmoplegia (bilateral CN III palsies, unilateral CN IV palsy), and subarachnoid hemorrhage—should prompt immediate neuroimaging (computed tomography or magnetic resonance imaging) to confirm the diagnosis.

Compression of the Oculomotor Nerve

Within the cavernous sinus, the oculomotor nerve is always at risk of compression by a tumor or an aneurysm of the ICA. A patient presenting with progressive extraocular muscle weakness is diagnosed here.

CASE 5-4 CN III Compression with Primary Aberrant Regeneration

Video Display

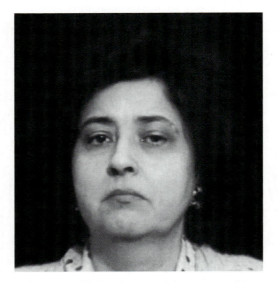

FIGURE 5-11 Forty-six-year-old woman with partial ptosis and a left oculomotor and abducens nerve palsy.

The patient is a 46-year-old woman from Portugal who developed double vision in all directions of gaze on waking one morning. The diplopia cleared within a few hours, except for vertical diplopia when she looked up. Six months later, in July 1986, she developed drooping of the left eyelid (Figure 5-11). She consulted an ophthalmologist and was referred to the neurovisual clinic and admitted to the Massachusetts General Hospital.

Past history negative for,

- *headache,*
- *face or eye pain,*
- *seizures,*
- *syncope,*
- *vertigo.*

Analysis of the History

- What are the major presenting symptoms?
- Where are the CNS lesion(s) likely to be?

CASE 5-4 SYMPTOMS

Symptoms	Location Correlation
Vertical diplopia looking up	Superior rectus muscle
	Inferior oblique muscle
Ptosis	Levator palpebrae superioris
	Oculomotor nerve

The analysis guides the clinical examination.

Examination

Neuro-ophthalmological

- Visual acuity 20/20 OU, full visual fields
- Normal fundus examination
- Pupils anisocoria OD 3 mm brisk to light and near
  OS 4 mm sluggish to light and near
  Unchanged with eyelid movements
- Eyelid OS
  Partial ptosis in primary gaze
  Complete ptosis on abduction
  Elevation of the ptotic lid on adduction
- Partial CN III palsy OS
  Paralysis superior rectus and inferior oblique
  Mild paresis medial rectus and inferior rectus
  Impaired convergence OS
- CN IV (superior oblique) normal
- CN V, impaired corneal reflex
- CN VI, lateral rectus paresis
- Bell's reflex (elevation of the eyes under closed lid) absent OS, present OD
- No exophthalmos
- Normal orbital resilience
- No ocular pulsation or bruit

The neurological examination was normal.

Localization and Differential Diagnosis

Unilateral CN III, V (VI first division) and VI nerve palsies localize the lesion to the ipsilateral cavernous sinus.

Abnormal movements of the ptotic eyelid indicate *aberrant regeneration of CN III,* diagnostic of a chronic compressive intracavernous mass—a meningioma or aneurysm.

What Diagnostic Tests Should Follow?

· Brain MRI
· Brain MRA

Test Results

Brain MRI showed a mass expanding the left cavernous sinus (Figure 5-12A–B).

Diagnosis: Left Cavernous Sinus Syndrome with primary aberrant regeneration of the oculomotor nerve.

Treatment

· Surgery
· Radiation therapy
· Conservative management with no biopsy

The patient elected conservative management. She returned for annual follow-ups for 5 years with no change in the examination.

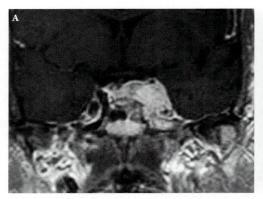 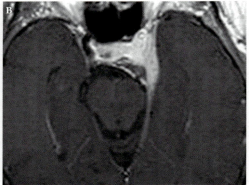

FIGURE 5-12 Brain magnetic resonance imaging. (A) Coronal T1 postcontrast image shows a middle fossa mass expanding the left cavernous sinus and obliterating Meckel's cave. (B) Axial T1 postcontrast image shows uniform enhancement of the mass and a dural tail extending posteriorly along the tentorium. The left internal carotid artery is severely narrowed.

Aberrant Regeneration

Atypical movements of the pupil, lid, or eye can occur after a CN III palsy. This phenomenon is called *aberrant regeneration* or *oculomotor synkinesis,* and it is caused by misdirection of regenerating axons[56] that, over time, find their own pathways to innervation.

When present in its entirety, the aberrant regeneration oculomotor syndrome features:

- *Gaze–lid dyskinesis.* Retraction and elevation of the eyelid on attempted downgaze (pseudo-von Graefe's sign)
- *Horizontal gaze-evoked dyskinesis.* Elevation of the eyelid on attempted adduction
- *Extraocular muscle dyskinesis.* Adduction on attempted elevation or depression (misdirection of fibers for superior or inferior rectus muscle to MR)
- *Limited vertical movements.* With occasional retraction of the globe on attempted vertical movement (due to simultaneous contraction of elevators and depressors)
- Pseudo *Argyll-Robertson pupil.* Light-near dissociation of the pupil; the pupil does not react to light stimulation but constricts on adduction (misdirection of fibers destined for MR muscle to pupillary sphincter muscles).[57]

The syndrome's characteristics are rarely present together in a single case, and, in Case 5-4, the size of the pupil and its reactivity remained stable in all positions of gaze.

There are two identifiable types of aberrant regeneration.

- *Primary* aberrant regeneration is a sign of an intracavernous meningioma[58] or aneurysm.[59] It is characterized by slowly progressive ocular motility and pupillary abnormalities consistent with aberrant regeneration of CN III without a preceding paralytic phase.
- *Secondary* aberrant regeneration can occur following a CN III palsy due to orbital trauma,[60] intracranial aneurysm,[61] compressive neoplasms, idiopathic CN III palsy,[62] basilar meningitis,[63] or following a midbrain stroke affecting the CN III fasciculus,[64] or transiently in temporal arteritis.[65]

Orbital Syndromes of the Oculomotor Nerve

Orbital lesions are commonly responsible for CN III pareses involving the pupil. They include inflammation, ischemia, infiltration, and compression by a tumor or metastasis. Visual loss due to compression of the optic nerve is the most important sign that clinically distinguishes an orbital apex syndrome from a cavernous sinus or SOF syndrome with and without proptosis and reduced orbital resilience. The opportunities for compression are considerable, given the path the nerve must take.

Superior Division Oculomotor Palsy

As the oculomotor nerve passes through the cavernous sinus, it divides into two branches, a superior division and a larger inferior division. The *superior division* runs in the orbit lateral to the optic nerve and ophthalmic artery to innervate the SR and LP muscles.[66,67] The larger *inferior division* innervates the MR, IR, and IO muscles, as well as the iris sphincter (the pupillary constrictor muscle) and ciliary body.[68,69]

A CT scan in the axial and coronal plane with bone windows provides the information needed to localize a lesion, which can occur as an isolated lesion of either branch. The case of "isolated" ptosis presented here illustrates this.

CASE 5-5 Superior Division Oculomotor Nerve Palsy

No Video Display

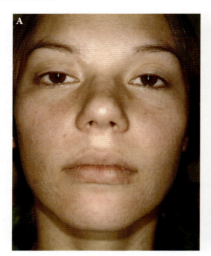 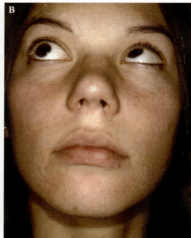

FIGURE 5-13 Twenty-year-old student with (A) Partial ptosis of the right eye. (B) Paresis of the right superior rectus muscle on upgaze to the right.

The patient is a 20-year-old student who consulted an ophthalmic surgeon for surgical correction of a partial left ptosis (Figure 5-13A). She had no diplopia, eye or periorbital pain, and no history of trauma. She was referred to the neurovisual clinic for a preoperative Tensilon test.

On examination, she had partial ptosis but also paresis of the superior rectus (Figure 5-13B) which had been overlooked in the ophthalmic examination because the eyelid was not held up when the eye movements were tested.

All other CN III muscles and the pupil innervated by the inferior division of CN III were normal.

What Tests Should Follow?

- Ophthalmological examination to rule out an orbital apex syndrome affecting vision
- Tensilon test
- CT of the orbit

Test Results

The ophthalmological examination was normal (visual acuity 20/20 OU and no proptosis). The Tensilon test was negative. A CT of the orbit showed an enhancing mass in the apex and minimal exophthalmus (Figure 5-14A). A left carotid angiogram showed displacement of the ophthalmic artery and a vascular tumor blush.

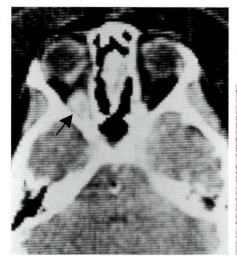
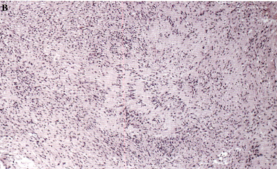

FIGURE 5-14 (A) Computed tomography (CT) of the orbit with contrast shows an enhancing right orbital apex mass. (B) Schwannoma with palisading Schwann cells. (Hematoxylin and eosin stain.)

Treatment

The mass was successfully surgically resected.

Diagnosis: Schwannoma (Figure 5-14B) of the Superior Division of the Oculomotor Nerve[70]

Special Explanatory Note

Schwannomas most commonly present with a history of proptosis that extends over a period of months or years, only rarely causing visual loss. The clinical diagnostic workup of an orbital lesion should include noninvasive imaging of the orbit either by echography (orbital ultrasound), CT, or MRI. Each modality has advantages and disadvantages, but the techniques are often complementary.[71–73]

On CT and MRI scans, schwannomas may be difficult to distinguish from primary optic nerve tumors, but this distinction must be made prior to surgical excision. Typically, neuroradiological features of schwannoma include a well-defined lesion that is isointense with the brain and enhances with gadolinium. Radiologically, they appear similar to cavernous hemangiomas, fibrous histiocytomas, and hemangiopericytomas. Surgical resection of schwannomas is the treatment of choice.[74]

Inferior Division Oculomotor Palsy

Inferior division third-nerve palsies are uncommon. Susac and Hoyt[75] reported three patients, two of whom were under 10 years of age, and the third 30 years old at onset. All three presented with painless diplopia.

One of the children, an 8-year-old girl, had a progressive palsy of the inferior division of the left CN III. Complete workup (including angiography) was normal. In the absence of a structural lesion, the authors suggested a postviral syndrome as the cause.

Traumatic Oculomotor Palsy

Traumatic CN III palsy is commonly due to a severe blow to the head causing skull fracture and loss of consciousness. Mild head trauma resulting in a CN III palsy may be an initial sign of a basal intracranial tumor,[76] and a high index of suspicion should prompt the examiner to image the brain.

THE TROCHLEAR NERVE

Cranial nerve four (CN IV) is the trochlear nerve. The trochlear nerve innervates the superior oblique muscle, the muscle responsible for depressing, adducting, and intorting the eye.

The Trochlear Nucleus

The trochlear nucleus is situated in the central gray matter of the midbrain, close to the median plane at the level of the inferior colliculus. The cell bodies are continuous anteriorly with the neurons of the oculomotor nucleus complex, with only a thinning out of the trochlear cells marking the separation. These cells are typical motor cells, with a few smaller cells, and they are surrounded laterally and ventrally by the MLF.

The Trochlear Fasciculus

The fascicles of the trochlear nerve emerge from the trochlear nucleus and pass laterally and posteriorly around the central gray matter and cross in the superior medullary velum (roof of the Sylvian aqueduct). They exit the brainstem *dorsally* below the inferior colliculi to form the trochlear nerve (Figure 5-15). This crossed innervation has important implications.

It is clinically impossible to differentiate a nuclear CN IV palsy from a fascicular CN IV palsy because of the extremely short course of the fascicles within the midbrain. The presence of an ipsilateral Horner's syndrome (with a contralateral CN IV paresis) in which sympathetic nerve fibers descending through the dorsolateral tegmentum of the midbrain close to the trochlear fascicles are involved, helps to localize a fascicular lesion.[77] A CN IV palsy with contralateral dysmetria suggests a lesion involving the cerebellar peduncle,[78] whereas a CN IV palsy plus a contralateral internuclear ophthalmoplegia localizes to the proximal fascicle and the MLF.[79]

Before the advent of MRI, reports of isolated or near isolated CN IV palsy from a brainstem stroke were rare, but neuroimaging now makes it easier to identify and localize the lesion.[80–82] One recent report, a 51-year-old man with a right CN IV palsy and variable upbeat nystagmus in primary gaze was found on MRI to have an infarct in the region of the left trochlear nucleus extending into the adjacent cerebellar peduncle, and asymmetry in the size of the superior oblique muscles.

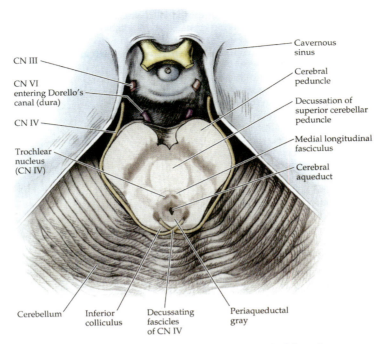

CN III

CN VI
entering Dorello's
canal (dura)

CN IV

Trochlear
nucleus
(CN IV)

Cavernous
sinus

Cerebral
peduncle

Decussation of
superior cerebellar
peduncle

Medial longitudinal
fasciculus

Cerebral
aqueduct

Cerebellum   Inferior   Decussating   Periaqueductal
colliculus   fascicles   gray
of CN IV

FIGURE 5-15 Section of the brainstem at the level of the inferior colliculus showing the decussation of the fascicles of the trochlear nerves (CN IV). Note CN IV exits the brainstem on the dorsal surface.

Reproduced with permission.[3]

The asymmetry was consistent with denervation atrophy of the right superior oblique muscle on MRI of the orbit.[83]

The Trochlear Nerve

The trochlear nerve follows the longest intracranial course of all the cranial nerves (75 mm). It runs in the subarachnoid space anteriorly and ventrally around the superior aspect of the cerebellar peduncles, then between the posterior cerebral artery and superior cerebellar artery (along with but laterally separated from CN III) and then runs forward along the free edge of the tentorium for 1–2 cm before penetrating the dura, below CN III's point of entry, to enter the cavernous sinus.

Within the lateral wall of the sinus, the nerve lies below CN III and above the ophthalmic division (VI) of the fifth (trigeminal) nerve (CN V). It then crosses over CN III and receives filaments from the carotid sympathetic plexus.

The nerve reaches the orbit in company with the frontal and lacrimal branches of the ophthalmic division of CN V and passes with them through the SOF outside the annulus of Zinn (Figure 4-1). The superior division of CN III—the nasociliary, the inferior division of CN III, and CN VI—all lie within the annulus (Figure 5-16). Mass lesions of the region of the SOF are clinically difficult to distinguish from those in the cavernous sinus.

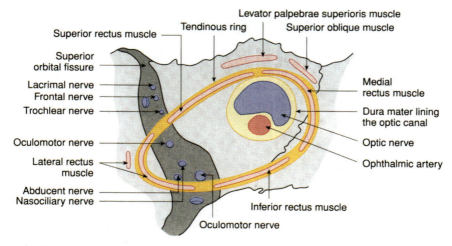

FIGURE 5-16 The anatomy of the superior orbital fissure and orbital apex, showing the common tendinous ring that gives origin to the four rectus muscles, the origins of levator palpebrae superioris and superior oblique, and positions of the nerves and blood vessels entering the orbital cavity.

Reproduced with permission.[84]

Traumatic Trochlear Palsy

The leading cause of a CN IV palsy is head trauma because the nerve's long course through the subarachnoid space leaves it particularly vulnerable to injury.[84]

■ **Clinical Points to Remember About the Trochlear Nerve**

- The fascicles of the trochlear nerve (CN IV) cross in the superior medullary velum.
- CN IV exits the brainstem dorsally below the inferior colliculi.
- The right trochlear nucleus innervates the left contralateral SO muscle.
- The left trochlear nucleus innervates the right contralateral SO muscle.
- The presence of an ipsilateral Horner's syndrome with a contralateral CN IV palsy localizes a midbrain fascicular CN IV palsy.
- Trauma is the commonest cause of a CN IV palsy.
- The three-step head tilt test is the best diagnostic test of a CN IV palsy (Chapter 4). ■

Bilateral CN IV Palsy

The key diagnostic feature of bilateral SO paresis (CN IV palsy) is an alternating hyperdeviation dependent on the direction of gaze, and, when the palsies are asymmetric, tilt of the head.[85] With post–head injury bilateral CN IV palsies, the lesion is likely to involve the anterior medullary velum, where the nerves emerge together. Whiplash forces transmitted to the brainstem by the free tentorial edge may injure the nerves at this site.

Paralysis of CN IV may also be due to compression by an aneurysm,[86] perineural spread of carcinoma,[87] multiple sclerosis,[88] and as a complication of neurosurgical procedures.[89]

THE ABDUCENS NERVE

Cranial nerve six (CN VI), the abducens nerve, innervates only the LR muscle that abducts the eye on lateral gaze.

The Abducens Nucleus

The abducens nucleus lies in the pontomedullary brainstem beneath the floor of the fourth ventricle, adjacent to the genu of the facial nerve. The neurons in the abducens nucleus are of four different types: motoneurons innervating the twitch muscle fibers in the lateral rectus, motoneurons innervating the nontwitch muscle fibers in the lateral rectus, abducens internuclear neurons (arranged around the periphery of the nucleus) innervating the contralateral MR muscle, and paramedian tract neurons that project to the cerebellar flocculus[90] (Figure 5-17).

The internuclear neurons project to the motoneurons of the MR muscle in the contralateral oculomotor nucleus to provide the mechanism for conjugate eye movements. Although motoneurons and internuclear neurons share the same burst-tonic firing pattern during eye movements,[91] the motor neurons activate only the lateral rectus. The ascending axons of the interneurons cross the midline, enter the MLF, and terminate in the MR motoneuron subgroups of CN III. Damage to the MLF causes paresis of the ipsilateral MR and an internuclear ophthalmoplegia (INO.[92a,92b] Vergence remains intact (Chapter 6).

An important congenital disorder of the abducens nucleus and nerve is Duane's syndrome, illustrated by the next case.[93]

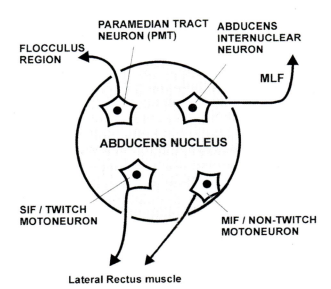

FIGURE 5-17 Diagram illustrating four different types of neurons within the abducens nucleus and their targets. SIF, singly innervated muscle fiber; MIF, multiply innervated muscle fiber; MLF, medial longitudinal fasciculus.

Reproduced with permission.[5]

CASE 5-6 Duane's Syndrome Type III

Video Display

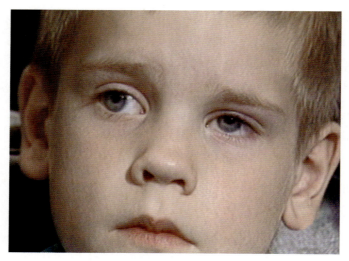

FIGURE 5-18 A seven-year-old boy with left Duane's syndrome type III. Note slight head turn to the right, tilt to the left, and left hypertropia.

The patient is a 7-year-old boy born 2 weeks premature in 1996 with transposition of the major arteries of the heart, four holes in the heart, and an absent spleen (Figure 5-18). He had cardiac surgery at age 2 days. At age 6 months, it was noted that the left eye did not move fully. At age 1 year, he had his second cardiac surgery. His development was excellent thereafter.

Examination

Ocular Motility

- A head turn to the right and slight tilt to the left
- Partial ptosis of the left eye and retraction of the globe on adduction
- Paresis of abduction and adduction
- Paresis of the superior oblique muscle with overaction of the inferior oblique muscle
- CN III and V normal

Localization and Differential Diagnosis

The defective abducens nerve function in this child is characterized by the paradoxical co-contraction of the ipsilateral medial and lateral rectus muscles, which are normally antagonistic and normally innervated by CN III and CN VI, respectively. He turned his head to the right to compensate for a left CN VI palsy and tilted his head to the left, ipsilateral to an associated CN IV palsy.

Special Explanatory Note

Duane's syndrome is classified into three types.[94] Narrowing of the palpebral fissure and abnormal retraction of the globe on attempted adduction are signs common to all three.

Type I, the most common, is characterized by limitation of abduction with normal adduction, indicating that abducens internuclear neurons are spared on the affected side since adducting saccades in the unaffected eye have normal velocities, and, during adduction, retraction of the globe results. Most patients with type I have no ocular misalignment.

Type II patients are characterized by limitation of adduction with normal abduction. The LR muscle contracts normally to abduct the eye, but contracts inappropriately in attempted adduction, producing defective adduction and globe retraction.

Type III is characterized by limitation of both adduction and abduction. The LR and MR muscles contract in both abduction and adduction and limit the motion of the eye in either direction. Type III Duane's may be difficult to distinguish from type I, but a minority of patients adopt a compensatory head turn to achieve binocularity.

In an autopsy case of Duane's type I, the sixth nerve was absent, the abducens nucleus was hypoplastic, and branches of the inferior division of CN III supplied the LR muscle. Within the hypoplastic abducens nucleus, the internuclear neurons were presumed to be spared. Clinical pathological studies[95,96] confirm the anomalous innervation of the LR muscle and MRI studies of patients with Duane's type I also confirm the absence of the abducens nerve,[97-100] with a normal appearing ipsilateral lateral rectus muscle on orbital imaging.[101]

Linkage studies in one family with Duane's syndrome localized a gene to chromosome 2q31, and mutations of this chromosome have been discovered in CHN1, a gene that encodes for alpha$_2$-chimaerin, a signaling protein that may play a role in ocular motor axon path finding.[102]

The Abducens Fasciculus

The fascicles of the abducens motoneurons run anteriorly in the pons through the medial lemniscus (Chaprer 6, Figure 6-4). CN VI fascicles exit the brainstem in a horizontal sulcus between the pons and medulla, lateral to the corticospinal tracts. Anterior paramedian lesions of the pons spare the abducens nucleus but affect the fascicles, resulting in ipsilateral CN VI and facial palsy with contralateral hemiplegia, usually due to ischemia.[103,104]

The Abducens Nerve

Once the abducens nerve leaves the brainstem, it climbs on the belly of the pons, running in the prepontine cistern to enter Dorello's canal beneath the petroclinoid ligament to enter the cavernous sinus. At this level (within the prepontine space), the nerve is exposed to compression by a basilar artery aneurysm or basal tumors (e.g., meningioma, chordoma, trigeminal schwannoma, acoustic neuroma).[105,106] Paresis of the abducens nerve (unilateral or bilateral) may also occur with increased intracranial pressure due to compression of the abducens nerve between the pons and the basilar artery or clivus or after lumbar puncture, shunting for hydrocephalus, or spinal anesthesia.

In the cavernous sinus, CN VI bends laterally around the intracavernous segment of the ICA and runs medial and parallel to the ophthalmic division (VI) of CN V. The ocular sympathetic fibers leave the ICA and join briefly with CN VI before joining the ophthalmic division (VI) of the trigeminal nerve. Unlike the oculomotor (CN III) and trochlear (CN IV) nerves, the abducens nerve does not lie within the lateral wall of the sinus, but runs within the body of the sinus.

A painless isolated abducens nerve palsy is a finding of clinical concern. The diagnostic approach to such a patient is presented here.

CASE 5-7 Unilateral Abducens Nerve Palsy

Video Display

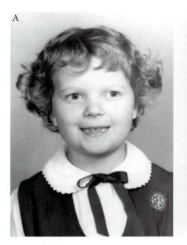 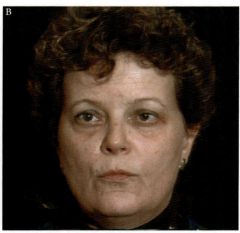

FIGURE 5-19 (A) Nonparalytic left exotropia in a girl aged 7 years. (B) At age 46, she presented with a left paralytic esotropia.

The patient is a 46-year-old woman referred by a glaucoma specialist in 1995 with new onset of horizontal diplopia at distance and a left esotropia measuring 30 diopters in primary gaze.

Past history:

- *Childhood strabismus, with the left eye deviated out (exotropia) at age 6 (Figure 5-19A).*
- *Unable to recall having one eye patched or doing eye exercises.*
- *No associated symptoms, such as headache, vertigo, deafness, or diplopia.*

Analysis of the History

- What are the major presenting symptoms?
- Where are the CNS lesion(s) likely to be?

CASE 5-7 SYMPTOMS

Symptoms	Location Correlation
Diplopia at distance	Lateral rectus muscle
Exotropia	Abducens nerve

The analysis guides the clinical examination.

Examination

Neuro-ophthalmological

- Visual acuity 20/40 OS(amblyopia) (20/20 OD)
- Pupils, visual fields, fundi normal
- Esotropia OS
- Paresis of the lateral rectus (CN VI)
- Full eye movements in all the other directions of gaze (CN III, CN IV)
- Corneal reflex normal (CN V [VI])
- No proptosis
- No ocular pulsation or bruit

The neurological examination was normal.

Localization and Differential Diagnosis

As a child, this patient had a nonparalytic strabismus (exotropia) (Chapter 4). As an adult, she developed a paralytic esotropia (deviation inwards of the eye with paresis of abduction on monocular viewing) diagnostic of an isolated abducens nerve (CN VI) palsy (Figure 5-19B).

What Diagnostic Tests Should Follow?

- CT of the orbit
- Brain MRI

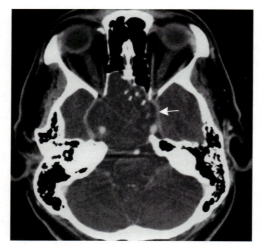

FIGURE 5-20 Axial computed tomography (CT) of the head shows a destructive central skull base lesion in the clivus expanding into the cavernous sinus (*arrow*) and encasing both internal carotid arteries.

Test Results

Computed tomography (CT) of the orbit, including base of skull, sella, and parasellar area without contrast, showed a lytic destructive lesion in the clivus with bony particles (destroyed bone) within the lesion (Figure 5-20). The lesion extended from the sella to the foramen magnum with extension laterally into the petrous apices and carotid canals. The lesion abutted the posterior part of the left and right cavernous sinus.

Brain MRI TI and T2, sagittal and coronal images pre- and post-gadolinium showed a destructive mass with mild patchy enhancement, significant expansion into the prepontine cistern with compression of the pons. Extension into Meckel's cave and left cavernous sinus and a convex bulging mass abutting the medial temporal lobe. The left and right cavernous internal carotid arteries were encased (Figure 5-21A–B).

Treatment

- Surgery
- Radiation therapy.

Biopsy of the tumor showed a chordoma with the characteristic appearance of cords of physaliferous cells with mucinous vacuoles. The tumor was inoperable. The patient received focal proton beam radiation therapy.

Remarkable for the absence of headache and diplopia, this patient's diagnosis might have been missed were it not for a glaucoma specialist who recognized the clinical signs of a significant palsy of the left abducens nerve and referred her.

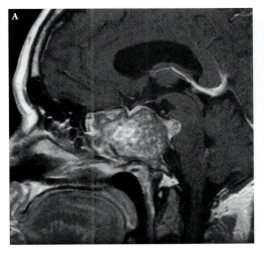
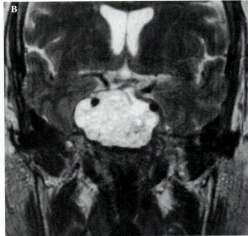

FIGURE 5-21 Brain MRI. (A) Sagittal post-contrast T1 image shows a prepontine hyperintense mass, destruction of the posterior clivus, and compression of the pons. (B) Coronal T2 image shows the lesion is extremely hyperintense (characteristic of most chordomas), and elevates and encases both internal carotid arteries.

MULTIPLE CRANIAL NERVE SYNDROMES

Cavernous Sinus Syndrome

The cavernous sinus is a plexus of various-sized veins that divide and coalesce. It contains CN III, IV, and VI; ophthalmic nerve (VI); the sympathetic carotid plexus; and the intracavernous ICA (Figure 5-22).

The same nerves pass through the SOF; thus, the clinical symptoms and signs of cavernous sinus syndrome characterised by eye pain (ophthalmic nerve VI) and ophthalmoplegia are

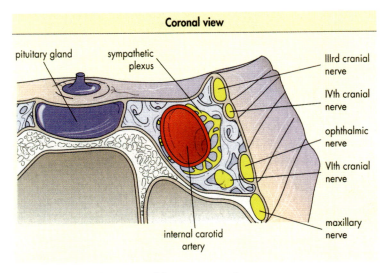

FIGURE 5-22 Anatomy of the cavernous sinus.

Reproduced with permission.[107]

typically not distinguishable from those of an SOF syndrome. The differential diagnosis of painful ophthalmoplegia is extensive. It includes trauma, intracavernous carotid artery aneurysm, carotid cavernous fistula, cavernous sinus thrombosis, primary and metastatic intracavernous tumors, meningeal carcinomatosis or lymphomatosis, infections such as mucormycosis or other fungal infection, herpes zoster, bacterial sinusitis, mucocele, and periostitis. Addionally, sarcoid, Wegener's granulomatosis, and orbital pseudotumor are important etiologies to keep in mind The Tolosa-Hunt syndrome is of particular importance to this list because of its simultaneous involvement of so many cranial nerves and its tendency to involve the orbit.[107]

Tolosa-Hunt Syndrome

The criteria for diagnosis of the Tolosa-Hunt syndrome proposed by Hunt in 1961[108] are as follows:

- Steady boring pain behind the eye
- Palsies localized to CN III, CN IV, the first division of CN V, and/or to CN VI and periarterial sympathetic fibers
- Symptoms lasting days or weeks
- Spontaneous remission and recurrence
- Absence of involvement of structures outside the cavernous sinus

Retrobulbar eye pain can precede the onset of cranial nerve signs by 3 days to up to a year—when the signs become evident they can be widespread. In one study[109] of 15 cases of Tolosa-Hunt, CN III was involved in six patients, CN V in five, CN IV in twelve, and CN VI and VII in four. The lower cranial nerves VIII, IX, and X were involved in three cases and XI and XII in two cases.

The pathological features of the syndrome are similar to those of orbital pseudotumor and orbital myositis, with a subgroup of cases showing a similar pathological process—a subacute granulomatous inflammation.[110–112] Steroid responsiveness is positive.[113]

In cases of Tolosa-Hunt, MRI axial and sagittal T1 images with gadolinium best visualize the extent of the enhanced infiltrating process in the cavernous sinus,[114–116] (Figure 5-23A) when the process extends forward into the orbital apex (Figure 5-23A–B).

A CTA may show narrowing of the carotid siphon, occlusion of the superior orbital vein, and nonvisualization of the cavernous sinus.

When possible, diagnosis should be confirmed by a transsphenoidal biopsy prior to treatment with corticosteroid. A course of steroid therapy usually results in dramatic relief from pain in under 24 hours to a few days with recovery of ophthalmoplegia. Follow up brain and orbit imaging in cases of the Tolosa-Hunt syndrome clearly illustrate the remarkable steroid response (Figure 5-23A–C).

A *cautionary note:* other causes of painful ophthalmoplegia, for example orbital myositis, B-cell lymphoma, meningioma, and metastases, all respond to steroid treatment. In the absence of a biopsy, which would confirm an inflammatory granulomatous process, patients with the Tolosa-Hunt syndrome should be followed up with serial MRI studies and continuing attention to steroid dosage.

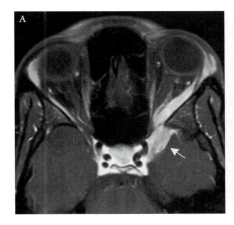
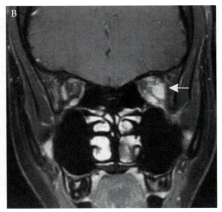
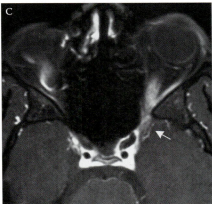

FIGURE 5-23 (A) Axial T1 image postcontrast shows hyperintense enhancing mass lesion centered in the left anterior cavernous sinus (*arrow*). It extends to the margin of the foramen ovale and through the orbital apex, with thickening and enhancement of the lateral rectus muscle. (B) Coronal T1 image of the orbit postcontrast shows enlarged and enhancing lateral rectus muscle (*arrow*). (C) Axial T1 image postcontrast 1 month post-corticosteroid therapy, shows marked decrease in the enhancing cavernous sinus mass and intraorbital extension (*arrow*).

Courtesy of Michael Preece, M.D.

Cavernous Sinus Thrombosis

Septic thrombosis of the cavernous sinus is a potentially life-threatening painful ophthalmoplegia that presents with periorbital pain, proptosis, headache, fever, and complete ophthalmoplegia involving CN III, IV, and VI or CN VI alone.[117,118] The organisms most often involved are *Staphylococcus aureus* (70% of cases) and *Streptococcus pneumoniae* or gram-negative bacilli. Direct spread of infection from the adjacent maxillary and sphenoid sinuses is the usual infection route. It may spread intracranially and into the contralateral cavernous sinus, with development of meningeal signs (nuchal rigidity) and persistent fever and delirium.

Orbital fungal infections, including aspergillosis, rhizopus, and organisms from the class of phycomycetes (mucormycosis), are dangerous. They are particularly threatening in diabetic patients.[119,120] A spinal tap may reveal abnormal CSF consistent with meningitis (i.e., elevated CSF protein and a neutrophilic pleocytosis), but fungi have a tendency to invade blood vessels, and central retinal or ophthalmic artery occlusion and visual loss maybe diagnostic.

The organisms can be identified, and antibiotic coverage for the bacterial infection guided, by a surgeon taking scrapings from the ethmoid bone for culture. Intravenous amphotericin and surgical debridement are the recommended treatments, with the extent of radical debridement dependent on the degree of visual loss and the extent of the infectious process. When severe, loss of the eye may be necessary to save life. Anticoagulation of patients with septic cavernous sinus thrombosis remains controversial but is still often recommended.

Carotid-Cavernous Fistula

A carotid-cavernous fistula (CCF) is an abnormal communication between the intracavernous ICA and the cavernous sinus. Carotid-cavernous fistulas are classified according to three criteria:

- Pathogenically, into spontaneous or traumatic fistulas
- Hemodynamically, into high-flow or low-flow fistulas
- Angiographically, into direct or dural fistulas[121–123]

A spontaneous CCF may develop following rupture of an intracavernous carotid aneurysm resulting in a direct shunt that fills the cavernous sinus with blood. When the blood drains anteriorly into the superior orbital vein, the vein expands and signs of orbital congestion develop: these include pulsatile proptosis, arterialization of the episcleral vessels producing generalized redness of the sclera (Figure 5-24), conjunctival chemosis, mechanical restriction of full eye movements, and/or ocular motor palsies.

The principal symptoms and signs of a high-flow CCF include a subjective bruit (80%), visual blurring (59%), headache (53%), diplopia (53%), and ocular or orbital pain (35%). A bruit may not be audible to the patient but is usually clinically audible if the examiner uses a bell stethoscope

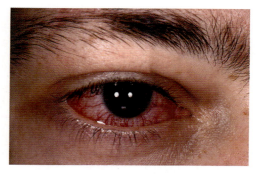

FIGURE 5-24 Arterialization of the episcleral veins in the eye of a patient with a high-flow ipsilateral carotid cavernous fistula.

Courtesy of R. Nick Hogan, M.D., Ph.D.

placed over the affected eyeball, with the contralateral eye open and fixed (to avoid eyelid blinking being misinterpreted as a bruit).

A post-traumatic, high-flow, carotid-cavernous sinus fistula in a 65-year-old woman with proptosis, eye pain, and a rushing noise in her left ear are illustrated in Figure 5-25A–B.

Traumatic CCF can present at the time of injury, or onset can be delayed for days or even weeks. Computed tomography or MRA readily confirms the diagnosis, and an interventional radiologist can seal the fistula by transarterial occlusion with platinum coils or liquid embolic material such as ethylene vinyl alcohol copolymer[124] (attachable balloons are no longer in use). Current endovascular techniques preserve the patency of the ICA and are successful in approximately 59–88% of patients.[125] Patients are usually delighted by the immediate cessation of the bruit, and signs of orbital congestion and ophthalmoparesis usually recover in 2–4 weeks.

Four types of fistulas are distinguishable angiographically.

- *Type A.* Direct high-flow shunt between the ICA and cavernous sinus.
- *Type B.* Dural shunt between meningeal branches of the ICA and cavernous sinus.
- *Type C.* Dural shunt between meningeal branches of the external carotid artery (ECA) and the cavernous sinus.
- *Type D.* Dural shunt between meningeal branches of both the ICA and ECA and the cavernous sinus.

Low-flow dural CCFs are less common than high-flow CCFs and are referred to as dural arteriovenous malformations (AVM).[126] A dural AVM is a "white-eyed shunt," there is no conjunctival arterialization or redness of the eye. Blood from the fistula drains posteriorly into the petrosal sinus,[127] signs of orbital congestion are absent, there is usually no audible bruit, and they rarely lead to vision-threatening complications. A dural AVM typically presents with an isolated palsy of CN VI or palsies of CN III, IV, V, and VI. They may close either spontaneously or following manual compression of the carotid artery.

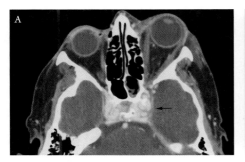 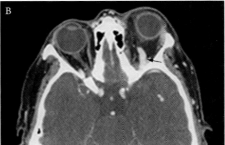

FIGURE 5-25 (A) Computed tomography angiography of a post-traumatic high-flow carotid-cavernous fistula shows left proptosis, mild asymmetric enlargement of the left extraocular muscles, and asymmetric hyperintense expansion and bulging of the left cavernous sinus. (*arrow*). (B) The blood is draining forward into an enlarged superior ophthalmic vein (*arrow*). Note proptosis of the left eye.

Courtesy of Michael Preece, M.D.

SELECTED REFERENCES

1. Warwick R. Representation of the extraocular muscles in the oculomotor nuclei of the monkey. *J Comp Neurol.* 1953;98:449–504.
2. Bienfang DC. Crossing axons in the third nerve nucleus. *Invest Ophthalmol.* 1975; 14:927–931.
3. Blumenfeld H. *Neuroanatomy Through Clinical Cases.* 2nd ed. Sunderland, MA: Sinauer Associates; 2010.
4. Buttner-Ennever JA, Akert K. Medial rectus subgroups of the oculomotor nucleus and their abducens internuclear input in monkey. *J Comp Neurol.* 1981;197:17–27.
5. Buttner-Ennever JA. The extraocular motor nuclei: organization and functional neuroanatomy. *Prog Brain Res.* 2006;151:95–125.
6. Liu GT, Carrazana EJ, Charness ME. Unilateral oculomotor palsy and bilateral ptosis from paramedian midbrain infection. *Arch Neurol.* 1991;48:983–986.
7. Martin TJ, Corbett JJ, Babikian PV, Crawford SC, Currier RD. Bilateral ptosis due to mesencephalic lesions with relative preservation of ocular motility. *J Neuro-ophthalmol.* 1996;16:258–263.
8. Saeki N, Yamaura A, Sunami K. Bilateral ptosis with pupil sparing because of a discrete midbrain lesion: magnetic resonance imaging evidence of topographic arrangement within the oculomotor nerve. *J Neuro-ophthalmol.* 2000;20:130–134.
9. Bryan JS, Hamed LM. Levator-sparing nuclear oculomotor palsy. Clinical and magnetic resonance imaging findings. *J Clin Neuro-ophthalmol.* 1992;12:26–30.
10. Growdon JH, Winkler GF, Wray SH. Midbrain ptosis. A case with clinicopathologic correlation. *Arch Neurol.* 1974;30:179–181.
11. Biller J, Shapiro R, Evans LS, Haag JR, Fine M. Oculomotor nuclear complex infarction. Clinical and radiological correlation. *Arch Neurol.* 1984;41:985–987.
12. Daroff RB. Oculomotor manifestation of brainstem and cerebellar dysfunction. In: Smith JL, ed. *Neuro-ophthalmology: Symposium of the University of Miami and Bascom-Palmer Eye Institute.* Vol 5. Hallandale: Huffman; 1971:104–121.
13. Leigh RJ, Zee DS. *The Neurology of Eye Movements.* 4th ed. New York: Oxford University Press; 2006.
14. Castro O, Johnson LN, Mamourian AC. Isolated inferior oblique paresis from brain-stem infarction. Perspective on oculomotor fascicular organization in the ventral midbrain tegmentum. *Arch Neurol.* 1990;47:235–237.
15. Ksiazek SM, Slamovits TL, Rosen CE, Burde RM, Parisi F. Fascicular arrangement in partial oculomotor paresis. *Am J Ophthalmol.* 1994;118:97–103.
16. Kwon JH, Kwon SU, Ahn HS, Sung KB, Kim JS. Isolated superior rectus palsy due to contralateral midbrain infarction. *Arch Neurol.* 2003;60:1633–1635.
17. Shuaib A, Israelian G, Lee MA. Mesencephalic hemorrhage and unilateral pupillary deficit. *J Clin Neuro-ophthalmol.* 1989;9:47–49.
18. Fortis AA, Nikolaou HD, Zidianakis VM, Maguina NM. Ischemic stroke in a young man following Ecstasy abuse: A case report. *Int J Emerg Inten Care Med.* 2005; 8(1):1092–4051.
19. Keane JR. Isolated brain-stem third nerve palsy. *Arch Neurol.* 1988;45:813–814.
20. Gauntt CD, Kashii S, Nagata I. Monocular elevation paresis caused by an oculomotor fascicular impairment. *J Neuro-ophthalmol.* 1995;15:11–14.
21. Hriso E, Masdeu JC, Miller A. Monocular elevation weakness and ptosis: an oculomotor fascicular syndrome? *J Clin Neuro-ophthalmol.* 1991;11:111–113.
22. Weber H. A contribution to the pathology of the crura cerebri. *Transactions of the Medical-Churirgical Society of London.* 1863;46:121–137.
23. Seo SW, Heo JH, Lee KY, Shin WC, Chang DI, Kim SM, Heo K. Localization of Claude's syndrome. *Neurology.* 2001;57(12):2304–2307.
24. Miller NR, Newman NJ, Biousse V, Kerrison JB, eds. *Walsh & Hoyt's Clinical Neuro-Ophthalmology THE ESSENTIALS.* 2nd ed. Philadelphia: Lippincott, Williams & Wilkins; 2008.
25. Claude H. Syndrome pedonculaire de la region du noyau rouge. *Revue Neurologique.* 1912;13:311–313.
26. Claude H, Loyez M. Ramollissement du noyau rouge. *Revue Neurologique.* 1912; 13:49–51.

27. Brew B, Sidtis J, Petito DK, Price RW. The neurologic complications of AIDS and human immunodeficieincy virus infection. In: Plum F, ed. *Advances in Contemporary Neurology*. F.A. Davis, Philadelphia; 1988;1:1–49.

28. Kerr F, Hollowell OW. Location of pupillomotor and accommodation fibres in the oculomotor nerve: experimental observations on paralytic mydriasis. *J Neurol Neurosurg Psychiat*. 1964;27:473–481.

29. Sunderland S, Bradley KC. Disturbances of oculomotor function accompanying extradural haemorrhage. *J Neurol Neurosurg Psychiat*. 1953;16:35–46.

30. Ropper AH. The opposite pupil in herniation. *Neurology*. 1990;40:1707–1709.

31. Chen R, Sahjpaul R, Del Maestro RF, Assis L, Young GB. Initial enlargement of the opposite pupil as a false localising sign in intraparenchymal frontal hemorrhage. *J Neurol Neurosurg Psychiat*. 1994;57(9):1126–1128.

32. Kole MK, Hysell SE. MRI correlate of Kernohan's notch. *Neurology*. 2000; 55(11):1751

33. Corbett JJ. The bedside and office neuro-ophthalmology examination. *Semin Neurol*. 2003;23:63–76.

34. Kupersmith MJ. *Neuro-vascular Neuro-ophthalmology*. Berlin: Springer-Verlag; 1993:69–108.

35. Kasoff I, Kelly DL. Pupillary sparing in oculomotor palsy from internal carotid aneurysm. Case report. *J Neurosurg*. 1975;42(6):713–717.

36. Kissel JT, Burde RM, Klingele TG, Zeiger HE. Pupil-sparing oculomotor palsies with internal carotid-posterior communicating artery aneurysms. *Ann Neurol*. 1983; 13(2):149–154.

37. Good EF. Ptosis as the sole manifestation of compression of the oculomotor nerve by an aneurysm of the posterior communicating artery. *J Clin Neuro-ophthalmol*. 1990;10:59–61.

38. Bartleson JD, Trautmann JC, Sundt TM. Minimal oculomotor nerve paresis secondary to unruptured intracranial aneurysm. *Arch Neurol*. 1986;43:1015–1020.

39. Crompton JL, Moore CE. Painful third nerve palsy: how not to miss an intra-cranial aneurysm. *Aust J Ophthalmol*. 1981;9(2):113–115.

40. Greenspan BN, Reeves AG. Transient partial oculomotor nerve paresis with posterior communicating artery aneurysm: A case report. *J Clin Neuro-ophthalmol*. 1990; 10:56–58.

41. Foroozan R, Slamovits TL, Ksiazek SM, Zak R. Spontaneous resolution of aneurysmal third nerve palsy. *J Neuro-ophthalmol*. 2002;22(3):211–214.

42. Grunwald L, Sund NJ, Volpe NJ. Pupillary sparing and aberrant regeneration in chronic third nerve palsy secondary to a posterior communicating artery aneurysm. *Br J Ophthalmol*. 2008;92:715–716.

43. Coppete JR, Lessell S. Dorsal midbrain syndrome from giant aneurysm of the posterior fossa: report of two cases. *Neurology*. 1983;33:732–736.

44. Ahn JY, Han IB, Yoon PH, Kim SH, Kim NK, Kim S, Joo JY. Clipping vs coiling of posterior communicating artery aneurysms with third nerve palsy. *Neurology*. 2006;66(1):121–123.

45. Nadeau E, Trobe JD. Pupil sparing in oculomotor palsy: a brief review. *Ann Neurol*. 1983;13:143–148.

46. Teuscher AU, Meienberg O. Ischaemic oculomotor nerve palsy. Clinical features and vascular risk factors in 23 patients. *J Neurol*. 1985;24(3):144–149.

47. Capo H, Warren F, Kupersmith MJ. Evolution of oculomotor nerve palsies. *J Clin Neuro-ophthalmol*. 1992;12(1):21–25.

48. Dreyfus PM, Hakim S, Adams RD. Diabetic ophthalmoplegia. Report of case with postmortem study and comments on vascular supply of human oculomotor nerve. *Arch Neurol Psychiat*. 1957;77:337–349.

49. Asbury AK, Aldredge H, Hershberg R, Fisher CM. Oculomotor palsy in diabetes mellitus: a clinicopathological study. *Brain*. 1970;93:555–566.

50. Weber RB, Daroff RB, Mackey EA. Pathology of oculomotor palsy in diabetes. *Neurology*. 1970;20:835–838.

51. Bailey TD, O'Connor PS, Tredici TJ, Shacklett DE. Ophthalmoplegic migraine. *J Clin Neuro-ophthalmol*. 1984;4:225–228.

52. Van Pelt W. On the early onset of ophthalmoplegic migraine. *Am J Dis Child*. 1964; 107:628–631.

53. Wong V, Wong WC. Enhancement of oculomotor nerve: a diagnostic criterion for ophthalmoplegic migraine? *Pediatr Neurol*. 1997;17:70–73.

54. Durkan GP, Troost BT, Slamovits TL, Spoor TC, Kennerdell JS. Recurrent painless oculomotor palsy in children. A variant of ophthalmoplegic migraine? *Headache*. 1981;21:58–62.

55. Warwar RE, Bhullar SS, Pelstring RJ, Fadell RJ. Sudden death from pituitary apoplexy in a patient presenting with an isolated sixth cranial nerve palsy. *J Neuro-ophthalmol*. 2006;26(2):95–97.

56. Bielschowsky A. Lectures on motor anomalies of the eyes: II. Paralysis of individual eye muscles. *Arch Ophthalmol.* 1935;13:33–59.

57. Sturm RJ, Smith JL. Aberrant regeneration of the oculomotor nerve: Monocular optokinetic response. *Trans Am Acad Ophthalmol Otolaryngol.* 1965;69:1054–1060.

58. Schatz NJ, Savino PJ, Corbett JJ. Primary aberrant oculomotor regeneration. A sign of intracavernous meningioma. *Arch Neurol.* 1977;34(1):29–32.

59. Cox TA, Wurster JB, Godfrey WA. Primary aberrant oculomotor regeneration due to intracranial aneurysm. *Arch Neurol.* 1979;36(9):570–571.

60. Sebag J, Sadun AA. Aberrant regeneration of the third nerve following orbital trauma. *Arch Neurol.* 1983;40:762–764.

61. Hepler RS, Cantu RC. Aneurysms and third nerve palsies. *Arch Ophthalmol.* 1967; 77:604–608.

62. Laguna JF, Smith MS. Aberrant regeneration in idiopathic oculomotor nerve palsy. *J Neurosurg.* 1980;52:854–856.

63. Sibony PA, Lessell S, Gittinger JW Jr. Acquired oculomotor synkinesis. *Surv Ophthalmol.* 1984;28(5):382–390.

64. Messe SR, Shin RK, Liu GT, Galetta SL, Volpe NJ. Oculomotor synkinesis following a midbrain stroke. *Neurology.* 2001;57:1106–1107.

65. Sibony PA, Lessell S. Transient oculomotor synkinesis in temporal arteritis. *Arch Neurol.* 1984;41:87–88.

66. Masucci EF, Kurtzke JF. Diabetic superior branch palsy of the oculomotor nerve. *Ann Neurol.* 1980;7(5):493.

67. Stefanis L, Przedborski S. Isolated palsy of the superior branch of the oculomotor nerve due to chronic erosive sphenoid sinusitis. *J Clin Neuro-ophthalmol.* 1993; 13:229–231.

68. Saul RF, Selhorst JB. Traumatic inferior division oculomotor palsy. *Neurology.* 1986; 36(suppl 1):250.

69. Ohtsuka K, Hashimoto M, Nakamura Y. Enhanced magnetic resonance imaging in a patient with acute paralysis of the inferior division of the oculomotor nerve. *Am J Ophthalmol.* 1997;124:406–409.

70. Leunda G, Vaquero J, Cabezudo J, Garcia-Uria J, Bravo G. Schwannoma of the oculomotor nerves. Report of four cases. *J Neurosurg.* 1982;57(4):563–565.

71. Cantore G, Ciappetta P, Raco A, Lunardi P. Orbital schwannomas: report of nine cases and review of the literature. *Neurosurgery.* 1986;19:583–588.

72. Konrad EA, Thiel HJ. Schwannoma of the orbit. *Ophthalmologica.* 1984;188:118–127.

73. Rootman J, Goldberg C, Robertson W. Primary orbital schwannomas. *Br J Ophthalmol.* 1982;66:194–204.

74. Schick U, Bleyen J, Hassler W. Treatment of orbital schwannomas and neurofibromas. *Br J Neurosurg.* 2003;17:541–545.

75. Susac JO, Hoyt WF. Inferior branch palsy of the oculomotor nerve. *Ann Neurol.* 1977;2:336–339.

76. Eyster EF, Hoyt WF, Wilson CB. Oculomotor palsy from minor head trauma. An initial sign of basal intracranial tumor. *JAMA.* 1972;220:1083–1086.

77. Guy J, Day AL, Mickle JP, Schatz NJ. Contralateral trochlear nerve paresis and ipsilateral Horner's syndrome. *Am J Ophthalmol.* 1989;107(1):73–76.

78. Brazis PW. Palsies of the trochlear nerve: diagnosis and localization-recept concepts. *Mayo Clin Proc.* 1993;68:501–509.

79. Vanooteghem P, Dehaene I, Van Zandycke M, Casselman J. Combined trochlear nerve palsy and internuclear ophthalmoplegia. *Arch Neurol.* 1992;49:108–109.

80. Galetta SL, Balcer LJ. Isolated fourth nerve palsy from midbrain hemorrhage: case report. *J Neuro-ophthalmol.* 1998;18:204–205.

81. Kim JS, Kang JK, Lee SA, Lee MC. Isolated or predominant ocular motor nerve palsy as a manifestation of brain stem stroke. *Stroke.* 1993;24:581–586.

82. Keane JR. Tectal fourth nerve palsy due to infarction. *Arch Neurol.* 2004;61(2):280.

83. Makki AA, Newman NJ. A trochlear stroke. *Neurology.* 2005;65(12):1989.

84. Snell RS, Lemp MA. *Clinical Anatomy of the Eye.* 2nd ed. Boston: Blackwell Scientific Publication; 1998.

85. Lee J, Flynn JT. Bilateral superior oblique palsies. *Br J Ophthalmol.* 1985;69:508–513.

86. Agostinis C, Caverni L, Moschini L, Rottoli MR, Foresti C. Paralysis of fourth cranial nerve due to superior-cerebellar artery aneurysm. *Neurology.* 1992; 42(2):457–458.

87. Wilcsek GA, Francis IC, Egan CA, Kneale KL, Sharma S, Kappagoda MB. Superior oblique palsy in a patient with a history of perineural spread from a periorbital squamous cell carcinoma. *J Neuro-ophthalmol.* 2000;20:240–241.

88. Jacobson DM, Moster ML, Eggenberger ER, Galetta SL, Liu GT. Isolated trochlear nerve palsy in patients with multiple sclerosis. *Neurology.* 1999;53(4):877–879.

89. Yoss RE, Rucker CW, Miller RH. Neurosurgical complications affecting the oculomotor, trochlear, and abducent nerves. *Neurology.* 1968;18:594–600.

90. Büttner-Ennever JA, Horn AKE, Scherberger H, D'Ascanio P. Motoneurons of twitch and nontwitch extraocular muscle fibers in the abducens, trochlear, and oculomotor nuclei of monkeys. *J Comp Neurol.* 2001;438:318–335.

91. Fuchs AF, Scudder CA, Kaneko CR. Discharge patterns and recruitment order of identified motoneurons and internuclear neurons in the monkey abducens nucleus. *J Neurophysiol.* 1988;60:1874–1895.

92a. Delgado-Garcia JM, Del Pozo F, Baker R. Behavior of neurons in the abducens nucleus of the alert cat. I. Motoneurons. *Neuroscience.* 1986a;17(4):929–952.

92b. Delgado-Garcia JM, Del Pozo F, Baker R. Behavior of neurons in the abducens nucleus of the alert cat. II. Internuclear neurons. *Neuroscience.* 1986b;17(4):953–973.

93. Duane A. Congenital deficiency of abduction, associated with impairment of adduction, retraction movements, contraction of the palpebral fissure and oblique movements of the eye. [Reprinted in abridged form in Arch Ophthalmol 1996; 114:1255–1257.] *Arch Ophthalmol.* 1905;34:133–159.

94. Huber A. Electrophysiology of the retraction syndromes. *Br J Ophthalmol.* 1974; 58:293–300.

95. Hotchkiss MG, Miller NR, Clark AW, Green WR. Bilateral Duane's retraction syndrome. A clinical-pathologic case report. *Arch Ophthalmol.* 1980;98:870–874.

96. Miller NR, Kiel S, Green WR, Clark AW. Unilateral Duane's retraction syndrome (type 1). *Arch Ophthalmol.* 1982;100:1468–1472.

97. Parsa CF, Grant PE, Dillon WP, du Lac S, Hoyt WF. Absence of the abducens nerve in Duane syndrome verified by magnetic resonance imaging. *Am J Ophthalmol.* 1998;125:399–401.

98. Kim JH, Hwang JM. Presence of the abducens nerve according to the type of Duane's retraction syndrome. *Ophthalmology.* 2005;112:109–113.

99. Demer JL, Ortube MC, Engle EC, Thacker N. High-resolution magnetic resonance imaging demonstrates abnormalities of motor nerves and extraocular muscles in patients with neuropathic strabismus. *J AAPOS.* 2006;10:135–142.

100. Kang NY, Demer JL. Comparison of orbital magnetic resonance imaging in Duane syndrome and abducens palsy. *Am J Ophthalmol.* 2006;142:827–834.

101. Appukuttan B, Gillanders E, Juo SH, Freas-Lutz D, Ott S, Sood R, Auken A, Bailey-Wilson J, Wang X, Patel R, Robbins C, Chung M, Annett G, Weinberg K, Borchert M, Trent J, Brownstein M, Stout J. Localization of a gene for Duane retraction syndrome to chromosome 2q31. *Am J Hum Genet.* 1999;65:1639–1646.

102. Miyake N, Chilton J, Psatha M, Cheng L, Andrews C, Chan W-M, Law K, Crosiwer M, Lindsay S, Cheung M, Allen J, Gutowski, et al. Human CHN1 mutations hyperactivate alpha2-chimaerin and cause Duane's retraction syndrome. *Science.* 2008;321:839–843.

103. Silverman IE, Liu GT, Volpe NJ, Galetta SL. The crossed paralyses: the original brainstem syndromes of Millard-Gubler, Foville, Weber, and Raymond-Cestan. *Arch Neurol.* 1995;52(6):635–638.

104. Donaldson D, Rosenberg NL. Infarction of abducens nerve fascicle as cause of isolated sixth nerve palsy related to hypertension. *Neurology.* 1988;38(10):1654.

105. Currie J, Lubin JH, Lessell S. Chronic isolated abducens paresis from tumors at the base of the brain. *Arch Neurol.* 1983;40(4):226–229.

106. Galetta SL, Smith JL. Chronic isolated sixth nerve palsies. *Arch Neurol.* 1989; 46:79–82.

107. Moster ML. Paresis of isolated and multiple cranial nerves and painful ophthalmoplegia. In: Yanoff M, Duker JS, eds. *Ophthalmology.* 2nd ed. Philadelphia, PA: Mosby; 2004;1323–1334.

108. Hunt WE, Meagher JN, LeFever HE, Zeman W. Painful ophthalmoplegia. Its relation to indolent inflammation of the cavernous sinus. *Neurology.* 1961;11:56–62.

109. Juncos JL, Beal MF. Idiopathic cranial polyneuropathy. A fifteen-year experience. *Brain.* 1987;110:197–211.

110. Hunt WE. Tolosa-Hunt syndrome: One cause of painful ophthalmoplegia. *J Neurosurgery.* 1976;44:544–549.

111. Tolosa E. Periarteritic lesions of the carotid siphon with the clinical features of a carotid infraclinoid aneurysm. *J Neurol Neurosurg Psychiat.* 1954;17:300–302.

112. Schatz JN, Farmer P. Tolosa-Hunt syndrome: the pathology of painful ophthalmoplegia. In: Smith JL, ed. *Neuro-ophthalmology: Symposium of the University of Miami and the Bascom Palmer Eye Institute.* Vol 6. St. Louis: CV Mosby; 1972;102–112.

113. Smith JL, Taxdal DSR. Painful ophthalmoplegia: the Tolosa-Hunt Syndrome. *Am J Ophthalmol.* 1966;61:1466–1472.

114. Thomas DJB, Charlesworth MC, Afshar F, Galton DJ. Computerised axial tomography and magnetic resonance scanning in the Tolosa-Hunt syndrome. *Br J Ophthalmol.* 1988;72:299–302.

115. Yousem DM, Atlas SW, Grossman RI, Sergott RC, Savino PJ, Bosley TM. MR imaging of Tolosa-Hunt syndrome. *AJNR Am J Neuroradiol.* 1989;10:1181–1184.

116. Goto Y, Hosokawa S, Goto I, Hirakata R, Hasuo K. Abnormality in the cavernous sinus in three patients with Tolosa-Hunt syndrome: MRI and CT findings. *J Neurol Neurosurg Psychiat.* 1990;53:231–234.

117. DiNubile MJ. Septic thrombosis of the cavernous sinuses. *Arch Neurol.* 1988; 45:567–572.

118. Bhatia K, Jones NS. Septic cavernous sinus thrombosis secondary to sinusitis: are anticoagulants indicated? A review of the literature. *J Laryngol Otol.* 2002; 116:667–676.

119. Galetta SL, Wulc AE, Goldberg HI, Nichols CW, Glaser JS. Rhinocerebral mucormycosis: management and survival after carotid occlusion. *Ann Neurol.* 1990;28(1):103–107.

120. Johnson EV, Kline LB, Julian BA, Garcia JH. Bilataeral cavernous sinus thrombosis due to mucormycosis. *Arch Neurol.* 1988;106:1089–1092.

121. Barrow DL, Spector RH, Braun IF, Landman JA, Tindall SC, Tindall GT. Classification and treatment of spontaneous carotid-cavernous sinus fistulas. *J Neurosurg.* 1985;62:248–256.

122. Keltner JL, Satterfield D, Dublin AB, Lee BCP. Dural and carotid cavernous sinus fistulas. Diagnosis, management and complications. *Ophthalmology.* 1987; 94:1585–1600.

123. Chuman H, Trobe JD, Petty EM, Schwarze U, Pepin M, Byers PH, Deveikis JP. Spontaneous direct carotid-cavernous fistula in Ehlers-Danlos syndrome type IV: two case reports and a review of the literature. *J Neuro-ophthalmol.* 2002; 22(2):75–81.

124. Bhatia KD, Wang L, Parkinson RJ, Wenderoth JD. Successful treatment of six cases of indirect carotid-cavernous fistula with ethylene vinyl alcohol copolymer (Onyx) transvenous embolization. *J Neuro-ophthalmol.* 2009;29(1):3–8.

125. Gemmete JJ, Ansari SA, Gandhi DM. Endovascular techniques for treatment of carotid-cavernous fistula. *J Neuro-ophthalmol.* 2009;29:62–71.

126. Hawke SHB, Mullie MA, Hoyt WF, Halinan JM, Halmagyi GM. Painful oculomotor palsy due to dural-cavernous sinus shunt. *Arch Neurol.* 1989; 46(11):1252–1255.

127. Stiebel-Kalish H, Setton A, Nimii Y, Kalish Y, Hartman J, Huna Bar-On R, Berenstein A, Kupersmith MJ. Cavernous sinus dural arteriovenous malformations: patterns of venous drainage are related to clinical signs and symptoms. *Ophthalmology.* 2002;109:1685–1691.

| 6 |

HORIZONTAL GAZE AND SYNDROMES OF THE PONS

THE PONS

The pons is both bridge and crossroads to the midbrain, the medulla, and the cerebellum. Limited dorsally by the fourth ventricle, it is attached to the cerebellum by the superior, middle, and inferior cerebellar peduncles. The ventral portion is referred to as the *basis pontis* or the *pontocerebellar portion*. The dorsal pons is referred to as the *tegmentum*.

The cerebral cortex and the cerebellum interact closely to generate not only eye movements but all other forms of motor behavior. Their interactions are dependent on a massive projection system in the brainstem that allows the exchange of signals between the two cortices. These projections terminate in the basis pontis and relay signals to several interconnected brainstem nuclei, including the pontine nuclei (PN)[1] and the rostral portion of the nucleus reticularis tegmenti pontis (NRTP),[2-4] which lie close to each other. Both the PN and the NRTP are intimately involved in the visual guidance of eye movements; the PN, specifically, relays signals to the vestibulocerebellum, the paraflocculus and ventral flocculus, and the oculomotor region of the dorsal vermis.[5]

The NRTP and the PN also receive signals from cortical and subcortical structures that play a role in the generation of saccadic eye movements: the frontal eye fields (FEF), the lateral intraparietal area, the medial parietal area,[6] and the superior colliculus (see Chapter 1). These connections suggest that the PN may be involved in information processing for saccadic eye movements in addition to their major function of controlling slow visually guided eye movements.

Pursuit-related visual signals descend the smooth pursuit pathway from the posterior parietal cortex and the medial superior temporal (MST) area,[7] which are involved in the processing of visual motion for smooth pursuit eye movements, and project to the dorsolateral PN (DLPN), which relay signals to the ventral paraflocculus of the cerebellum, the final cerebellar target. In its own turn, the ventral paraflocculus projects to the medial vestibular nucleus (MVN), fastigial nucleus, and y-group.

The DLPN also receives non–visual-related signals, and many neurons in the DLPN keep firing during smooth pursuit eye movements even in the absence of visual cues. This is a hallmark of visual-tracking neurons in the MST area,[8-10] as well as of pursuit-related neurons in the FEF,[11] which suggest that pursuit-related neurons in the DLPN are essentially faithful transmitters of cerebrocortical signals. Many DLPN pursuit neurons can also be driven by saccadic eye movements. Lesions of the DLPN can cause an impairment of pursuit initiation and of steady-state smooth pursuit,[12] with the impairment affecting pursuit toward the side of the lesion. Pursuit in other directions can also be affected.

Patients with ischemia of the ventral pons have major pursuit deficits, especially in ipsilateral pursuit.[13,14] Recovery is usually incomplete, and this may reflect more widespread damage of pursuit-related circuits in the ventral pons.

Horizontal Gaze

The critical structures in the pontine tegmentum important for horizontal gaze are:

- The paramedian pontine reticular formation (PPRF)
- The abducens nucleus (AN)
- The medial longitudinal fasciculus (MLF) and axons in passage-carrying pursuit, vestibular, and gaze-holding signals to the AN

The medial portions of the nucleus reticularis magnocellularis (or nucleus centralis pontis oralis and caudalis) have been designated the *paramedian pontine reticular formation,*[15] and contain a key class of brainstem neurons that generate all types of saccades: horizontal, vertical and torsional (Figure 1-14). The projection from the PPRF to the abducens nerve (cranial nerve [CN] VI) nucleus and the projection of the MLF to the contralateral oculomotor (CN III) nucleus in the midbrain[16] are shown in Figure 6-1.

The excitatory burst neurons (EBNs) lie in the nucleus reticularis pontis chordalis (NRPC) and fire to generate horizontal saccadic eye movements. Omnipause cells are located at the midline of the PPRF in the nucleus raphe interpositus (rip) and project to excitatory and inhibitory burst neurons (IBNs) for horizontal and vertical saccades. The omnipause cells stop firing milliseconds before and during saccades. The IBNs lie in the nucleus paragigantocellularis dorsalis (PGD) caudal to the abducens nucleus (AN) in the pontine tegmentum. The IBN receive excitatory input from the ipsilateral EBN and inhibitory inputs from omnipause cells. They project to the contralateral AN to inhibit the antagonist muscles.[17]

Pontine nuclei involved in eye movement control are shown in Figure 6-2.[18]

The pontine tegmentum contains almost all the nuclei that ultimately control horizontal gaze, and the (AN) is the most important among them. The AN contains motoneurons that innervate the lateral rectus muscle, and internuclear neurons whose axons cross the midline and ascend the contralateral MLF to project to the medial rectus subnucleus, in the contralateral oculomotor (CN III) nucleus, to activate the muscle for adduction of the eye in lateral gaze.

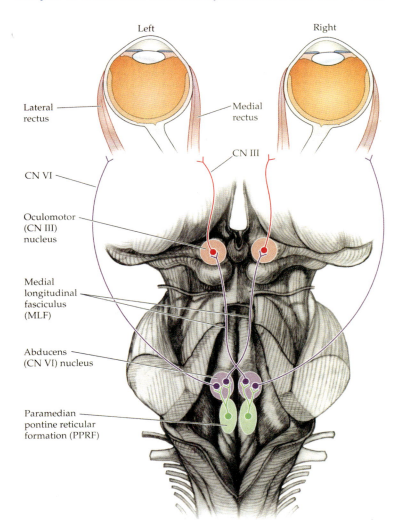

Left

Right

Lateral rectus

Medial rectus

CN III

CN VI

Oculomotor (CN III) nucleus

Medial longitudinal fasciculus (MLF)

Abducens (CN VI) nucleus

Paramedian pontine reticular formation (PPRF)

FIGURE 6-1 Brainstem pathways for control of horizontal eye movements.

Reproduced with permission.[16]

Input from the horizontal semicircular canals, carried by the vestibular nerve (CN V III), to the MVN in the medulla, where they synapse, send an excitatory connection to the contralateral AN and an inhibitory connection to the ipsilateral AN. To generate saccades, signals originate from EBNs in the ipsilateral PPRF rostral to the AN and from contralateral IBNs. Vestibular and optokinetic inputs reach the AN from the MVN in the medulla. Disease affecting the MVN causes an impairment of gaze holding and an inadequately sustained eye position. This disorder result is in a drift of the eyes back from an eccentric position to the central primary position of gaze and corrective quick phases that produce gaze-evoked nystagmus (Chapter 10, Figure 1-16).

All the nuclei projecting to the AN also project to the cell groups of the paramedian tracts (PMT). Scattered in the midline fiber tracts in the pons and medulla, these neurons receive inputs from all structures that project to ocular motoneurons. The PMT neurons also project

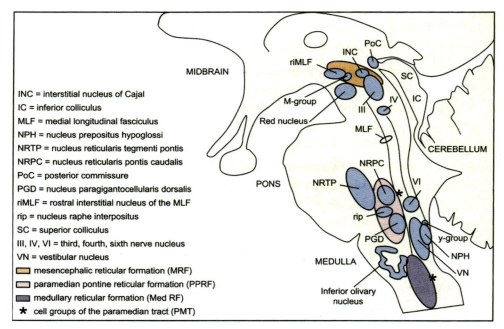

FIGURE 6-2 Pontine nuclei involved in eye movement control.

Reproduced with permission.[18]

to the vestibulocerebellum, enabling the cerebellum to receive feedback and motor signals relayed to the AN.[19,20]

The Medial Longitudinal Fasciculus

The MLF is the major internuclear pathway (CN VI nucleus to CN III nucleus) for axons from the abducens internuclear neurons. These neurons carry horizontal saccade signals to the medial rectus subnucleus in the oculomotor nuclear complex, for contraction of the medial rectus muscle to adduct the eye on lateral gaze.

The MLF contains axons from the vestibular nuclei that carry signals to the rostral interstitial nucleus of the MLF for the vertical vestibulo-ocular reflex (VOR), smooth pursuit, gaze-holding, and the otolith-ocular reflex. The MLF also contains axons that descend to the oculomotor (CN III) and trochlear (CN IV) nuclei, as well as to the interstitial nucleus of Cajal (INC) the neural integrator for vertical gaze.

The ascending tract of Deiters (ATD) carries projections from important position-vestibular-pause (PVP) neurons in the MVN, that encode head velocity and eye position but are silent (pause) during saccades. The PVP neurons appear to change their activity depending on whether the vestibular stimulation is passive, as in steady fixation, or active, as part of a gaze change. Position-vestibular-pause neurons project to the medial rectus subnucleus of the oculomotor nuclear complex. The functional significance of the ATD pathway is not yet clear but may possibly relate to VORs associated with near viewing.

DIAGNOSTIC PONTINE SIGNS

Horizontal Gaze Deviation

Horizontal gaze deviation to the contralateral side may present acutely following an ipsilateral lesion of the PPRF or AN. In these cases ipsilaterally directed saccades and quick phases are small and slow and do not carry the eyes past the midline.

Horizontal Gaze Palsy

Horizontal saccadic gaze palsy suggests a lesion of the PPRF. The examiner should ask the patient to look right and back to center, left and back to center, while noting the speed of the saccade and whether eccentric gaze is complete. The VOR is intact when the eyes can be driven across the midline to the side of the gaze palsy by the oculocephalic (doll's head) maneuver and by ice water calorics (see Case 6-4).

A horizontal global gaze palsy involving saccades, pursuit, and vestibular eye movements localizes to the AN and the oculocephalic reflex is absent.

Worth remembering: the critical importance of the VORs contribution to the evaluation of eye movements in patients with a horizontal gaze palsy (Figure 6-3).

Peripheral Facial Palsy: Bell's Palsy

For diagnostic purposes, it is important to keep in mind the proximity of the nuclei of the trigeminal nerve (CN V), the abducens nerve (CV VI), the facial nerve (CN VII), and the vestibular

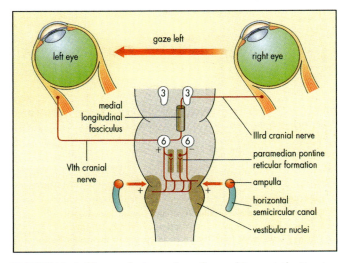

FIGURE 6-3 The vestibulo-ocular reflex and its contribution to ocular movements.

From reference.[21]

nerve (CN VIII), which are all clustered together in the pontine tegmentum. The anatomy of the pons, highlighted in Figure 6-4, helps predict involvement of adjacent nuclei in lesions of the pontine tegmentum[22] (see, notably, Cases 6-3 and 6-4).

Internuclear Ophthalmoplegia

A lesion of the MLF causes an ipsi lateral adduction palsy which is the cardinal sign of internuclear ophthalmoplegia (INO) (see Cases 6-6 and 6-7).

Ocular Bobbing

Ocular bobbing (rhythmic, downward jerks, followed by slow return of the eyes to mid-positon) and it variants can be caused by pontine hemorrhage or infarction, cerebellar hemorrhage compressing the pons and subarachnoid hemorrhage from aneurysms of the posterior circulation (see Case 6-5).

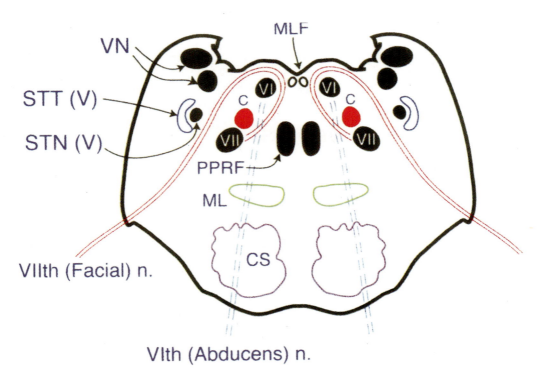

FIGURE 6-4 Diagram of axial section through the pons at the level of the sixth nerve nuclei. VI, sixth nerve; VII, seventh nerve; C, central tegmental tract; CS, corticospinal tract; VN, vestibular nuclei; ML, medial lemniscus; MLF, medial longitudinal fasciculus; PPRF, parapontine reticular formation; STT (V), spinal trigeminal tract of the fifth nerve; STN (V), spinal trigeminal nucleus of the fifth nerve. Note the proximity of the central tegmental tract (C [in red]) to the PPRF.

Reproduced with permission.[22]

CONGENITAL PONTINE SYNDROMES

Möbius Syndrome

A newborn with Möbius syndrome can be identified by facial appearance—congenital facial diplegia, which is the hallmark sign; a high nasal bridge; micrognathia with limited mandibular movement; small mouth; expressionless face; mild ptosis; and a deficit of horizontal gaze. The abducens nerve weakness is almost always bilateral and asymmetrical. The clinical findings correlate with developmental failure or degeneration of the involved cranial nerve nuclei (Figure 6-5).

The syndrome,[23] also known as the Möbius sequence,[24] has been associated with exposure to cocaine or misoprostol in utero.[25,26]

Magnetic resonance imaging (MRI) of Möbius cases has demonstrated brainstem hypoplasia with straightening of the floor of the fourth ventricle, indicating an absence of the facial colliculus.[27] Brainstem calcification is also reported.[28] Several gene foci have been identified, and the nomenclature now refers to Möbius syndromes 1, 2, and 3.[29]

A subset of children with "straight" eyes and absent horizontal gaze use convergence substitution to look to the side. The presence of horizontal gaze palsy rather than bilateral sixth-nerve palsy in these children suggests a primary injury involving the caudal brainstem nuclei.

Autopsy cases implicate at least four modes of developmental pathology: destructive degeneration of brainstem nuclei (the most common type), hypoplasia or absence of central brainstem nuclei, peripheral nerve involvement, and myopathy.[30]

In the case of congenital hypoplasia of the pons presented here the ocular motility signs indicating pontine involvement were missed.

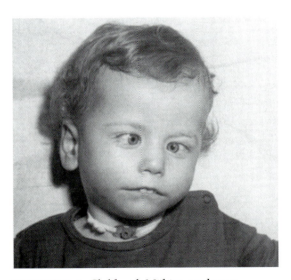

FIGURE 6-5 Child with Möbius syndrome with bilateral weakness of cranial nerves VI and VII. Recurrent swallowing impairment resulted in multiple episodes of pneumonia, which necessitated tracheostomy.

Reproduced with permission.[31]

CASE 6-1 Congenital Horizontal Gaze Palsy and Progressive Scoliosis

Video Display

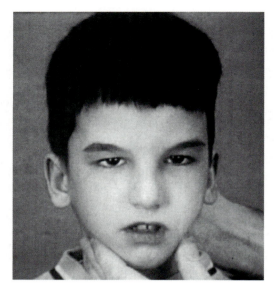

FIGURE 6-6 An eight-year-old boy with absent conjugate horizontal gaze and scoliosis.

The patient is an 8-year-old boy referred in 1976 with a rare autosomal recessive disorder (Figure 6-6) characterized by

- *congenital absence of conjugate horizontal eye movements,*
- *preservation of vertical gaze and convergence,*
- *progressive scoliosis developed in early childhood.*

He had been misdiagnosed as a case of congenital ocular motor apraxia.

CASE 6-1 SYMPTOMS

Symptoms	Location Correlation
Absent horizontal gaze	Paramedian pontine reticular formation
	Abducens nucleus

Analysis of the History

- What are the major presenting symptoms?
- Where are the central nervous system (CNS) lesion(s) likely to be?

Examination

The analysis guides the clinical examination.

Ocular Motility

- Esotropia (nonparalytic) of the left eye (OS)
- Absent conjugate horizontal saccadic, pursuit, and vestibular eye movements
- Normal vertical eye movements
- Normal convergence—he converged his eyes when attempting to look to the right or left side
- Absent optokinetic nystagmus
- No nystagmus or head oscillations

The neurological examination was normal.

Localization and Differential Diagnosis

This boy has signs typical of a congenital pontine syndrome in association with scoliosis: a complete paralysis of horizontal gaze (affecting saccades and pursuit), preservation of convergence, and failure of vestibular stimulation to move the eyes laterally, signifying disruption of the VOR arc at the level of the AN.[32]

Special Explanatory Note

Patients with congenital horizontal gaze palsy may adopt several adaptive strategies to compensate for their handicap. They substitute rapid head movements (head saccades) for eye saccades to change gaze rapidly, or they use their intact vergence system to move both eyes into adduction and then cross-fixate, using the right eye to view objects seen on the left and vice versa, as this boy did (see also Case 8-1, Chapter 8).

What Diagnostic Tests Should Follow?

- Brain MRI
- MRI of the spine

The MRI features in horizontal gaze palsy progressice scoiliosis (HGPPS) were reported in 2002 by Pieh et al.[33] In two affected offspring of consanguineous parents, the imaging showed dysplasia of the brainstem, absence of the facial colliculi, and a deep midline pontine cleft—the split-pons sign—and a butterfly configuration of the medulla.

Jen et al.[34] conducted a genome scan of two unrelated consanguineous families in the same year and mapped an HGPPS gene to a 30-cM region of chromosome 11q 23-q25—ROBO3/11q23.

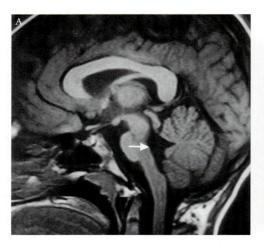
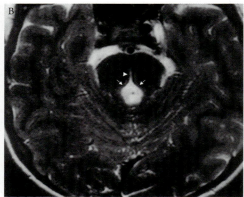

FIGURE 6-7 Brain magnetic resonance imaging (MRI) in a child with horizontal gaze palsy and progressive scoliosis. (A) Sagittal T1 image shows expansion of the floor of the fourth ventricle (*arrow*). The pons and medulla oblongata have a reduced volume. (B) Axial T2 image at the level of the pons shows absence of the facial colliculi, with tent-shaped configuration of the floor of the fourth ventricle (*arrows*). A deep midsagittal cleft extends ventrally from the fourth ventricular floor, producing the split pons sign (*arrowhead*).

Reproduced with permission.[35]

Test Results

Neither brain MRI nor genetic correlation were available when this patient was seen. Neuroimaging in a similar case, a 13-year-old girl with early-onset thoracolumbar scoliosis and associated deformities is shown here (Figure 6-7A–B).[35]

Special Explanatory Note

Neuroimaging studies are critical in this syndrome. All HGPPS patients to date have shown very similar findings of hypoplasia of the pons and cerebellar peduncles, with both anterior and posterior midline clefts of the pons and medulla.

Diffusion tensor imaging and electrophysiological studies have shown ipsilateral corticospinal and dorsal column medial lemniscus tract innervation, indicating defective crossing of some brainstem neuronal pathways,[36] a characteristic of this syndrome.

Genetic studies in HGPPS have led to the identification of mutations in the gene *ROBO3,* which is responsible for neuronal and axonal guidance during development of the brainstem.[37,38] Loss of *ROBO3* function disrupts midline crossing by axons, which accounts for congenital absence of horizontal gaze and may also account for neurogenic progressive scoliosis. Congenital absence of horizontal gaze, progressive scoliosis, and severe dysplasia of the brainstem are the specific markers of this syndrome.

Although they were not present in this case, additional facial and ocular motor signs associated with HGPPS are shown in Table 6-1.

TABLE 6-1: Facial and Ocular Motor Signs Associated with Horizontal Gaze Palsy with Progressive Scoliosis

Horizontal gaze palsy with absent saccadic pursuit and vestibular eye movements
Horizontal, elliptical, or pendular nystagmus
Convergence nystagmus
Head oscillations in the presence of nystagmus
Saccadic vertical pursuit
Intermittent slow blinking of one or both eyes
Retraction of the nonfixing eye during vergence movements
Facial myokymia and spasm
Facial weakness
Absent response to ice-water calorics
Normal forced ductions

ACQUIRED SYNDROMES OF THE PONS

Diseases of the CNS affecting brainstem pathways for horizontal gaze in the pons cause classic ocular motor syndromes (Figure 6-8A–B). Among them paresis of abduction due to an abducens nerve (CNV1) palsy (lesion 1) unilateral horizontal gaze palsy due to disease affecting the

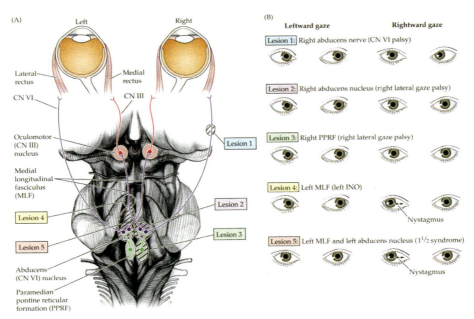

FIGURE 6-8 Effects of lesions in brainstem pathways for horizontal eye movements. (A) Location of lesions. (B) Eye movements during leftward and rightward gaze with lesions shown in (A).

Reproduced with permission.[16]

ipsilateral AN (lesion 2), unilateral horizontal gaze palsy due to a unilateral lesion of the PPRF (lesion 3), internuclear ophthalmoplegia (INO) (lesion 4) an INO plus a horizontal gaze palsy—Fisher's one-and-a-half syndrome (lesion 5), and other oculomotor syndromes including paralytic pontine exotropia, and paralytic pontine esotropia.

Examination of this figure helps clarify the impact of different lesions in the pons on horizontal gaze. It is also worth remembering that ipsilateral horizontal palsy may be due to a single unilateral lesion affecting the ipsilateral

- PPRF only;
- the ipsilateral AN only; both
- the ipsilateral PPRF and the AN.
- If two lesions are the cause, the motoneuron root fibers of the ipsilateral AN to the lateral rectus muscle and the contralateral MLF internuclear fibres to the medial rectus muscle are involved.

Paramedian Pontine Reticular Formation

The signs of a unilateral lesion of the PPRF (Figure 6-9) are:

- A horizontal *saccadic* gaze palsy to the side of the lesion
- Conjugate deviation of the eyes to the contralateral side in the acute stage
- Gaze-evoked nystagmus to the contralateral side with quick phases directed away from the side of the lesion
- Smooth pursuit eye movements with preservation of the VOR[39,40]

The eyes can be driven to the side of the gaze palsy by turning the head rapidly from side to side (doll's head maneuver) to stimulate the oculocephalic reflex[41] and/or by ice water calorics.

The signs of pontine involvement in the case presented here are unmistakeable and their significance extreme.

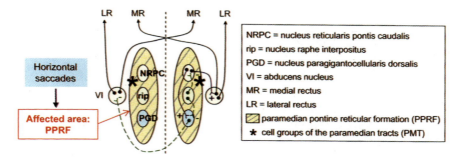

FIGURE 6-9 Lesions in the paramedian pontine reticular formation.

Reproduced with permission.[18]

CASE 6-2 Bilateral Sixth-Nerve Palsy: Pontine Glioma

Video Display

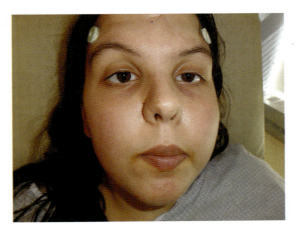

FIGURE 6-10 Young woman with bilateral esotropia.

The patient is a 21-year-old pregnant woman who first noted a sensation that she was about to fall (dizziness), headache, and unilateral facial numbness at the end of December when her delivery was 1-week overdue (Figure 6-10). Her father recalled that she complained of light-headedness and a sensation that she was spinning in the room (vertigo). She had gone to the ER of her local hospital on several earlier occasions, had been treated for dehydration and sent home. Her vertigo persisted, and she developed an unsteady gait.

The patient delivered a healthy baby on January 6, 2012 and was reevaluated at her local hospital on January 11, at which time she was using a walker for fear of falling. A brain MRI showed a brainstem lesion. She was discharged home with home physiotherapy on January 20. She fell, however, while stepping unsteadily out of the shower (mechanical fall, no head trauma, no loss of consciousness) and was hospitalized on January 24. A follow-up MRI showed a persistent abnormality, and she was transferred to the Massachusetts General Hospital.

On admission, she had

- *generalized headache,*
- *vertigo described as a persistent sensation of herself spinning anti-clockwise and being pulled to the left,*
- *numbness of her left face,*
- *clumsiness of the left arm and leg.*

Analysis of the History

· What are the major presenting symptoms?
· Where are the CNS lesion(s) likely to be?

CASE 6-2 SYMPTOMS

Symptoms	Location Correlation
Vertigo (anti-clockwise rotation)	Vestibular system
Numbness of the left side of her face	Trigeminal nucleus or nerve CN V
Clumsiness of the left arm and leg	Cerebellum or cerebellar pathways
Unsteady gait	

The analysis guides the clinical examination.

Examination

Neurological

· Afebrile and fully oriented
· No nuchal rigidity
· No papilledema
· Pupils 3 mm OU—brisk to light and near
· No pronator drift with 5/5 motor strength throughout
· Symmetric hyperreflexia with extensor plantar responses
· Incoordination left finger-nose and heel-knee-shin and gait ataxia
· Impaired light touch and pain sensation left face

Ocular Motility

· Esotropia OU
· Spontaneous upbeat nystagmus
· Bilateral horizontal gaze weakness with oblique gaze-evoked nystagmus (horizontal and downbeat)
· Full upgaze with upbeat nystagmus
· Full downgaze with downbeat nystagmus
· Saccadic pursuit in all directions
· Horizontal saccades overshoot (hypermetria) right gaze to center, left gaze to center
· Normal convergence

Localization and Differential Diagnosis

Headache, vertigo, bilateral horizontal gaze palsy and unilateral facial numbness, localize to the pons and pontomedullary junction. Downbeat nystagmus, saccadic hypermetria and gait/limb ataxia localize to the cerebellum or cerebellar pathways. This constellation of symptoms and signs, despite the absence of papilledema, suggest a lesion of the pons and obstructive hydrocephalus.

What Diagnostic Tests Should Follow?

· Brain MRI to look for a brainstem lesion and/or obstructive hydrocephalus

Test Results

Brain MRI with and without contrast showed a T2 hyperintense expansile lesion predominantly within the right mid pons extending into the middle cerebrallar peduncles greater on the right, superiorly into the right midbrain and caudally to the pontine-medullary junction (Figure 6-11A–C).

The studies also showed:

· Narrowing of the distal cerebral aqueduct and fourth ventricle without evidence of hydrocephalus
· No herniation
· Narrowing of the prepontine cistern without compression of the basilar artery

What Is the Differential Diagnosis in This Case?

The differential diagnosis rests between acute disseminated encephalomyelitis (ADEM) and pontine glioma. Acute disseminated encephalomyelitis is a CNS white matter disorder that can present as a solitary mass lesion of the pons but usually does not enlarge the brainstem.[42] Empirical treatment with steroids may resolve or shrink the lesion.

Treatment

With this possibility in mind, the patient received IV methylprednisolone 1 g/day for 5 days prior to consideration of a brain biopsy, knowing that a delay in diagnosis of less than a week would have no impact on her overall prognosis if a pontine glioma turned out to be the diagnosis. On completion of the course of steroids, there was no change in the patient's symptoms and signs, and no change in the imaging features of the brainstem mass.

Is a Brain Biopsy Indicated?

The MRI appearance of a typical pontine glioma—a characteristic T1 nonenhancing diffuse mass expanding the brainstem—has caused opinion to change on diagnostic

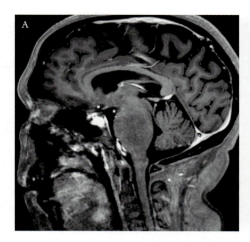
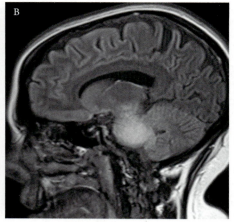
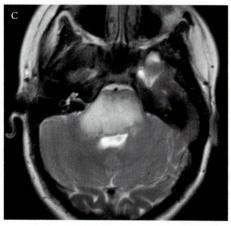

FIGURE 6-11 Magnetic resonance imaging (MRI) of the brain. (A) Sagittal T1 post contrast image shows extension of a pontine mass into the superior medulla and inferior midbrain with effacement of the prepontine cistern. (B) Sagittal fluid-attenuated inversion recovery (FLAIR) image shows hyperintense expansile lesion within the right mid pons extending into the middle cerebellar peduncle. (C) Axial T2 image shows the hyperintense lesion extending into the cerebellar peduncles and partially effacing the fourth ventricle.

biopsies since there is little evidence that a biopsy yields information that alters therapy.[43] Nevertheless a biopsy was performed in this case.

Biopsy Results

Biopsy of the nodular cerebellar portion was sampled successfully through a computed tomography (CT)-guided stereotactic VarioGuide needle through a single burr hole in the right suboccipital region. Pathology showed a highly pleomorphic, densely cellular, and mitotically active malignant brainstem glioma.

Diagnosis: Pontine Glioma

Treatment

· Surgery
· Radiation therapy

Radical surgical removal of a brainstem glioma is not feasible. Radiation therapy is the treatment of choice because it offers initial relief of symptoms associated with the rapid progression of this disease, and may allow survival for 12–15 months. Adding chemotherapy has provided little long-term benefit.

The patient received radiation therapy as an outpatient and tolerated it well.

The Abducens Nucleus

Unilateral lesions of the AN produce

- An *ipsilateral lateral rectus palsy* (due to involvement of the lateral rectus motoneurons), An *ipsilateral conjugate horizontal gaze palsy* involving saccades, pursuit, and the VOR to the same side (due to involvement of the abducens internuclear neurons, which activate the subnucleus of the contralateral medial rectus muscle) (Figure 6-12).
- Vergence is spared.
- The horizontal oculocephalic reflex is absent.[44–46]

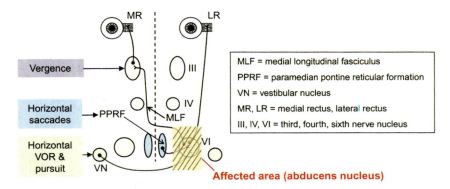

FIGURE 6-12 Lesions of the abducens nucleus.

Reproduced with permission.[18]

CASE 6-3 Unilateral Horizontal Gaze Palsy and Peripheral Facial Weakness

Video Display

The patient is a 56-year-old woman who was treated for adenocarcinoma of the breast 2 years before she developed horizontal diplopia, deviation of her left eye inward and facial weakness (Figure 6-13A–B). Her oncologist referred her for a neuro-ophthalmic evaluation.

Analysis of the History

- What are the major presenting symptoms?
- Where are the CNS lesion(s) likely to be?

CASE 6-3 SYMPTOMS

Symptoms	Location Correlation
Horizontal diplopia	Lateral rectus muscle
Esotropia	Abducens nerve

The analysis guides the clinical examination.

Examination

Ocular Motility

- Left peripheral facial weakness (Bell's palsy)
- Esotropia of the left eye (OS)
- Horizontal saccadic and pursuit gaze palsy to the left
- Normal horizontal gaze to the right with gaze-evoked nystagmus
- Full vertical eye movements
- Horizontal oculocephalic reflex, absent abduction OS
- Normal convergence, right eye induced to cross the midline

The neurological examination was normal.

Localization and Differential Diagnosis

Horizontal gaze palsy involving saccades, pursuit, and vestibular eye movements localizes to the AN in the pons (Figure 6-13C–D), esotropia to a fascicular abducens (CN VI) nerve palsy (Figure 6-13C), intact convergence (Figure 6-13E) and an ipsilateral peripheral facial palsy to involvement of the genu of the facial nerve (CN VII) (see Figure 6-4).

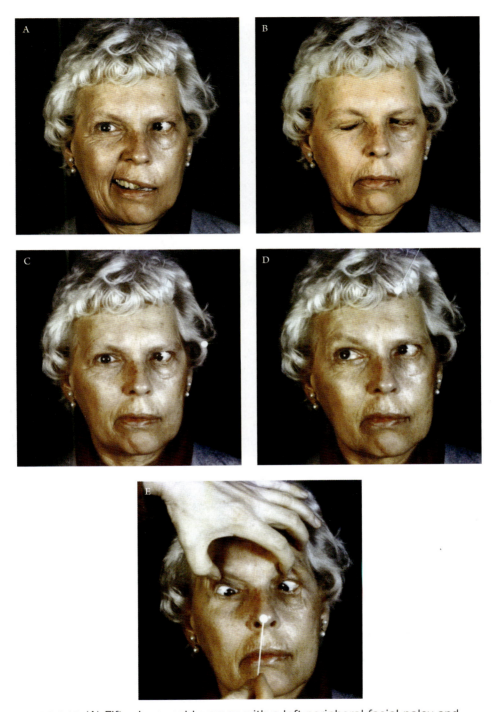

FIGURE 6-13 (A) Fifty-six-year-old woman with a left peripheral facial palsy and inability to retract the angle of the mouth. (B) Inability to close the left eye. (C) Left esotropia: fascicular sixth-nerve palsy and a left horizontal gaze palsy on attempted left gaze to a white headed pin. (D) Full horizontal gaze looking right. (E) Convergence movements induce the right eye to cross the midline to converge.

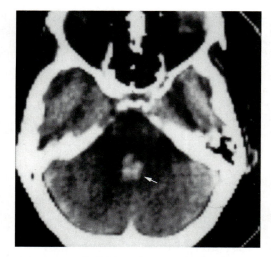

FIGURE 6-14 Axial head computerised tomography (CT) shows hemorrhage in the fourth ventricle (*arrow*).

What Tests Should Follow?

· Brain CT
· Bone scan

Test Results

A head CT showed a hemorrhage in the fourth ventricle (Figure 6-14). A bone scan was positive for multiple metastases.

Treatment

· Oncology consultation/chemotherapy

The patient was advised of the findings and elected no further therapy. She was followed for several months and wished to donate her body to enable clinicopathological correlation of the brainstem lesion with the CT images. Her family withheld their permission when she died.

Special Explanatory Note

Vergence is spared in lesions of the AN because vergence commands are sent from vergence neurons directly to the medial rectus motoneurons in the oculomotor nucleus without passing through the AN or the MLF.

Horizontal gaze nystagmus directed to the intact contralateral side, with quick phases directed away from the side of the lesion, may be due to interruption either of fibers in passage from the MVN that provide an eye position signal to the contralateral AN or to interruption of fibers from cell groups of the PMT, which lie at the rostral end of the AN.

CASE 6-4 Right Horizontal Gaze Palsy, Internuclear Ophthalmoplegia, and Unilateral Numbness of the Face

Video Display

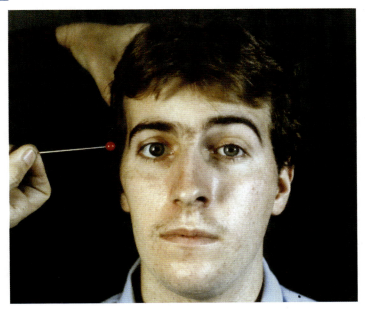

FIGURE 6-15 Young man with a right horizontal conjugate gaze palsy and internuclear ophthalmoplegia.

The patient is a 19-year-old sophomore who presented in 1983 with numbness of the left hand, involving initially just the fingers, and numbness and weakness of the right side of the face. He described the numbness in his hand as "intensely asleep." The facial numbness involved the perioral region.

Over the next 5 days prior to admission (PTA), the numbness spread to the entire left side of his body and extended over a greater area of the right face to involve the cheek and right side of his tongue.

One day PTA, he developed a right peripheral facial palsy, mild occipital headache, and unsteadiness standing and walking. He was admitted to a local hospital. The brain scan revealed a mass in the region of the fourth ventricle that was thought to represent a brain tumor. He was transferred to the Massachusetts General Hospital.

Analysis of the History

· What are the major presenting symptoms?
· Where are the CNS lesion(s) likely to be?

CASE 6-4 SYMPTOMS

Symptoms	Location Correlation
Right facial numbness	Trigeminal nerve nucleus or CN V
Right peripheral facial weakness	Facial nerve CN VII
Left hemisensory loss	Pons/medulla

The analysis guides the clinical examination.

Examination

Neurological

- Alert, oriented ×3
- Normal speech
- Pupils equal and briskly reactive to light and near
- Right hemifacial concentric perioral numbness/paresthesia
- Right peripheral facial weakness
- Motor strength: mild left pronator drift, 4/5 throughout
    Left ataxic hemiparesis
    Symmetric 2+ reflexes with flexor plantar responses

Ocular Motility

- Right horizontal gaze palsy (saccades, pursuit, and vestibular eye movements)
- Right internuclear ophthalmoplegia on gaze left[1]
- Clockwise rotary gaze-evoked nystagmus on gaze right
- Normal convergence
- Full vertical eye movements
- Horizontal oculocephalic reflex failed to drive the eyes across the midline to the right

[1] Fisher's one-and-a half syndrome (see later section for discussion).

Localization and Differential Diagnosis

Ataxic hemiparesis is a classic pontine syndrome usually diagnosed as lacunar infarction during the pre-CT era and often found in patients with paramedian infarcts.

Right hemifacial sensory loss (CN V nucleus) ipsilateral INO and horizontal gaze palsy—Fisher's one-and-a-half-syndrome, absent oculocephalic reflex (abducens nucleus), and peripheral facial palsy (CN VII fasciculus) localize to the ipsilateral pontine tegmentum (Figure 6-15).

What Diagnostic Tests Should Follow?

· Head CT (MRI not available)
· Vertebral angiogram

Test Result

Head CT showed a right pontomedullary hemorrhage. Vertebral angiogram showed no evidence of a vascular malformation.

Treatment

· Surgery to drain the hemorrhage

A suboccipital craniectomy was performed to drain the hemorrhage.

Postoperatively, only the ataxic hemiplegia recovered.

Between 1983 and 1988, the patient had three further bleeds. He was readmitted in 1988 with progressive ataxia of the left extremities. Brain MRI, T1 and T2 images in the axial and sagittal plane showed a hyperintense lesion in the pons with slight extension into the inferior aspect of the midbrain on the right side consistent with hemorrhage into a cavernous angioma (Figure 6-16A–B).

The bleeds were attributed to venous seepage of blood and not to arterial bleeding.

Treatment

Focal proton beam therapy was recommended. The patient received a total dose of 1,700 rads delivered by two portals, one on each side of the head. Despite radiation treatment, he continued to have recurrent bleeds and, after his 11th bleed in 1999, he developed bilateral horizontal gaze palsy and pendular vertical oscillations without a palatal tremor.

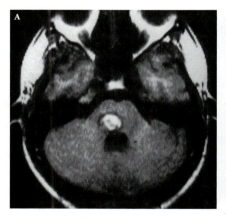 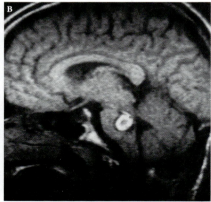

FIGURE 6-16 Magnetic resonance imaging (MRI) of the brain. (A) Axial T1 image and (B) Sagittal T1 image show a hyperintense lesion (methemoglobin) in the pons consistent with hemorrhage into a cavernous angioma.

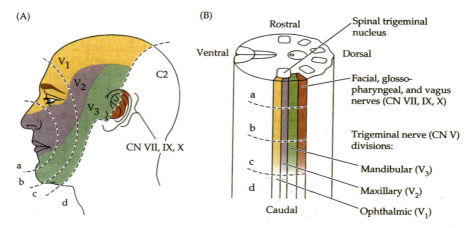

FIGURE 6-17 Somatotopic maps of the spinal trigeminal nucleus. (A) Concentric regions (a–d) emanating from the mouth are indicated as they correspond with rostral to caudal regions of the spinal trigeminal nucleus. (B) Regions of spinal trigeminal tract supplying each trigeminal nerve division, as well as CN VII, IX, and X. In addition, rostral to caudal regions of the nucleus and tract (a–d) are indicated, corresponding to the concentric regions shown in (A).

Reproduced with permission.[16]

Special Explanatory Note

This patient had an extensive lesion in the pontine tegmentum affecting the spinal nucleus of the trigeminal nerve (CN V) causing concentric facial sensory loss, and also affecting the AN (CN VI), PPRF, MLF and the fascicles of the facial nerve CN VII.

A somatotopic map of the spinal trigeminal nucleus (Figure 6-17A–B) shows clearly the anatomy of concentric rings of sensory loss (formed like a slice of onion) radiating from the perioral area represented rostrally in the spinal CN V nucleus, with areas farther from the mouth represented more caudally (Figure 6-17A).

Regions of the spinal trigeminal tract supplying each trigeminal nerve division as well as CN VII, IX and X are also illustrated. The mandibular division (V3) is represented dorsally, the ophthalmic division (V1) is represented ventrally, and the maxillary division (V2) lies in between (Figure 6-17B).

CASE 6-5 Bilateral Horizontal Gaze Palsy: Pontine Infarction

Video Display

The patient is a 73-year-old woman with known bipolar disease and hyperthyroidism who presented with sudden onset of nausea and vomiting in the early hours of the morning on the day of admission. She vomited approximately 10 times during the night. She got up at 8 A.M. to go downstairs to feed her dog. She felt woozy and needed to hold onto the banister rail. She collapsed when she walked into the kitchen but did not lose consciousness.

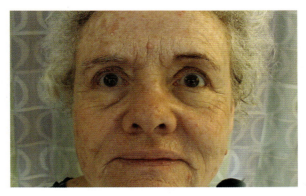

FIGURE 6-18 Elderly woman with bilateral horizontal gaze palsy.

Her vision was blurred, and she had difficulty seeing the numbers on her cell phone. About 20 minutes later, friends came and found her on the floor. She complained of double vision, dizziness, and fatigue. She was taken to Nantucket Hospital, where she was found to have hypertension, tachycardia, vertical nystagmus, and eyes fixed in the midline (Figure 6-18).

Head CT showed no infarct or hemorrhage, and her lab studies were unremarkable. She received intravenous (IV) thiamine and normal saline and was transferred to the Massachusetts General Hospital. On admission, she was reported by the Stroke Team to have ocular bobbing with the fast phase down. Symptomatic inquiry was negative for headache, deafness, neck pain, tinnitus, spinning vertigo, impaired swallowing, and weakness of the limbs.

Analysis of the History

- What are the major presenting symptoms?
- Where are the CNS lesion(s) likely to be

CASE 6-5 SYMPTOMS

Symptoms	Location Correlation
Dizziness	
Vertical nystagmus	Vestibular pathways
Ocular bobbing	Pons

The analysis guides the clinical examination.

Examination

Neurological

- Fully alert, oriented, and attentive
- Normal speech

- Memory 3/3, registration 2/3, recall at 5 minutes
- No facial weakness
- Motor strength 5/5 throughout; symmetric 2+ reflexes with flexor plantar responses
- Coordination: mild tremor at rest bilaterally aggravated by elevating the arms
- Sensory system: intact apart from mild decreased vibration sense at the ankle

Ocular Motility Examination on Day 4

- Bilateral horizontal saccadic and pursuit gaze palsy with <3–4 degrees of movement past the midline to either side
- Slow saccadic upgaze without nystagmus
- Normal saccadic downgaze
- Normal convergence
- Saccadic vertical pursuit
- No skew deviation
- Absent horizontal oculocephalic reflex
- Normal vertical oculocephalic reflex

Localization and Differential Diagnosis

This patient's signs are difficult to localize. Bilateral horizontal global gaze palsy (with no facial weakness) and absent oculocephalic reflex should indicate involvement of the PPRF and adjacent pathways.

What Diagnostic Tests Should Follow?

The caloric test evaluates the VOR[47] by introducing warm or cold water into the external auditory meatus. Warm water introduced into the external auditory meatus warms the endolymph and stimulates the horizontal semicircular canal, causing the eyes to move slowly away from the irrigated meatus. Normally, the eyes will move quickly back to the irrigated side, producing a fast phase of a caloric-evoked nystagmus toward the *same* (ipsilateral) side as the warm water stimulus.

Introduction of cold (ice) water into an external auditory meatus cools the endolymph and mimics a lesion. The horizontal semicircular canal is inhibited on the cold water side. The opposite vestibular complex causes the eyes to move slowly toward the irrigated ear and horizontal nystagmus (quick phase) beating toward the *opposite* (contralateral) ear.

Test Results

Irrigation of the right ear showed the following:

- A very delayed latency to the onset of deviation of the eyes toward the irrigated ear.
- Eyes became dysconjugate—the right eye deviated fully to the right (abducted), the left eye remained essentially in primary gaze and adducted only 5 degrees.
- No nystagmus.
- Tonic dysconjugate gaze deviation was prolonged, with the right eye returning slowly to primary gaze (Figure 6-19A).

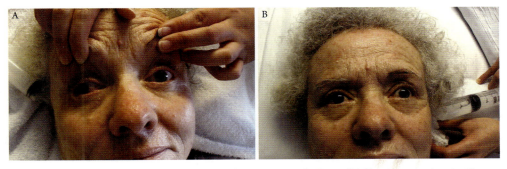

FIGURE 6-19 The patient's response to ice-water calorics. (A) Post ice-water in the right ear, eyes dysconjugate, full abduction right eye, impaired adduction left eye. (B) Post ice-water in the left ear, no deviation of the eyes, absent vestibulo-ocular reflex.

Irrigation of the left ear showed the following:

· No conjugate deviation of the eyes to the side of the irrigated ear
· No nystagmus (Figure 6-19B)

What specifically can ice-water calorics tell us?[48] The test may show:

· *Normal response.* Tonic conjugate deviation of the eyes toward the cold stimulus and nystagmus quick phases toward the contralateral ear.
· Impaired abduction suggesting a sixth-nerve palsy.
· Impaired adduction implying either an INO or a third-nerve palsy.
· Occasionally, there is an impaired response in patients with metabolic obtundation or drug intoxication (in barbiturate coma, eyes may deviate downward).
· In brain death, no response.

The patient was extremely cooperative and allowed us to repeat the test the next day to confirm the findings of a left horizontal gaze palsy and paresis of adduction of the left eye consistent with a left INO.

The combination of a left horizontal gaze palsy and a left INO is termed *a one-and-a-half syndrome* (see next section).

What Diagnostic Tests Should Follow?

· Brain MRI

Test Results

Brain MRI DWI showed restricted diffusion represented by hypersdensity in the posterior central pns bilaterally in the floor of the fourth venricle, consistent with bilateral infarcts 12 hours to 2 weeks in age.

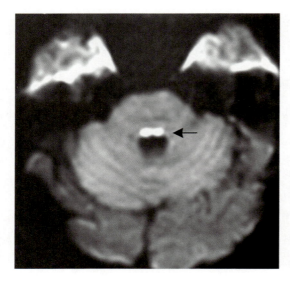

FIGURE 6-20 Magnetic resonance imaging (MRI) of the brain. Axial DWI image shows restricted diffusion represented by hyperintensity (*arrow*) in the posterior central pons bilaterally in the floor of the fourth ventricle consistent with bilateral infarcts.

The presence of infarction involving both sides of the pontine tegmentum in the floor of the fourth ventricle can be explained by Fisher's observation that one perforating paramedian tegmental artery bifurcates into terminal branches at the level of the abducens nuclei, thereby supplying both sides of the paramedian pontine tegmentum[49] (analogous to the artery of Percheron supplying both sides of the ventral midbrain).

Treatment

· Blood pressure control
· A "baby" asprin daily

■ **Clinical Points to Remember About Caloric Testing with Ice Water**

- Inspect the tympanic membrane with an auriscope.
- Keep in mind that caloric stimulation is a test of horizontal canal (HC) function.
- Position the patient so that the HCs are oriented vertically to maximize the effect of gravity on the endolymph—about 30 degrees up from the supine position.
- With the patient's eyes open (elevate the eyelids in obtunded patients), irrigate each ear by inserting a small suction catheter into the external auditory canal, connecting it to a 50 mL syringe filled with ice water.
- Irrigate the ear and watch for horizontal deviation of the eyes to the side of the stimulation and nystagmus with the fast phase toward the contralateral ear—which typically begins just before the end of stimulation, reaches a peak approximately 60 seconds post stimulation, and then slowly decays.
- Wait a minimum of 5 minutes from the end of one response to the next stimulation to avoid additive effects.

- In the absence of a response, repeat the irrigation of the ear with a second 50 mL bolus of ice water.
- For a brief period during the test, fixation can be permitted so as to evaluate the suppression of nystagmus by fixation.[50,51]
- Patients generally tolerate this test well. ■

In comatose patients, caloric irrigation with ice water is used to test whether the brainstem is intact (Chapter 1). Comatose patients with loss of brainstem function have no quick phases, and consequently there is no nystagmus, only a tonic drift of the eyes toward the irrigated ear. However, if the brainstem is intact, patients in a persistent vegetative state due to severe damage to the cerebral hemispheres will have nystagmus with caloric stimulation.

Ocular Bobbing

Ocular bobbing,[52] a transient feature in the acute stage of the patient's stroke in Case 6-5, is a classic sign of an intrinsic pontine lesion, usually hemorrhage. It consists of intermittent, brisk conjugate downward movements of the eyes through an arc of a few mm followed by a slow return to primary position.

Ocular bobbing has also been reported with cerebellar lesions. Figure 6-21A shows the MRI of a patient who developed ocular bobbing due to acute hemorrhagic infarction of the cerebellum with swelling that compressed the pons. Figure 6-21B shows the waveforms and names used for variants of ocular bobbing.[53]

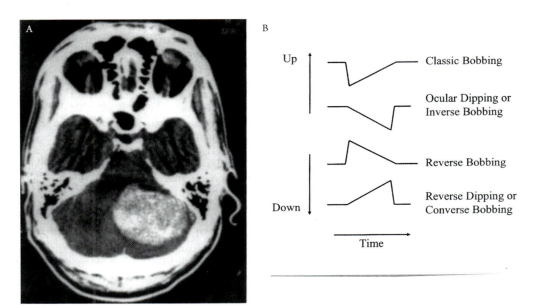

FIGURE 6-21 (A) Magnetic resonance imaging of a patient who developed ocular bobbing, showing acute hemorrhagic infarction of the cerebellum with swelling that compressed the pons. (B) Waveforms and names used for variants of ocular bobbing.

Reproduced with permission.[53]

Although a range of disorders is associated with ocular bobbing,[54-60] its variants are less reliable for localization. Two are worth noting:

- *Reverse ocular bobbing,*[61] which consists of rapid deviation of the eyes upward and a slow return to the horizontal. It is associated with metabolic disorders such as hepatic encephalopathy.
- *Reverse ocular dipping,*[62] which consists of a slow upward drift of the eyes followed by a rapid return to central position. It is associated with pontine infarction and with AIDS.

Neither of these variants can as yet be precisely localized. Notably, patients may develop more than one type of bobbing during the course of their illness, and this suggests a common underlying pathophysiology.[63]

Ping-pong gaze, which is not a bobbing variant, is an extremely rare condition, and the affected patient is usually obtunded.[64] The eye movement consists of slow horizontal, conjugate deviation of the eyes alternating every few seconds. It occurs with bilateral infarction of the cerebral hemispheres or of the cerebral peduncles, and it has also been attributed to diffuse cerebral ischemia following cardiac surgery.[65]

Transient horizontal oscillations with a periodicity similar to ping-pong gaze may be induced in patients with bilateral hemispheric lesions by rapid horizontal head rotation, and a transient saccadic form may occur in a persistent vegetative state.[66]

Periodic alternating gaze deviation, in which gaze deviations change direction every 2 minutes, has been reported in hepatic coma.[67]

Medial Longitudinal Fasciculus

Lesions of the MLF between the AN and the oculomotor nucleus interrupt the input from the internuclear neurons (in AN) to the medial rectus subnucleus (CN III) to activate the medial rectus muscle (Figure 6-22).

This classic neurologic syndrome is called an *internuclear ophthalmoplegia.* The side of the INO is the side of the lesion in the MLF, and the side on which the ipsilateral eye shows paralysis of adduction for all conjugate eye movements, usually (but not always) with preservation of convergence and with horizontal nystagmus in the contralateral eye when this eye is in abduction. When damage to the MLF is partial, adduction paralysis is replaced during the recovery phase by an impaired adductive saccade; that is to say, with a clear slowing of adduction from eccentric gaze laterally.[68]

During the recovery phase, nystagmus often affects both eyes but remains predominant in amplitude in the contralateral eye (which is in abduction), resulting in *dissociated nystagmus.*

Bilateral INO is common because the two MLFs are in close proximity in the dorsal pontine tegmentum as they ascend to the midbrain. Convergence may be affected in bilateral INO, after midbrain as well as pontine lesions, usually resulting in the so-called *wall-eyed bilateral INO* (WEBINO) syndrome, in which the pathophysiological mechanism of convergence impairment is not yet well understood. The pathophysiology of the abduction nystagmus observed in INO also remains unclear. It is postulated that an adaptive mechanism involving quick phases could account for this nystagmus, reflecting the brain's attempt to compensate for the adduction weakness.

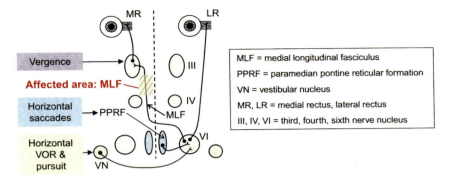

FIGURE 6-22 Lesions of the medial longitudinal fasciculus: internuclear ophthalmoplegia.

Reproduced with permission.[18]

Unilateral INO is often accompanied by skew deviation, with hypertropia on the side of the lesion. Skew deviation, a supranuclear vertical misalignment of the eyes, is due to damage to the central otolithic pathway passing within or close to the MLF. Vertical (gaze-evoked) nystagmus is common in bilateral INO, resulting from damage to the vestibulo-ocular motor pathways passing through the MLF.

The etiology of INO is a study in itself. Infarction of the MLF is the commonest cause of a unilateral INO, and multiple sclerosis (MS) is the commonest cause of a bilateral INO.[69] However, there is an extensive list of causes that should include postradiation demyelination,[70] AIDS,[71,72] carcinomatous infiltration,[73] remote effect of occult malignancy,[74] and head trauma.[75-77] A large number of unusual cases have been reported by Keane[78] and others.[79,80]

CASE 6-6 Bilateral Internuclear Ophthalmoplegia

Video Display

The patient is a 25-year-old woman (Figure 6-23) who was in excellent health until 4 days PTA in 1970 when she noted blurred vision and horizontal double vision on lateral gaze to right and left. Past history was negative for strabismus as a child, prism glasses, trauma, or previous episodes of transient neurological symptoms. Family history was negative for neurological diseases.

The diplopia history revealed that she had:

- A single image with one eye covered
- No diplopia in primary gaze
- No diplopia reading
- Images side-by-side

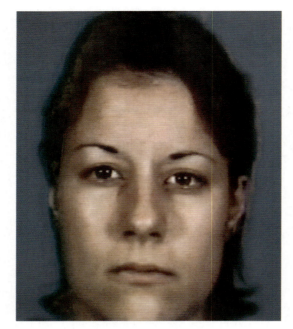

FIGURE 6-23 A twenty-five-year-old woman with multiple sclerosis.

- No drooping of the eyelids
- No eye pain or headache
- No past history of diplopia, ptosis, or muscle fatigue
- On no medications

Analysis of the History

- What are the major presenting symptoms?
- Where are the CNS lesion(s) likely to be?

CASE 6-6 SYMPTOMS

Symptoms	Location Correlation
Horizontal diplopia on lateral gaze	Medial rectus
	Lateral rectus

The analysis guides the clinical examination.

Examination

Ocular Motility

- Visual acuity 20/20 OU
- Visual fields, pupils, and fundus examination normal
- Paresis of adduction of the right eye on gaze left
- Abducting nystagmus of the left eye on gaze left
- Paresis of adduction of the left eye on gaze right
- Abducting nystagmus of the right eye on gaze right
- Normal convergence
- Upbeat nystagmus on upgaze
- Downbeat nystagmus on downgaze

The neurological examination was normal.

Localization and Differential Diagnosis

Bilateral INO with normal convergence localizes to a lesion of the MLF at the pontine or midbrain level. Because vergence disorders with INO are so variable, they preclude accurate localization based on absent or preserved convergence. In a young adult with no history of recent trauma or risk factors for stroke, a demyelinating lesion of the MLF is the first etiology to suspect.

What Diagnostic Tests Should Follow?

- Brain MRI (was not available at the time)
- Spinal tap

The patient declined a spinal tap.

Multiple sclerosis was the suspected diagnosis in this case, and it was discussed with the patient and her parents.

Brain MRI should be the first test performed to evaluate a patient with bilateral ION and suspected MS, always bearing in mind that additional clinically silent white matter demyelinating plaques may be detected and add support to the diagnosis of MS in addition to ruling out other brainstem diseases that can cause an INO, for example a cavernous angioma (Case 6-4). The patient was followed over the next several weeks. She recovered full eye movements within 8 weeks, consistent with a diagnosis of MS. Based on the natural history of MS at that time, she had a risk of converting to clinical MS within 2 years.

> ■ **Clinical Points to Remember About INO**
>
> - Internuclear ophthalmoplegia is due to a lesion of the MLF.
> - It is characterized by weakness of adduction (medial rectus muscle) and abducting nystagmus in the contralateral eye on lateral gaze.
> - Paresis of adduction on conjugate lateral gaze is ipsilateral to a lesion of the MLF after the MLF crosses the midline caudally in the pons.
> - The adduction deficit is frequently manifested as slowing of adduction saccades—an "adduction lag" best observed in horizontal saccades from full gaze right to full gaze left.
> - Convergence may be preserved because vergence inputs to the oculomotor nucleus bypass the MLF. In acute INO, an increase in accommodative vergence may cause an esophoria,[81] and, in bilateral INO, an exophoria, which is referred to as WEBINO.[82] The exophoria does not necessarily involve loss of vergence.
> - In the abducting eye, abducting saccades are hypometric with centripetal drifts of the eye and abducting nystagmus due to impaired ability to inhibit the affected medial rectus.
> - Dissociated vertical nystagmus caused by interruption of pathways mediating the vertical VOR may result in downbeat nystagmus with a greater torsional component in the eye contralateral to a unilateral INO.
> - Skew deviation (commonly seen in unilateral INO) is due to interruption of central projections in the otolith pathway ascending in the MLF to the midbrain. The higher eye (hypertropia) is usually on the side of the MLF lesion.
> - Small-amplitude saccadic intrusions may interrupt fixation.
> - The so-called *posterior INO of Lutz*, in which abduction (but not adduction) is impaired during saccades and pursuit (but not during ice water caloric vestibular stimulation) is rare.[83] ■

CASE 6-7 Internuclear Ophthalmoplegia in Childhood

Video Display

This patient is a 4.5-year-old boy whose parents noticed that his right eye had been drifting for 4 months. He was referred to the clinic for evaluation.

On examination, his pediatrician noted:

- Paresis of adduction of the right eye on gaze left
- Abducting nystagmus of the left eye
- Paresis of adduction of the left eye on gaze right
- Abducting nystagmus of the right eye
- Normal convergence
- Full vertical up and downgaze (Figure 6-24A–C)

The neurological examination was normal.

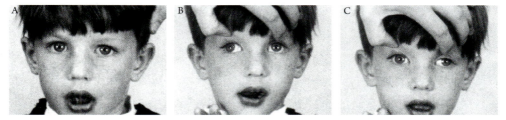

FIGURE 6-24 A child, aged 4.5 years, with bilateral internuclear ophthalmoplegia. (A) In primary gaze. (B) On gaze right, left adduction weakness. (C) On gaze left, right adduction weakness.

Imaging Studies

- This case pre-dated the arrival of CT and MRI.
- It is a rare and instructive case diagnosed by plain skull xrays and by pneumo-encephalography (PEG).

Skull x-rays revealed widening of the suture lines suggestive of chronic increased intra-cranial pressure (despite the absence of papilledema). Pneumoencephalography failed to fill the ventricular system Gas and pantopaque ventriculography disclosed symmetri-cal enlargement of the lateral ventricles, an expanded third ventricle, a dilation of the anterior end of the fourth ventricle, and a block at the posterior end of the aqueduct (i.e., obstructive hydrocephalus) (Figure 6-25A–B).

Treatment

A posterior fossa craniotomy revealed an inoperable tumor arising from the anterior floor of the fourth ventricle, and a biopsy of the tumor was positive for a medulloblas-toma. A ventriculo-peritoneal shunt was placed.

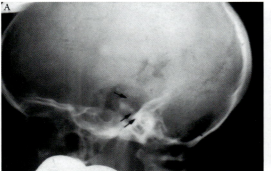
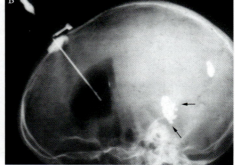

FIGURE 6-25 (A) Pneumoencephalogram shows blockage of the cerebral aqueduct (*arrows*). (B) Pantopaque ventriculography shows enlargement of the third ventricle (*arrows*) and hydrocephalus.

Reproduced with permission.[84]

The boy received radiation therapy with a total dose of 5,000 rads to the area of the mass. The spine was irradiated with 2,500 rads as a precautionary measure because of the statistical frequency of spinal seeding.

Prognosis

Follow-up 11 months later showed no change in the eye movements. He had only mild ataxia. The patient was lost to follow-up.

Special Explanatory Note

This case was responsible for a retrospective study of childhood INO in six children—three boys and three girls aged, 4.5, 7.5, 9.5, 10, 16, and 17 years.[84] The presence of INO in childhood indicated malignant disease, and 4 of the 6 children reported died, 2 from glioma, and 2 from medulloblastoma.

The One-and-a-Half Syndrome

Internuclear ophthalmoplegia is a confirmed component of the *one-and-a half syndrome*, described by Fisher in 1967 in a 79-year-old woman with a right hemiplegia and abnormal horizontal eye movements.[85] Her left eye did not move to the right past the midline. The right eye was exotropic (deviated to the right—the side of the hemiplegia) but able to be moved toward the left. Two days later, the patient deteriorated, and the left eye became fixed in a central position and did not move or develop nystagmus with ice-water irrigation of either ear canal. On head rotation and ice-water irrigation of the right ear, the right eye abducted but no other ocular movement occurred.

Fisher attributed these signs to a pontine conjugate gaze palsy to the left and a left INO—a one-and-a half syndrome of a conjugate gaze palsy in one direction plus one-half of a gaze palsy in the other (Figure 6-26).

Fisher's patient had basilar artery thrombosis, and, at autopsy, infarction of the lower three-quarters of the left side of the pons involving the PPRF, AN, and MLF was found.

In 1983, all cases of the one-and-a-half syndrome reported up to then were reviewed, and 20 new cases (the Boston series) added.[86] The anatomical location of the lesion had been confirmed at autopsy in seven patients, six of whom had a single unilateral lesion in the pontine tegmentum, ipsilateral to the gaze palsy, involving the PPRF and the ipsilateral MLF, but sparing the AN.

The etiology of 49 cases of the one-and-a-half syndrome is shown in Table 6-2.

Paralytic Pontine Exotropia and Esotropia

Exotropia in association with the one-and-a-half syndrome was first described by Fisher and later termed *paralytic pontine exotropia*.[87] One MS case in the Boston series presented with this combination. The patient was a 23-year-old woman who developed numbness and weakness of the right side of the face and horizontal diplopia worse at distance.

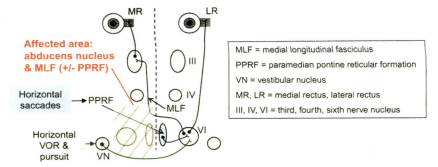

FIGURE 6-26 Combined lesions in the abducens nucleus and medial longitudinal fasciculus: one-and-a-half syndrome.

Reproduced with permission.[18]

Examination documented

- A 60-diopter left exotropia
- Partial right horizontal gaze palsy
- A right INO with gaze-evoked nystagmus in the abducting left eye
- Impaired convergence
- Absent horizontal optokinetic nystagmus
- Full vertical gaze with saccadic smooth pursuit
- Ice-water calorics and oculocephalic stimulation failed to move the right eye fully to the left.

The contralateral exotropia (right horizontal gaze palsy, left exotropia) was attributed to tonic activation of the unaffected contralateral PPRF (Figure 6-27A–E).

Paralytic pontine esotropia associated with the one-and-a half syndrome is due to a coexisting abducens nerve fascicular palsy. A man with MS illustrates this syndrome (Figure 6-28A–D).

TABLE 6–2: Etiology of the one-and-a-Half Syndrome

	Reported Cases	Boston Series	Total
Brainstem infarct	12	4	16
Multiple sclerosis	2	14	16
Pontine glioma	2	1	3
Arteriovenous malformation	1	0	1
Pontine hemorrhage	8	0	8
Basilar artery aneurysm	0	1	1
Cerebellar astrocytomas	2	0	2
Metastatic melanoma	1	0	1
Ependymoma fourth ventricle	1	0	1
	29	20	49

Reproduced with permission.[86]

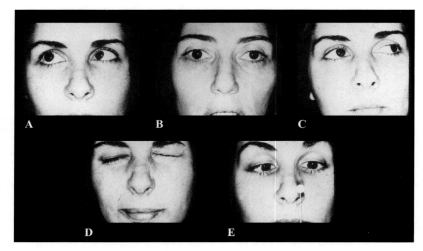

FIGURE 6-27 Paralytic pontine contralateral exotropia. (A) Horizontal conjugate gaze paresis looking right. (B) Exotropia left eye (contralateral) in the primary position of gaze. (C) Right internuclear ophthalmoplegia looking left. (D) Right "peripheral-type" ipsilateral facial palsy. (E) Impaired convergence.

Reproduced with permission.[86]

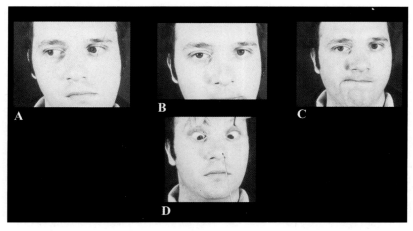

FIGURE 6-28 Paralytic pontine esotropia. (A) Mild left adduction weakness—internuclear ophthalmoplegia—looking right. (B) Esotropia left eye (ipsilateral) in the primary position of gaze due to paresis of abduction. (C) Horizontal conjugate gaze palsy attempting to look left. (D) Normal convergence.

Reproduced with permission.[86]

■ **Clinical Points to Remember About the One-and-a-Half Syndrome**

- The syndrome consists of a conjugate gaze palsy in one direction plus one-half of a gaze palsy in the other.
- It is usually due to a unilateral lesion in the dorsal pontine tegmentum involving the ipsilateral PPRF and the internuclear fibers of the MLF.
- Multiple sclerosis is the commonest cause in young adults.
- Pontine infarction is the commonest cause in patients over 50 years of age.
- The commonest associated oculomotor sign is gaze-evoked upbeat nystagmus, followed by impaired saccadic vertical pursuit and skew deviation.
- Paralytic pontine exotropia, which precisely localizes to the pons, is a one-and-a-half syndrome with contralateral exotropia.
- Paralytic pontine esotropia with a one-and-a-half syndrome is due to an ipsilateral fascicular abducens nerve palsy.
- A vertical one-and-a-half syndrome can present as a downgaze palsy in both eyes, with monocular paresis of elevation in the ipsilateral eye, intact vertical oculocephalic movements, and normal conjugate horizontal gaze. ■

SELECTED REFERENCES

1. Thier P, Mock M. The oculomotor role of the pontine nuclei and the nucleus reticularis tegmenti pontis. *Prog in Brain Res.* 2006;151:293–320.
2. Crandall WF, Keller EL. Visual and oculomotor signals in nucleus reticularis tegmenti pontis in alert monkey. *J Neurophysiol.* 1985;54:1326–1345.
3. Fries W. Pontine projection from striate and prestriate visual cortex in the macaque monkey: an anterograde study. *Vis Neurosci.* 1990;4:205–216.
4. Distler C, Mustari MJ, Hoffmann KP. Cortical projection to the nucleus of the optic tract and dorsal terminal nucleus and to the dorsolateral pontine nucleus in macaques: a dual retrograde tracing study. *J Comp Neurol.* 2002;444:144–158.
5. Ron S, Robinson DA. Eye movements evoked by cerebellar stimulation in the alert monkey. *J Neurophysiol.* 1973;39:1004–1022.
6. Thier P, Anderson RA. Electrical microstimulation distinguishes distinct saccade-related areas in the posterior parietal cortex. *J Neurophysiol.* 1998;80:1713–1735.
7. Newsome WT, Wurtz RH, Komatsu H. Relation of cortical areas Mt and MST to pursuit eye movements II. Differentiation of retinal from extraretinal inputs. *J Neurophysiol.* 1998;60(2):604–620.
8. Thier P, Erickson RG. Responses of visual-tracking neurons from cortical area MST1 to visual, eye and head motion. *Eur J Neurosci.* 1992;4:539–553.
9. Ilg UJ, Thier P. Visual tracking neurons in primate area MST are activated by smooth-pursuit eye movements of an "imaginary" target. *J Neurophysiol.* 2003;90:1489–1502.
10. MacAvoy MG, Gottlieb JP, Bruce CJ. Smooth pursuit eye movement representation in the primate frontal eye field. *Cereb Cortex.* 1991;1(1):95–102.
11. May JG, Keller EL, Suzuki DA. Smooth-pursuit eye movement deficits with chemical lesions in the dorsolateral pontine nucleus of the monkey. *J Neurophysiol.* 1988;59(3):952–977.
12. Thier P, Bachor A, Faiss W, Dichgans J, Koenig E. Imperfect visual tracking eye movements due to an ischemic lesion of the basilar pons. *Ann Neurol.* 1991; 29:443–448.
13. Gaymard B, Pierrot-Deseilligny C, Rivaud S, Velut S. Smooth pursuit eye movement deficits after pontine nuclei lesions in humans. *J Neurol Neurosurg Psychiat.* 1993;56:799–807.

14. Hirose G, Furui K, Yoshioka A, Sakai K. Unilateral conjugate gaze palsy due to a lesion of the abducens nucleus. Clinical and neuroradiological correlations. *J Clin Neuro-ophthalmol.* 1993;3(1):54–58.

15. Büttner-Ennever JA, Büttner U. The reticular formation. In: Buttner-Ennever JA, ed. *Neuroanatomy of the Oculomotor System.* New York: Elsevier; 1988:119–176.

16. Blumenfeld H. *Neuroanatomy Through Clinical Cases.* 2nd ed. Sunderland, MA: Sinauer Associates; 2010.

17. Büttner U, Büttner-Ennever JA. Present concepts of oculomotor organization. *Progress in Brain Research.* 2006;151:1–42.

18. Wong AMF. *Eye Movement Disorders.* New York: Oxford University Press; 2008.

19. Büttner-Ennever JA, Horn AK, Schmidtke K. Cell groups of the medial longitudinal fasciculus and paramedian tracts. *Rev Neurol (Paris).* 1989;145:533–539.

20. Büttner-Ennever JA, Horn AKE. Pathways from cell groups of the paramedian tracts to the floccular region. *Ann NY Acad Sci.* 1996;781:532–540.

21. Lavin PJM, Donahue SP. Disorders of Supranuclear Control of Ocular Motility. In: Yanoff, M, Duker JS, eds. *Ophthalmology.* 2nd ed. St. Louis: Mosby; 2004;197:1305–1304.

22. Liu GT, Volpe NJ, Galetta SL. *Neuro-ophthalmology: Diagnosis and Management.* 2nd ed. Philadelphia: Saunders/Elsevier; 2010.

23. Möbius PJ. Ueder angeborenen doppelseitge abducens-facialis-lahmung. *Munch Med Wochenschr.* 1888;35:91–94.

24. Saint-Martin C, Clapuyt P, Duprez T, Ghariani S, Verellen G. Möbius sequence and severe pons hypoplasia: a case report. *Pediatr Radiol.* 1998;28(12):932.

25. Ghabrial R, Versace P, Kourt G, Lipson A, Martin F. Möbius syndrome: features and etiology. *J Pediatr Ophthalmol Strabismus.* 1998;35(6):304–311.

26. Swaiman KF. Neurologic examination of the older child. In: Swaiman KF, Ashwal S, Ferriero DM, eds. *Pediatric Neurology: Principles & Practice.* Vol 1, 4th ed. St. Louis: Mosby Elsevier; 2006;CH 2:17–35.

27. Pedraza S, Gamez J, Rovira A, Zamora A, Grive E, Raguer N, Ruscalleda J. MRI findings in Möbius syndrome: correlation with clinical features. *Neurology.* 2000; 55(7):1058–1060.

28. Dooley JM, Stewart WA, Hayden JD, Therrien A. Brainstem calcification in Möbius syndrome. *Pediatr Neurol.* 2004;30(1):39–41.

29. Kremer H, Kuyt LP, van den Helm B, van Reen M, Leunissen JA, Hamel BC, Jansen C, Mariman EC, Frants RR, Padberg GW. Localization of a gene for Möbius syndrome to chromosome 3q by linkage analysis in a Dutch family. *Hum Mol Genet.* 1996;5(9):1367–1371.

30. Towfighi J, Marks K, Palmer E, Vannucci R, Möbius syndrome. Neuropathologic observations. *Acta Neuropathol.* 1979;48:11–17.

31. Connolly AM, Iannaccone ST. Anterior horn cell and cranial motor neuron disease. In: Swaiman KF, Ashwal S, Ferriero DM, eds. *Pediatric Neurology: Principles & Practice.* Vol 2. 4th ed. St. Louis: Mosby Elsevier, 2006;Ch 75:1859–1885.

32. Sharpe JA, Silversides JL, Blair RD. Familial paralysis of horizontal gaze. Associated with pendular nystagmus, progressive scoliosis, and facial contraction with myokymia. *Neurology.* 1975;25:1035–1040.

33. Pieh C, Lengyel D, Neff A, Fretz C, Gottlob I. Brainstem hypoplasia in familial horizontal gaze palsy and scoliosis. *Neurology.* 2002;59:462–463.

34. Jen J, Coulin CJ, Bosley TM, Salih MA, Sabatti C, Nelson SF, Baloh RW. Familial horizontal gaze palsy with progressive scoliosis maps to chromosome 11q23–25. *Neurology.* 2002;59(3):432–435.

35. Rossi A, Catala M, Biancheri R, Di Comite R, Tortori-Donati P. MR imaging of brain-stem hypoplasia in horizontal gaze palsy with progressive scoliosis. *Am J Neuroradiol.* 2004;25:1046–1048.

36. Sicotte NL, Plaitakis A, Salamon G, et al. Brainstem axon crossing defects in horizontal gaze palsy with progressive scoliosis assessed with diffusion tensor imaging and neurophysiological testing. *Neurology.* 2005;64(suppl 1):A2.

37. Jen JC, Chan WM, Bosley TM, Wan J, Carr JR, Rub U, Shattuck D, Salamon G, Kudo LC, Ou J, Lin DD, Salih MA, Kansu T, Al Dhalaan H, Al Zayed Z, MacDonald DB, Stigsby B, Plaitakis A, Dretakis EK, Gottlob I, Pieh C, Traboulsi EI, Wang Q, Want L, Andrews C, Yamada K, Demer JL, Karim S, Alger JR, Geschwind DH, Deller T, Sicotte NL, Nelson SF, Baloh RW, Engle EC. Mutations in a human ROBO gene disrupt hindbrain axon pathway crossing and morphogenesis. *Science.* 2004;304(5676):1509–1513.

38. Bosley TM, Salih MA, Jen JC, Lin DD, Oystreck D, Abu-Amero KK, MacDonald DB, Al Zayed Z, Al Dhalaan H, Kansu T, Stigsby B, Baloh RW. Neurologic features of horizontal gaze palsy and progressive scoliosis with mutations in ROBO3. *Neurology.* 2005;64:1196–1203.

39. Johnston JL, Sharpe JA. Sparing of the vestibulo-ocular reflex with lesions of the paramedian pontine reticular formation. *Neurology.* 1989;39(6):876.

40. Kommerell G, Henn V, Bach M, Lucking CH. Unilateral lesion of the paramedian pontine reticular formation. Loss of rapid eye movements with preservation of vestibulo-ocular reflex and pursuit. *Neuro-ophthalmol.* 1987;7:93–98.

41. Solomon D, Ramat S, Tomsak RL, Reich SG, Shin RK, Zee DS, Leigh RJ. Saccadic palsy after cardiac surgery: Characteristics and pathogenesis. *Ann Neurol.* 2008; 63(3):355–365.

42. Tateishi K, Takeda K, Mannen T. Acute disseminated encephalomyelitis confined to brainstem. *J Neuroimaging.* 2002;12:67–68.

43. Albright AL, Packer RJ, Zimmer man R, Rorke LB, Boyett J, Hammond GD. Magnetic resonance scans should replace biopsies for the diagnosis of diffuse brainstem gliomas: a report from the Children's Cancer Group. *Neurosurgery.* 1993;33:1026–1029.

44. Meienberg O, Büttner-Ennever JA, Kraus-Ruppert R. Unilateral paralysis of conjugate gaze due to lesion of the abducens nucleus: clinico-pathological case report. *Neuro-ophthalmology.* 1981;2:47–52.

45. Müri RM, Chermann JE, Cohen L, Rivaud S, Pierrot-Deseilligny C. Ocular motor consequences of damage to the abducens nucleus area in humans. *J Neuro-ophthalmol.* 1996;16(3):191–195.

46. Miller NR, Biousse V, Hwang T, Patel S, Newman NJ, Zee DS. Isolated acquired unilateral horizontal gaze paresis from a putative lesion of the abducens nucleus. *J Neuro-ophthalmol.* 2002;22(3):204–207.

47. Fitzgerald G, Hallpike CS. Studies in human vestibular function: 1. Observations of the directional preponderance of caloric nystagmus resulting from cerebral lesions. *Brain.* 1942;65:115–137.

48. Sills AW, Baloh RW, Honrubia V. Caloric testing. II. Results in normal subjects. *Ann Otol Rhinol Laryngol.* 1977;86(suppl 43):7–23.

49. Fisher CM. Neuroanatomic evidence to explain why bilateral internuclear ophthalmoplegia may result from occlusion of a unilateral pontine branch artery. *J Neuro-ophthalmol.* 2004;24:39–41.

50. Baloh RW, Solingen L, Sills AW, Honrubia V. Caloric testing. I. Effect of different conditions of ocular fixation. *Ann Otol Rhinol Laryngol.* 1977;86(suppl 43):1–6.

51. Lightfoot GR. The origin of order effects in the results of the bi-thermal caloric test. *Int J Audiol.* 2004;43(5):276–282.

52. Fisher CM. Ocular bobbing. *Arch Neurol.* 1964;11:543–546.

53. Leigh RJ, Zee DS. Diagnosis of central disorders of ocular motility. In: Leigh RJ, Zee DS, eds. *The Neurology of Eye Movements.* 4th ed. New York: Oxford University Press, 2006;Ch 12:598–718.

54. Susac JO, Hoyt WF, Daroff RB, Lawrence W. Clinical spectrum of ocular bobbing. *J Neurol Neurosurg Psychiat.* 1970;33:771–775.

55. Hammeroff SB, Garcia-Mullin R, Eckholdt J. Ocular bobbing. *Arch Ophthalmol.* 1969;82:774–780.

56. Daroff RB, Waldman AL. Ocular bobbing. *J Neurol Neurosurg Psychiat.* 1965; 28:375–377.

57. Nelson JR, Johnston CH. Ocular bobbing. *Arch Neurol.* 1970;22:348–356.

58. Katz B, Hoyt WF, Townsend J. Ocular bobbing and unilateral pontine hemorrhage. *J Clin Neuro-ophthalmol.* 1982;2:193–195.

59. Gaymard B. Disconjugate ocular bobbing. *Neurology.* 1993;43:2151.

60. Goldschmidt TJ, Wall M. Slow-upward ocular bobbing. *J Clin Neuro-ophthalmol.* 1987;7(4): 241–243.

61. Brusa A, Firpo MP, Massa S, Piccardo A, Bronzini E. Typical and reverse bobbing: a case with localizing value. *Eur Neurol.* 1984;23:151–155.

62. Mehler MF. The clinical spectrum of ocular bobbing and ocular dipping. *J Neurol Neurosurg Psychiat.* 1988;51:725–727.

63. Titer EM, Laureno R. Inverse/reverse ocular bobbing. *Ann Neurol.* 1988;23:103–104.

64. Larmande P, Dongmo L, Limodin J, Ruchoux M. Periodic alternating gaze: a case without any hemispheric lesion. *Neurosurgery.* 1987;20:481–483.

65. Diesing TS, Wijdicks EF. Ping-pong gaze in coma may not indicate persistent hemispheric damage. *Neurology.* 2004;63:1537–1538.

66. Johkura K, Komiyama A, Tobita M, Hasegawa O. Saccadic ping-pong gaze. *J Neuro-ophthalmol.* 1998;18:43–46.

67. Averbuch-Heller L, Meiner Z. Reversible periodic alternating gaze deviation in hepatic encephalopathy. *Neurology.* 1995;45:191–192.

68. Smith JL, Cogan DG. Internuclear ophthalmoplegia: a review of 58 cases. *Arch Ophthalmol.* 1959;61:687–694.

69. Müri RM, Meienberg O. The clinical spectrum of internuclear ophthalmoplegia in multiple sclerosis. *Arch Neurol.* 1985;42:851–855.

70. Lepore FE, Nissenblatt MJ. Bilateral internuclear ophthalmoplegia after intrathecal chemotherapy and cranial irradiation. *Am J Ophthalmol.* 1981;92:851–853.

71. Hamed LM, Schatz NJ, Galetta SL. Brainstem ocular motility defects and AIDS. *Am J Ophthalmol.* 1988;106:437–442.

72. Pfister HW, Einhaupl KM, Büttner U Dissociated nystagmus as a common sign of ocular motor disorders in HIV-infected patients. *Eur Neurol.* 1989;29:277–280.

73. Ford CS, Cruz J, Biller J, Laster W, White DR. Bilateral internuclear ophthalmoplegia in carcinomatous meningitis. *J Clin Neuro-ophthalmol.* 1983; 3:127–130.

74. Pillay N, Gilbert JJ, Ebers GC, Brown JD. Internuclear ophthalmoplegia and "optic neuritis": paraneoplastic effects of bronchial carcinoma. *Neurology.* 1984; 34:788–791.

75. Gray M, Forbes RB, Morrow JI. Primary isolated brainstem injury producing internuclear ophthalmoplegia. *Br J Neurosurg.* 2001;15:432–434.

76. Mueller C, Koch S, Toifl K. Transient bilateral internuclear ophthalmoplegia after minor head trauma. *Dev Med Child Neurol.* 1993;35:163–166.

77. Muthukumar N, Veeraraijkumar N, Madeswaran K. Bilateral internuclear ophthalmoplegia following mild head injury. *Childs Nerv Syst.* 2001;17:366–369.

78. Keane JR. Internuclear ophthalmoplegia. Unusual causes in 114 of 410 patients. *Arch Neurol.* 2005;62:714–717.

79. Bolanos I, Lozano D, Cantu C. Internuclear ophthalmoplegia: causes and long-term follow-up in 65 patients. *Acta Neurol Scand.* 2004;110:161–165.

80. Rucker JC, Jen J, Stahl JS, Natesan N, Baloh RW, Leigh RJ. Internuclear ophthalmoparesis in episodic ataxia type 2. *Ann NY Acad Sci.* 2005;1039:571–574.

81. Averbuch-Heller L, Rottach KG, Zivotofsky AZ, Suga H, Suarez H, Pettee JI, Remler BF. Torsional eye movements in patients with skew deviation and spasmodic torticollis: responses to static and dynamic head roll. *Neurology.* 1997;48:506–514.

82. Komiyama A, Takamatsu K, Johkura K, Hasegawa O, Fukutake T, Hirayama K. Internuclear ophthalmoplegia and contralateral exotropia. Nonparalytic pontine exotropia and WEBINO syndrome. *Neuro-ophthalmology.* 1998;19:33–44.

83. Lutz A. Ueber die Bahnen der Blickwendung und deren Dissoziierung. *Klin Monatsble Augenheilkd.* 1923;70:213–235.

84. Cogan DG, Wray SH. Internuclear ophthalmoplegia as an early sign of brainstem tumors. *Neurology.* 1970;20:629–633.

85. Fisher CM. Some neuro-ophthalmological observations. *J Neurol Neurosurg Psychiat.* 1967;30:383–392.

86. Wall M, Wray SH. The one-and-a-half syndrome: a unilateral disorder of the pontine tegmentum: a study of 20 cases and review of the literature. *Neurology.* 1983; 33:971–980.

87. Sharpe JA, Rosenberg MA, Hoyt WF, Daroff RB. Paralytic pontine exotropia. A sign of acute unilateral pontine gaze palsy and internuclear ophthalmoplegia. *Neurology.* 1974;24:1076–1081.

7

VERTICAL GAZE AND SYNDROMES OF THE MIDBRAIN

THE MIDBRAIN

The midbrain lies midway between the diencephalon, where it connects with the thalamus and hypothalamus, and the junction with the pons caudal to the trochlear nuclei (Figure 7-1). The roof of the midbrain—the tectum—is formed by two pairs of bumps on the dorsal surface. These are the superior colliculi and the inferior colliculi, which lie dorsal to the cerebral aqueduct. The ventral surface of the midbrain is formed by the cerebral peduncles.[1]

The midbrain is relatively short. The oculomotor nuclear complex and the red nucleus lie in the rostral midbrain at the level of the superior colliculi. The trochlear nuclei and brachium conjunctivum (decussation of the superior cerebellar peduncles) lie more caudally, at the level of the inferior colliculi. The tectum ventral to the cerebral aqueduct makes up the bulk of the mesencephalic reticular formation, a central core of nuclei which runs through the entire length of the brainstem. The central midbrain reticular formation is continuous rostrally with the diencephalon and caudally with the pontine reticular formation. The mesencephalic reticular formation and the diencephalic nuclei maintain an alert conscious state, and the caudal reticular formation of the pons and medulla work together to carry out important motor reflex and autonomic functions.[2,3]

The concept of a fragile region in the rostral midbrain-diencephalic junction where focal lesions can cause somnolence and even coma is clinically important (Figure 7-2). Recognition of levels of consciousness helps diagnostically and the mnemonic AAA for awake, alert, attentive, keeps them in mind.

The paramedian diencephalic syndrome is a triad of signs: hypersomnia, supranuclear vertical gaze palsy, and an acute confusional state typical of posterior thalamosubthalamic paramedian artery infarction.[4] Hypersomnia or hypersomnolence (excessive sleeping) is the clinical alert that the thalamus and/or the diencephalic nuclei are involved.

The case presented here began with the patient oversleeping and being late for work.

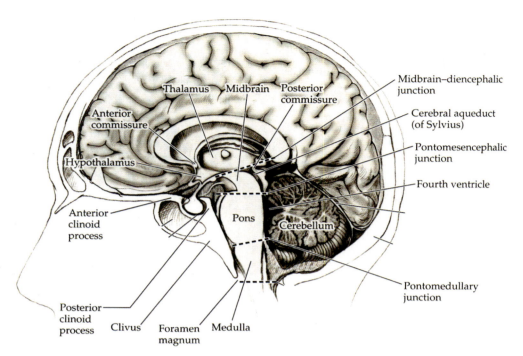

FIGURE 7-1 Midsagittal view of the brainstem in situ.

Reproduced with permission.[1]

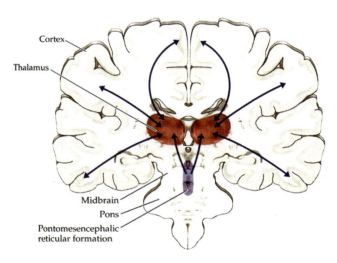

FIGURE 7-2 Coronal view. Projections to the cortex arise from outputs of the pontomesencephalic reticular formation relayed by the thalamic intralaminar nuclei.

Reproduced with permission.[1]

CASE 7-1 The Paramedian Diencephalic Syndrome: Supranuclear Vertical Gaze Palsy and Hypersomnolence

Video Display

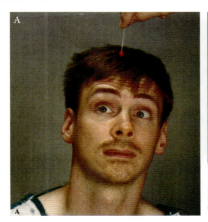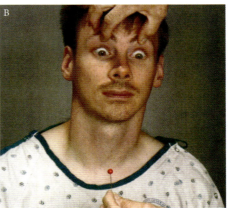

FIGURE 7-3 Young man with (A) upgaze palsy and (B) downgaze palsy.

The patient is a healthy, 36-year-old lieutenant commander in the Coast Guard who felt perfectly well when he went to bed at 2 A.M. on the day of admission, July 15, 2007 (Figure 7-3). He awoke that morning around 9 A.M. having overslept, a rare event for him. He noticed immediately that his vision was "all askew" due to vertical diplopia. On his way to work, he felt tilted to the left and a little off balance, tending to veer to the left. His left face was slightly drooped, and the left arm and leg were clumsy. When he arrived at his office, he was unable to type. The fingers of his left hand were clumsy, and he failed to hit the keys accurately. His colleagues insisted that he go to the hospital, and he arrived at the ER at 11:30 A.M. At that time, he complained of fatigue and attributed this to working at his computer almost nonstop for 2 weeks to design a software program.

Symptomatic inquiry was negative for: headache, vertigo, speech disturbance, chest pain, shortness of breath, or palpitations; positive for recent dental work and night sweats.

Analysis of the History

· What are the major presenting symptoms?
· Where are the central nervous system (CNS) lesion(s) likely to be?

CASE 7-1 SYMPTOMS

Symptoms	Location Correlation
Overslept	Reticular activating system
Vertical diplopia	Vestibular pathways
Left facial and mild hemiparesis	Corticospinal tract

The analysis guides the clinical examination.

Examination

Neurological

- BP 110/60, heart rate 53, normal rhythm
- Somnolent and inattentive
- Oriented × 3
- Obeyed three-step commands
- Mild left facial droop
- No pronator drift and normal motor strength throughout
- Deep tendon reflexes 1+ symmetric, plantar responses flexor
- Coordination normal
- Gait normal
- Sensory system intact

Ocular Motility

- Pupils mid-dilated, 5 mm OU, light/near dissociation
- Global supranuclear vertical paralysis of gaze (only 15 degrees up, 5 degrees down from midposition)
- Convergence normal
- Optokinetic nystagmus (OKN) with rotation of the stripes down showed convergence retraction nystagmus as he attempted to look up to refixate the stripes. Lateral view confirmed retraction of the globe
- Horizontal gaze full
- A left ocular tilt reaction (OTR) contralateral to the lesion
    - Head tilt to the left
    - Hypotropia of the undermost, left eye
    - Hypertropia of the ipsilateral right eye
- Gaze evoked nystagmus to the right
- Ocular dysmetria:
    - Right gaze to center overshoot (hypermetric)
    - Left gaze to center undershoot (hypometric)
- Vertical oculocephalic movements normal
- Bell's reflex—eyes deviated up under tightly closed lids

Localization and Differential Diagnosis

When confronted by an abundance of localizing signs, listing their topographical localization helps to assess the rostral-caudal extent of the lesion in the diencephalic/mesencephalic area. In this patient, somnolence was a major localizing symptom, and the structures likely to be involved are:

- Thalamus
- Diencephalon/mesencephalic reticular formation
- Pretectal pupillary nuclei
- Excitatory burst neurons (EBNs) in the rostral interstitial nucleus of the medial longitudinal fasciculus (riMLF)
- Interstitial nucleus of Cajal (INC) and/or their projections

Mesencephalic lesions in or around the INC cause a skew deviation and the ocular tilt reaction (OTR). The head tilt is contralateral to the side of the lesion, and the hypertropia is ipsilateral to the lesion, with the ipsilateral eye intorting and the contralateral eye extorting.

What Diagnostic Tests Should Follow?

- Blood studies
- Brain magnetic resonance imaging (MRI)
- Computed tomography angiogram (CTA)

Test Results

Initially, there was concern for a diagnosis of endocarditis, given the history of recent dental work and night sweats. A complete blood count and erythrocyte sedimentation rate (ESR) were normal.

The blood cultures ×3 were negative, and the hemocoagulable panel was normal.

Brain MRI showed a diffusion weighted (DWI) hyperintensity and corresponding ADC hypointensity in the right anterior medial thalamus, extending into the right parasagittal midbrain adjacent to the red nucleus and a very faint fluid-attenuated (FLAIR) hyperintensity corresponding to the restricted diffusion image in the right thalamus (Figure 7-4A–B).

A CTA of the head showed a hyperdensity in the right anterior medial thalamus, consistent with infarction; no arterial occlusion(s) or dissection were noted.

Special Explanatory Note

Diffusion-weighted MR imaging is very sensitive and specific for acute cerebral ischemia and contributes to the early detection of such lesions. The emergency studies may not, however, include sagittal views, and, without them, accurate topographic correlation of the caudal extent of a unilateral medial thalamic infarct is incomplete. Subsequent sagittal images showed extension of the infarct into the diencephalon and dorsal midbrain, resulting in a closer correlation of the anatomy with the clinical syndrome (Figure 7-5A–B).

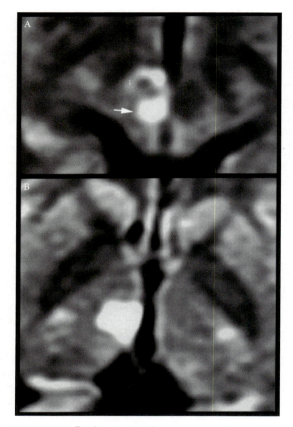

FIGURE 7-4 Brain magnetic resonance imaging (MRI). (A) Diffusion weighted image (DWI) hyperintensity (*arrow*) in the right parasagittal midbrain adjacent to the red nucleus. (B) Extending into the right thalamus.

What Other Diagnostic Studies Are Indicated?

· A work-up for an embolic source
· Echocardiogram

Test Results

A transthoracic and transesophageal echocardiogram revealed a patent foramen ovale (PFO) with right-to-left shunting by Doppler.

Chest x-ray and CT showed a right pulmonary embolus and infarction of the lung. A CT of the abdomen/pelvis was normal.

Ultrasound and MR venography (MRV) of the lower extremities and pelvis were normal, showing no deep vein thrombosis (DVT).

Diagnosis: Unilateral Embolic Infarction of the Right Paramedian Midbrain and Thalamus

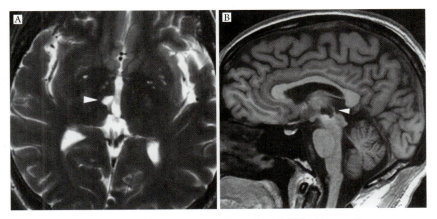

FIGURE 7-5 Brain magnetic resonance imaging (MRI), 3 months post stroke. (A) Axial T2 image shows a hyperintensity in the right thalamic-parasagittal midbrain region (*arrowhead*). (B) Sagittal T1 image shows cystic encephalomalacia in the thalamic-diencephalic infarcted area (*arrowhead*).

Additional diagnoses included right lower lobe pulmonary embolus and infarction, and a patent foramen ovale.

Special Explanatory Note

A PFO (an abnormal communication between the right and left atria) is found in about 10% of the general asymptomatic population younger than 45 years. In patients with an otherwise unexplained ischemic stroke in the same age group, the prevalence of PFO detected by air contrast echocardiography with Valsalva maneuver rises significantly to 40–50%. This suggests that a paradoxical embolism (of venous origin) through an abnormal right-to-left shunt is a potential source of embolic cerebral infarction, and this possibility is illustrated by this case. Embolic infarcts characteristically occur during activity in the awake state, and the presence of a deficit is unusual on waking. Conversely, thalamic stroke causes hypersomnia, and hypersomnia resulted in the patient oversleeping.

Treatment

· Anticoagulation
· Closure of the PFO

The patient was treated with warfarin sodium (Coumadin) 5 mg q.i.d and enoxaparin (Lovenox) 70 mg SC b.i.d.

On day 5, he had no vertical diplopia and the OTR had resolved. The patient returned 3 months after his acute stroke for closure of the PFO. On examination, he had:

· Normal pupils
· Full up- and downgaze with slow saccades on upgaze only

- Contraversive lateropulsion of the eyes to the left on gaze down from a position of full upgaze
- Normal vertical pursuit

He complained of persistent somnolence and had adopted the habit of setting three alarm clocks to wake him in the morning.

Special Explanatory Note

The top of the rostral basilar artery syndrome, which this case illustrates, is well recognized,[5-8] and several cases of bidirectional vertical gaze palsy due to a unilateral midbrain lesion have been reported.[9-12]

Two further cases with neuroimaging correlation are informative. The first case is a 47-year-old woman who developed a sudden supranuclear vertical gaze palsy with complete loss of vertical saccades, pursuit, and vestibular eye movements[13] (Figure 7-6A–E).

An MRI showed a unilateral midbrain infarct involving the riMLF and the INC, and sparing the posterior commissure (PC). The lesion is presumed to have interrupted the pathways involved in vertical gaze just before they decussate, causing an anatomically unilateral but functionally bilateral lesion (Figure 7-7A–B).

The second case is a 64-year-old man admitted to hospital with an acute myocardial infarction.[14] On his second hospital day, he developed diplopia and became drowsy. Examination showed a skew deviation, vertical upgaze saccades absent above the midposition, and slow and limited to about 15 degrees on downgaze. Vertical pursuit was saccadic and limited. Oculocephalic maneuvers increased the range of vertical eye movements, but they were still limited. Convergence was limited to a few degrees. Horizontal saccades and vestibular ocular reflex (VOR) movements appeared normal. Brain CT with contrast (15 days after the stroke) demonstrated an infarction in the right midbrain tegmentum that was attributed to embolism at the top of the basilar artery from a mural thrombus post myocardial infarction. The patient was maintained on anticoagulation for a period of 2 weeks and then he stopped taking it. He died suddenly at home, 6 weeks after his stroke.

At autopsy, the bidirectional palsy of vertical saccades was attributed to a discrete wedge-shaped infarct in the right rostral midbrain, dorsomedial to the rostral border of the red nucleus. Its caudal extent reached 1 mm below the level of the habenulopeduncular tract (tractus retroflexus of Meynert), and it extended 10.5 mm rostrally in two discrete bands into the medial thalamus, adjacent to the wall of the third ventricle (Figure 7-8).

The infarction destroyed the prerubral region containing the riMLF, the rostral 1 mm of the INC, the nucleus of Darkshevich (ND), the ventral portion of the nuclei of the posterior commissure, and parts of the dorsomedial and parafascicular thalamic nuclei. The PC, left midbrain tegmentum, and oculomotor nuclei were spared. The infarction was in the distribution of the right posterior thalamosubthalamic paramedian artery of Percheron.[15-17]

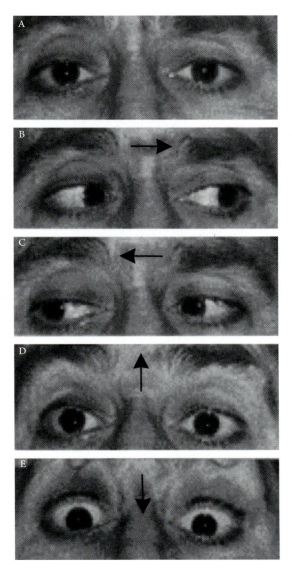

FIGURE 7-6 Position of the patient's eyes in (A) straight-ahead position, (B) left gaze, (C) right gaze, (D) attempted upgaze, and (E) attempted downgaze.

Reproduced with permission.[13]

The Pretectum and Posterior Commissure

The pretectum is the area of the dorsal brainstem that lies directly rostral to the superior colliculus (before the tectum). It is situated between the midbrain and the diencephalon and extends to either side of the PC.[18,19] It contains two oculomotor-related nuclei that receive

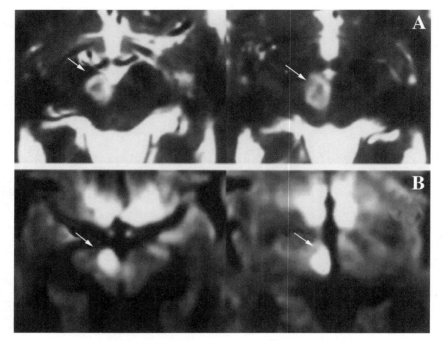

FIGURE 7-7 (A) Axial T2 and (B) diffusion weighted magnetic resonance imaging (MRI) of the midbrain. The arrows indicate the ischemic lesion at caudal (*left*) and rostral (*right*) midbrain levels.

Reproduced with permission.[13]

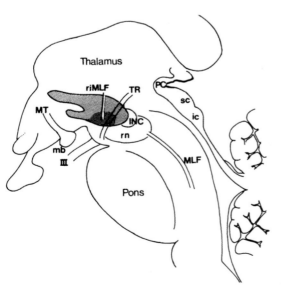

FIGURE 7-8 Extent of infarction, depicted in a right parasagittal plane. Within the area of infarction (light shading) lies the riMLF (dark shading). PC, posterior commissure; MT, mammillothalamic tract; mb, mammillary body; TR, tractus retroflexus of Meynert (habenulopeduncular tract); INC, interstitial nucleus of Cajal; III, oculomotor nerve; rn, red nucleus; sc, superior colliculus; ic, inferior colliculus; MLF, medial longitudinal fasciculus; riMLF, rostral interstitial nucleus of MLF.

Reproduced with permission.[14]

retinal input—the nucleus of the optic tract (NOT) and the pretectal olivary nucleus (PON).[20] Neurons in NOT encode retinal error position, velocity, and acceleration.[21] Specific connections of NOT play a role in optokinetic nystagmus, smooth pursuit eye movements, and the adaptation of the horizontal VOR. The PON plays a critical part in the pupillary light reflex, light-evoked blinks, rapid eye movement (REM) sleep and modulating subcortical nuclei involved in circadian rhythms.

The PC, with the pretectum extending to either side of it, marks the transition from midbrain to diencephalon. It is the major pathway by which axons important for controlling vertical gaze cross to the contralateral riMLF and INC, where they mix with scattered cells that constitute the nucleus of the PC (nPC). The nPC contains burst neurons for upward saccades and projects through the PC to the riMLF, INC, the M-group, and the intralaminar thalamic nuclei (Figure 7-9).[22]

Lesions of the PC and nPC are traditionally equated with supranuclear paralysis of upgaze, light-near dissociated pupils, and paralysis of convergence. The definitive localization of these signs was not achieved until the 1960s, when the critical importance of the pretectum was confirmed clinicopathologically in humans[23] and in the monkey,[24] and the use of the term "pretectal syndrome" was recommended, rather than "syndrome of the PC" to describe the ocular findings.

It is worth noting, however, that isolated interruption of the PC can produce the entire "pretectal" syndrome of upward gaze palsy, pupillary light-near dissociation, lid retraction, convergence-retraction nystagmus, skew deviation, and upbeat nystagmus.[25]

Other names for the pretectal syndrome include Parinaud's syndrome (widely used, although Parinaud was not the first to confirm the syndrome's pretectal localization[26,27] and only two of his seven cases can be considered to have the full syndrome triad of absent upgaze, fixed pupils, and convergence paralysis). The condition is sometimes known as Koerber-Salus-Elschnig syndrome, also named for the authors of early and different reports of convergence retraction nystagmus.[28–30] Keane clarified the ensuing confusion by adopting "pretectal syndrome" to describe the constellation of signs resulting from damage to the PC,[31–33] and I have followed suit.

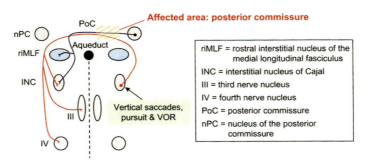

FIGURE 7-9 Lesions in the posterior commissure and the nucleus of the posterior commissure: vertical gaze palsy and pretectal syndrome.

Reproduced with permission.[33]

The Rostral Interstitial Nucleus of the Medial Longitudinal Fasciculus

The riMLF is a paired cluster of neurons lying adjacent and immediately rostral to the INC lateral to the periaqueductal gray, ventral to the ND, and dorsomedial to the rostral pole of the red nucleus. The riMLF has been referred to as the nucleus of the prerubral field by Graybiel.[34]

The riMLF contains the premotor EBNs essential for the generation of vertical and torsional saccades. Equal numbers of EBNs for up- and downgaze are intermingled within the nucleus. Excitatory burst neurons discharge only during saccades. Their anatomical projections to motoneurons differ in the degree to which they control upward versus downward saccades. Excitatory burst neurons encoded for upgaze project *bilaterally* to the INC, the adjacent mesencephalic reticular formation, and the oculomotor (CN III) nucleus to innervate vertically acting elevator extraocular muscles (superior rectus and inferior oblique). A purely *ipsilateral* projection from downward EBNs in the riMLF to the INC, the oculomotor, and the trochlear nuclei innervates ipsilateral motoneurons for the depressor muscles—the inferior rectus and superior oblique (Figure 7-10). This anatomical arrangement is reflected clinically in that lesions of the mesencephalon (generally bilateral) can cause either a selective supranuclear paralysis of upgaze or downgaze, or a combined upgaze and downgaze palsy.[35–38]

Torsional saccades are also generated by EBNs in the riMLF. The right riMLF encodes ipsilateral torsional saccades with a *clockwise* torsional component. The left riMLF encodes ipsilateral torsional saccades with a *counter-clockwise* torsional component[39] (Figure 7-11A–B) Lesions of the riMLF lead to slowing or absence of vertical or torsional saccades.

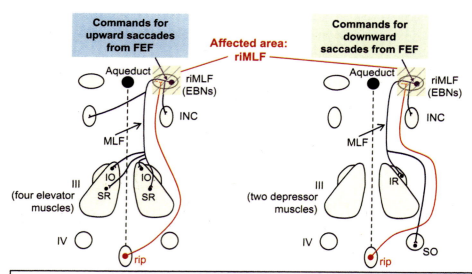

FEF = frontal eye field; riMLF = rostral interstitial nucleus of the medial longitudinal fasciculus
EBNs = excitatory burst neurons; INC = interstitial nucleus of Cajal; rip = nucleus raphe interpositus
MLF = medial longitudinal fasciculus; III, IV, VI = third, fourth, sixth nerve nucleus
SR, IR = superior and inferior rectus; IO, SO = inferior and superior oblique

FIGURE 7-10 Lesions in the rostral interstitial nucleus of the medial longitudinal fasciculus. Commands for upward saccades. Commands for downward saccades.

Reproduced with permission.[33]

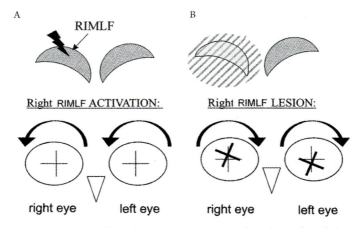

FIGURE 7-11 Effect of right rostral interstitial nucleus of medial longitudinal fasciculus (riMLF) activation (A) and lesion (B) on eye movements. (A) Activation leads to ipsitorsional saccades (extorsion of the right eye and intorsion of the left eye). (B) A lesion causes a tonic contralesional torsion and a skew deviation (hypotropia of the left eye). In addition, a torsional nystagmus beating contralesionally can be seen.

Reproduced with permission.[39]

The riMLF is involved only in saccade generation; for this reason, it is the vertical/torsional counterpart of the pontine paramedian reticular formation.

Small lesions restricted to the riMLF cause a visible torsional nystagmus, with the fast phase beating to the contralateral side; vertical saccades are only mildly affected (slow) after a unilateral lesion.[40–42] Bilateral riMLF lesions abolish all vertical and torsional saccades and quick phases, with other types of eye movements preserved.

The Interstitial Nucleus of Cajal

The INC is the neural integrator (i.e., gaze holder) during vertical and torsional movements. A separate population of neurons is responsible for eye–head coordination in the roll plane. Projections from the INC travel in the PC to the contralateral oculomotor and trochlear nuclei, as well as to the contralateral INC, Ascending projections go directly to the ipsilateral riMLF and nucleus of the contralateral thalamus.

Neurons in the INC also project to motoneurons of the neck and trunk muscles and appear to play a role in coordinating combined eye-head movements in torsional and vertical planes.

An ocular tilt reaction, skew deviation (contralateral hypotropia), excyclotorsion of the contralateral eye (incyclotorsion of the ipsilateral eye), and contralateral head tilt is the diagnostic sign of an INC lesion (Figure 7-12). With bilateral INC lesions, all vertical movement—saccades, pursuit, and VOR—are impaired.

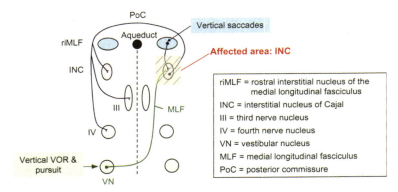

FIGURE 7-12 Lesions in the interstitial nucleus of Cajal.

Reproduced with permission.[33]

DIAGNOSTIC MIDBRAIN SIGNS

Supranuclear Paralysis of Upgaze

Supranuclear gaze palsies result from interruption of the neural pathways that carry commands for voluntary saccades and pursuit before they can reach the eye movement "generators" in the brainstem (Figure 7-13).[43]

Supranuclear paralysis of upgaze is the most common and the most important sign of pretectal syndromes (Figure 7-14A). Paresis initially affects upward saccades, but, if pursuit is tested correctly, it is almost always found to be affected. Full vertical eye movements with neck flexion (oculocephalic reflex) and normal Bell's reflex (Figure 7-14B) are evidence that the palsy is supranuclear in origin. Supranuclear upgaze palsy may occur alone with normal pupils and convergence (Figure 7-14C), in combination with other pretectal signs, or in combination with downgaze paresis (see Cases 7-1 and 7-5). Sustained gaze-evoked upbeat nystagmus rarely precedes the limitation of voluntary upgaze.

Monocular supranuclear paralysis of upgaze palsy is rare. It is characterized by inability of one eye to look up, regardless of whether the eye is abducted or adducted. This disorder has been diagnosed as monocular supranuclear upgaze palsy. It is attributed to a discrete lesion in the pretectal region close to the contralateral oculomotor nucleus, involving both crossed and uncrossed central neural connections to the subnuclei of the superior rectus and inferior oblique muscles.[44-47]

An alternative explanation may be appropriate in some cases of monocular upgaze palsy when both elevator muscles are involved (double-elevator palsy)—it may be caused by a lesion selectively involving the oculomotor fascicles supplying the inferior oblique and superior rectus muscles, which lie adjacent to where the third-nerve fascicles exit the brainstem[48-50] (see Chapter 4, Case 4-3).

Pretectal Pupils

The pupillary light reflex pathway (Figure 7-15) carries light-related signals that leave the optic tract, enter the brachium of the superior colliculus at the level of the midbrain, and synapse at the

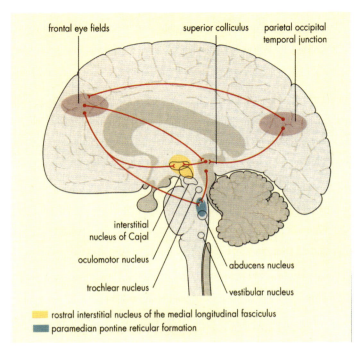

FIGURE 7-13 Supranuclear control of eye movements.

Reproduced with permission.[43]

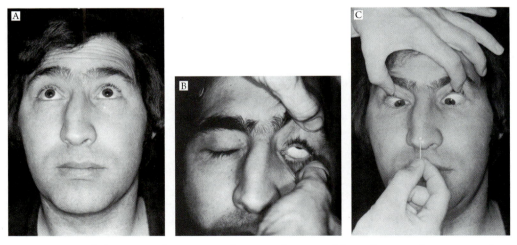

FIGURE 7-14 (A) Supranuclear upgaze palsy. Note elevation of the eyebrows and overaction of the frontalis muscle. (B) Normal Bell's reflex, eyes deviated up during forced eye closure. (C) Normal convergence.

Reproduced with permission.[53]

The Pupillary Light Reflex Pathway

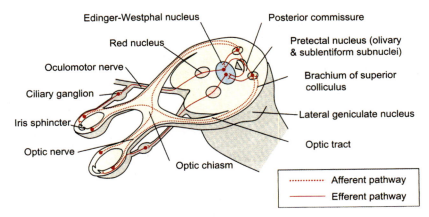

FIGURE 7-15 The pupillary light reflex pathway. Light-near dissociation of the pupils in pretectal syndrome.

Reproduced with permission.[33]

pretectal nucleus (olivary and sublentiform subnuclei). The pretectal nuclues also receives input from the superior colliculus, which carries descending accomadation-related signals from the retina and cortical ares to the pretectal nucleus. The pretectal nucleus projects to the Edinger-Westphal nucleus (EWN), in the ventral midbrain.

The light reflex fibers enter the EWN caudally and fibres for the near response (accomadative) enter the EWN more rostrally.

Pretectal pupils (midbrain pupils) are bilateral, moderately dilated (5–6 mm mydriasis), with decreased or absent pupillary light reaction and an intact near response (*light-near dissociation*).[51,52]

In patients with paralysis of convergence, the examiner should hold a near target close to the eye and observe the constriction of the pupil to accommodation for near[53] (Figure 7-16A–B).

Ectopic pupils[54]—with the pupil not in the center of the iris—are attributed to random inhibition of portions of the EWN causing segmental relaxation in the iris sphincters, eccentric oval dilation of the pupils, and the clinical appearance of misplaced pupils.

In a reported case of coma, the pupils were noted to dilate spontaneously, independently, and eccentrically. Sporadic cycles of dilation and constriction, each lasting 5–15 minutes, occurred during the last 3 days of life. The pupil aperture expanded regularly to an oval shape and independently shifted off-center, upward, and outward in the right eye and downward and outward in the left eye. Then the pupils reconstricted, became round, and returned to center. In this miotic phase, both pupils were nearly equal in size. At autopsy, the right thalamus contained a hemorrhagic lesion that extended into the mesencephalon, bilaterally involving the rostral tectum, periaqueductal gray, lateral midbrain tegmentum, and ventral lateral midbrain. The authors used the term *midbrain corectopia* to describe the pupillary disorder[55] (Figure 7-17A–B).

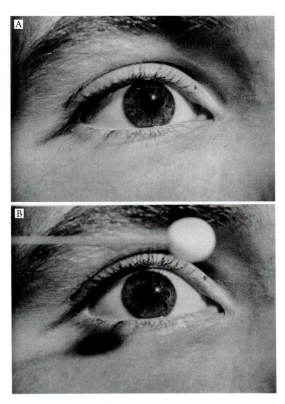

FIGURE 7-16 (A) Pupillary are flexia to light. (B) Pupillary constriction with accommodation to a near target (pinhead) placed directly in front of the eye.

Reproduced with permission.[53]

Eyelid Disorders

Collier's "tucked lid" sign[56]—eyelid retraction—is invariably associated with supranuclear paralysis of upgaze and is attributed to compression of levator inhibitory fibers in the PC that originate in the M-group (Chapter 2) (see Case 7-3).

Collier's sign is exacerbated on attempted upgaze, and, in some cases, there is lid lag on downgaze. This neurogenic lid sign can result from either a unilateral lesion of the nPC or from interruption of the PC, both of which result in decreased inhibition of levator neurons in the central caudal nucleus of the oculomotor complex.

Bilateral ptosis is associated with supranuclear downgaze paralysis and paralysis of convergence. The combination of ptosis and paralysis of downgaze was first reported by Büttner-Ennever et al.[57] in 1989, in a 73-year-old woman with a single midbrain glioma. Other ocular motor functions were intact. At autopsy, a tumor was found to be growing around the third ventricle and aqueduct, causing moderate hydrocephalus, but it had also invaded a network of neural elements involved in eyelid control that lie in the supraoculomotor area of the mesencephalic reticular

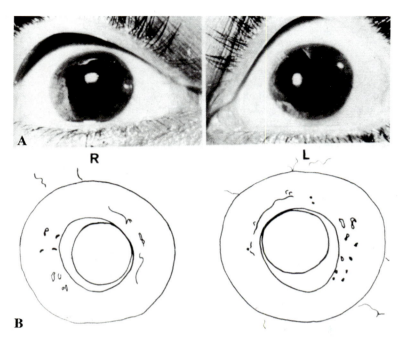

FIGURE 7-17 Midbrain corectopia. (A) Right pupil (R) is in miotic phase, and left pupil (L) is in corectopic phase. (B) Limits of both phases of each pupil are depicted. Paired irregular markings on the iris drawings indicate central-to-peripheral shift of iris crypts during change from miotic to corectopic position of the pupils.

Reproduced with permission.[55]

formation, immediately dorsal to the oculomotor nucleus. The lesion likely involved emerging efferent projections from the medial portions of the riMLF to the CN III and CN IV nuclei. Lesions producing supranuclear downgaze palsy are almost always bilateral[58,59] (see Case 7-4).

Worth noting: the term *midbrain ptosis* refers to a lesion of the central caudal nucleus of the oculomotor nucleus and is usually associated with a unilateral CN III palsy[60] (Chapter 2).

Vergence Disorders

Paralysis of convergence, the third "Parinaud" sign, the other two are absent upgaze and light-near dissociated puplis, is an inability to converge the eyes (with consequent crossed diplopia) when the eyes change focus from far to a near target. In ventral midbrain lesions, convergence is usually absent in the presence of a supranuclear downgaze palsy and sometimes present in dorsal midbrain lesions when only paralysis of upgaze is involved.[61] (Figure 7-14C).

In some patients, convergence is excessive and causes convergence spasm (Chapter 1). Patients with the pretectal syndrome associated with increased intracranial pressure may have divergence insufficiency (Figure 7-13, Chapter 1) which can mimic partial bilateral CN VI palsies[62,63] (see Chapter 6, Case 6-2).

Classic descriptions of the pretectal syndrome report a range of other vergence disorders, including rhythmical convergence spasm,[64] pure convergence nystagmus,[65,66] pure retraction nystagmus (nystagmus retractorius), and the last two combined.[67]

Convergence retraction nystagmus is perhaps the most distinctive associated pretectal sign, but it is not a true form of nystagmus since there is no slow phase. It consists of closely spaced, alternating, adducting saccades[68] and is usually elicited by an attempted upward saccade with cofiring of horizontal and vertical extraocular muscles leading to retraction of the globe.

Convergence retraction nystagmus may be present before upgaze becomes grossly limited. It can be elicited by asking the patient to rapidly look up when using an optokinetic drum (or tape) with the stripes rotating down (Figure 7-18A). Normal downward eye movements will be followed by rapid convergence or retractory movements, or both, instead of normal upward quick phases. The presence of retraction of the globe is best seen viewing the patient's eye from the side (Figure 7-18B).

Convergence retraction nystagmus also occurs when convergence and focusing on a near object are attempted, on attempted downward saccades, and spontaneously as a paroxysmal burst of motor activity. When convergence retraction nystagmus is pronounced, any saccadic attempt, either horizontal or vertical, causes a convergent jerk of the eyes followed by a slower divergent drift back to primary gaze. Attempts to make vertical saccades produce bursts of low-amplitude, rapid eye movements, called *lightning* movements.[69,70] Patients with these signs complain of slowness focusing and difficulty reading.

Excessive convergence and increased tone may limit abduction and mimic a partial abducens nerve palsy, the so-called *pseudo-abducens palsy* described by Fisher[71] in which the abducting eye moves more slowly than the adducting eye.

One or both eyes may have an abduction deficit. The sign is frequently bilateral and accompanied by "hyperconvergence." Close inspection of eye movements in the abducting eye show that there are small inward-directed movements of the eye as it abducts. Often the contralateral eye is hyperadducted. Oculocephalic or caloric stimulation usually produces full abduction.[72,73]

Pseudo-abducens palsy may account for some patients with pretectal lesions presenting early with a chief complaint of difficulty in reading. This is due to a transient inability to find and focus both eyes on the beginning of the next line when a horizontal saccade is made.

Pretectal pseudobobbing, or V-pattern convergence nystagmus, occurs in the same clinical context as convergence retraction nystagmus. It is characterized by nonrhythmic, repetitive downward and inward (convergent) eye movements at a rate ranging from 1:3 seconds to 2:1 second and an amplitude of one-fifth to one-half of the full voluntary range of downward eye movement. Each movement is typically preceded by a blink.

V-pattern convergence nystagmus is usually seen in stuporous or comatose patients with an abnormal pupillary light reflex and intact horizontal eye movements. This nystagmus may represent a variation of spontaneous convergence nystagmus, a sign of acute hydrocephalus that requires prompt surgical attention.[74]

Oculogyric crisis is a dramatic and now very rare disturbance of gaze whose hallmark is forceful, tonic involuntary upward deviation and convergence of the eyes. The attack may present as no more than a mild intermittent upward movement, or it may be evident as a pronounced and sustained spasm of eye deviation, frequently associated with backward (retrocollic) or horizontal (torticollic) head positions. Recurrent attacks lasting from a few seconds to an hour or two were pathognomic of postencephalic Parkinson's disease (PD). Affected patients experience severe eye

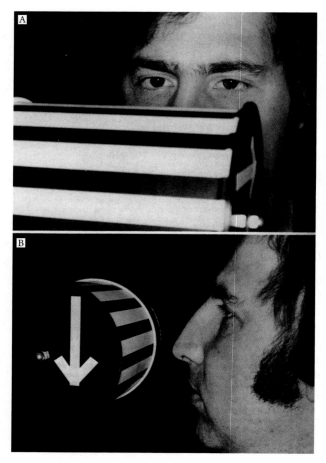

FIGURE 7-18 Vertical optokinetic nystagmus. (A) With
the striped drum rotated with lines going down.
Note convergence of the eyes in a patient with
convergence-retraction nystagmus as he looks up to fixate on
a stripe. (B) Retraction of the globe is best seen looking at the
eye from the side.

Reproduced with permission.[53]

pain during the period of upward deviation and great difficulty looking down, except when they
combine a blink and downward saccade.

Postencephalitic PD is also now a rare disorder,[75,76] and oculogyric crisis more typically occurs
in patients with tardive dyskinesia[77,78]—a side effect of neuroleptic (antipsychotic) treatment with
drugs including carbamazepine,[79] pentazocine,[80] cetirizine,[81] intramuscular haloperidol,[82] and
ziprasidone.[83] The pathogenesis of these ocular spasms is unknown. In the drug-induced form,
upward deviation of the eyes is associated with peculiar obsessive thoughts, but the spasms can be
terminated with an atropinic medication.[84]

Oculogyric crisis can usually be distinguished from the brief ocular deviations seen in
Tourette's syndrome, Rett's syndrome,[85] and Lesch-Nyhan disease.[86] A delayed oculogyric crisis
has been reported after bilateral putaminal hemorrhage.[87]

CASE 7-2 The Pretectal Syndrome: Supranuclear Upgaze Palsy

No Video Display

Supranuclear paralysis of upgaze should always raise the possibility of a pineal region tumor and concomitant hydrocephalus.

The patient is a 44-year-old man who presented with a 3-month history of headache and transient visual obscurations. On examination in the ER, he had papilledema and impaired upgaze. He was admitted as an emergency.

Analysis of the History

- What are the major presenting symptoms?
- Where are the CNS lesion(s) likely to be?

CASE 7-2 SYMPTOMS

Symptoms	Location Correlation
Headache	Increased intracranial pressure
Visual obscurations	Optic disc edema

The analysis guides the clinical examination.

Examination

Neuro-ophthalmological

- Alert and very cooperative
- Visual acuity 20/25 OD 20/30 OS
- Normal visual fields
- Fundus examination showed bilateral papilledema
- Pupils equal 5mm both eyes (OU)
  Slow constriction to light, down to 4 mm OU
  Brisk constriction to near, down to 3 mm OU
- Impaired vertical saccadic upgaze
- Normal vertical downgaze
- Normal horizontal gaze
- Normal pursuit eye movements in all directions of gaze
- Convergence normal
- Convergence retraction nystagmus
- Normal deviation of the eyes up under closed lids—Bell's reflex

Localization and Differential Diagnosis

Headache, light-near dissociation of the pupils, and papilledema are indicative of raised intracranial pressure and obstructive hydrocephalus.

What Diagnostic Tests Should Follow?

- Brain MRI (as an emergency)

Test Results

Brain MRI showed an enhancing mass in the pineal region, approximately 2 cm in diameter, and obstructive hydrocephalus with dilation of the ventricular system (Figure 7-19A–B).

Diagnosis: Obstructive Hydrocephalus due to a Pineal Region Tumor

Treatment

- Surgical intervention to relieve increased intracranial pressure
- Cerebrospinal fluid (CSF) cytology looking for dysgerminoma cells
- Tumor markers

A third-ventriculostomy was done endoscopically and biopsy of the pineal region mass was positive for malignant germinoma. CSF cytology was negative for dysgerminama cells.

Tumor markers from blood and CSF were within normal limits. There was no elevation of alpha-fetoprotein or beta-human chorionic gonadotrophin (β-HCG), which is present in embryonal carcinomas, malignant teratoma, and in up to 10% of germinomas in either of the sample fluids.

Diagnosis: Pineal Germinoma

The patient received chemotherapy (carboplatin and etoposide) prior to radiation therapy to the tumor (craniospinal irradiation is reserved for patients with documented CSF spread with malignant cells on cytology).

Special Explanatory Note

Pineal tumors are relatively rare.[88] In a study of 22 cases of tumor of the pineal region, the infundibular region, or both, the average age at presentation was 19, the range being 6–35 years. The ratio of males to females was 15:7, a predominance supported by others.

The duration of symptoms prior to tumor diagnosis ranged from 6 weeks to 4 years (average approximately 7 months).[53]

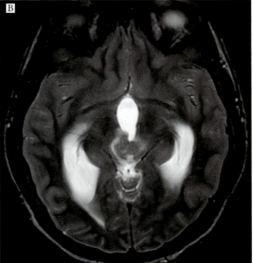

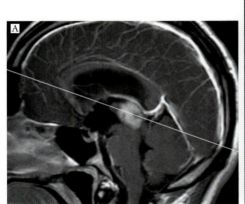

FIGURE 7-19 Brain magnetic resonance imaging (MRI). (A) Sagittal T1 postcontrast image shows an enhancing mass centered in the region of the pineal gland with mild mass effect on the adjacent tectal plate. (B) Axial T2 image shows marked effacement of the cerebral aqueduct and enlarged third and lateral ventricles—signs of marked hydrocephalus.

The leading symptoms and signs of pineal region lesions, in order of prevalence, are shown in Table 7-1.

Pineal cysts, as distinct from tumors associated with pretectal syndromes, can be an incidental finding on brain MRI evaluating other symptoms—for example, migraine headaches. Magnetic resonance imaging will show fluid in a pineal cyst, isodense with the same signal characteristics as CSF (low density on T1-weighted and high density on T2-weighted images).

Asymptomatic cysts can be followed serially. Five personal cases, followed for 4–8 years (3 years is adequate), showed no change in the size of the cyst during follow-up. Surgical intervention is only indicated in patients who have symptoms of increased intracranial pressure and/or signs of the full-blown pretectal syndrome—supranuclear upgaze palsy, light-near dissociation of the pupils, absent convergence, and often Collier's sign.

An exceptional case of pineal apoplexy was reported by Apuzzo et al.[89] in a patient on anticoagulants, with a prothrombin level above the "safe" level of hypercoagulability, who hemorrhaged into a pineal cyst. He became disoriented and confused and had marked limitation of upgaze. Pneumoencephalography showed the cystic mass encroaching on the posterior recess of the third ventricle. It was excised completely, and the patient made a full recovery.

Extrinsic disorders of the midbrain that affect vertical gaze are shown in Table 7–2.

TABLE 7-1: Ocular Symptoms and Signs in 22 Cases of Tumor of the Pineal Region

		No of Patients
Symptoms	Headache	15
	Diplopia	7
	"Blurred vision"	4
Signs	Pupils light-near dissociation	13
	Supranuclear upward gaze palsy	12
	Convergent-retraction nystagmus	10
	Skew deviation	5
	Accommodative control disorder	3
	Convergence paretic	3
	Sixth-nerve palsy (nonlocalizing)	3
	Fourth-nerve palsy (bilateral)	1
	Downward gaze palsy	0
	Collier's sign	0
	Third-nerve palsy	0
	Fundi: Normal	8
	Papilledema	10
	Optic atrophy	4

Modified and reproduced with permission.[53]

TABLE 7-2: Extrinsic Disorders of the Midbrain Affecting Vertical Gaze

Pineal region tumors
Vascular malformations and aneurysms
Hydrocephalus (failed ventricular shunt)
Parasitic cysts

Modified and reproduced with permission.[43]

CASE 7-3 The Sylvian Aqueduct Syndrome and Hydrocephalus

Video Display

The Sylvian aqueduct syndrome[90,91] is a term that should be used only when the *rostral* end of the aqueduct is obstructed and signs of the pretectal syndrome are present.

In March 1985 a 33-year-old man called the police to his apartment at 3 A.M. on the morning of admission (Figure 7-20). They found the apartment in a state of disarray. The man had been down on the floor for some hours—he was only just able to open the door to let them in.

He was admitted to hospital, able to walk but very somnolent, and he had extensive bruising over large areas of the right side of his body.

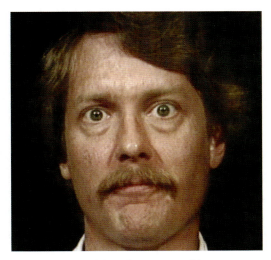

FIGURE 7-20 A thirty-three-year-old man with the Sylvian aqueduct syndrome and Collier's "tucked" lid sign.

Analysis of the History

- What are the major presenting symptoms?
- Where are the CNS lesion(s) likely to be?

CASE 7-3 SYMPTOMS

Symptoms	Location Correlation
Found down	Cerebro-vascular accident
Somnolent	Reticular activating system Thalamus

The analysis guides the clinical examination.

Examination

Examination in the ER

- Afebrile, BP 150/88, pulse regular
- Somnolent but arousable to loud voice and tactile stimuli
- Oriented ×2 with fluent speech
- Remote memory appeared intact
- Obeyed one-step commands
- Fundus—no papilledema
- Supranuclear upgaze palsy

- Light-near dissociation of the pupils
- Mild right hemiplegia, face, arm and leg
- Reflexes 3+ on the right, 2+ on the left
- Extensor plantar responses
- Sensory testing unreliable

Localization and Differential Diagnosis

Headache, somnolence, supranuclear upgaze palsy, and light-near dissociation of the pupils are acute signs of pressure on the pretectum. The differential diagnosis is between hemorrhage versus infarction of the thalamus and/or midbrain.

Special Explanatory Note

Patients "found down" are at risk of developing rhabdomyolysis, a term used to describe the rapid necrosis of striated muscle fibers crushed by the weight of the body lying inert for many hours and usually accompanied by myoglobinuria. Myoglobin and other muscle proteins may enter the bloodstream and appear in the urine, which becomes discolored—appearing burgundy red or brown. The affected muscles become painful and tender within a few hours, and power of contraction is diminished. When rhabdomyolysis is extensive the patient is at risk of renal damage and anuric renal failure requiring dialysis.

What Diagnostic Tests Should Follow?

- Creatine kinase level
- Creatinine level
- Electrocardiogram
- Chest X-ray
- Brain CT, noncontrast

Test Results

Blood studies showed a markedly elevated creatine kinase (CK) level of 19,700U (upper limit of normal varies from 65 to 200U (CK is a sensitive measure of muscle damage and when elevated kidney function should be evaluated by checking the serum creatinine level (normal 0.6 to 1.1 mg/dl)) The white blood count showed an accompanying leukocytosis. The electrocardiogram and the chest x-ray were normal.

A noncontrast CT showed a left thalamic hemorrhage with minimal midline shift, blood within the lateral, third and fourth ventricles, and hydrocephalus.

What Emergency Procedures Should Follow?

- Neurosurgical consult

An urgent neurosurgery consult was obtained because of the patient's markedly decreased level of consciousness, alternating between periods of extreme somnolence and sleep-like behavior with periods of alertness.

A right ventriculostomy was placed, which drained bloody ventricular fluid under normal pressure. The patient received decadron-LA and mannitol to lower the intracranial pressure. On day 4, the ventriculostomy was removed.

Examination on Day 4

- Alert and fully cooperative
- Visual acuity 20/25 OU
- Bilateral lid retraction—Collier's sign
- Light-near dissociation of the pupils
- Global supranuclear paralysis of upgaze (saccades and pursuit)
- Convergence retraction nystagmus
- Normal convergence
- Vertical oculocephalic reflex normal
- Bell's reflex normal—eyes deviated up under closed lids

Diagnosis: Thalamic Hemorrhage rupturing into the venticles and cerebral aqueduct with Obstructive Hydrocephalus

Treatment-Conservative management in the ICU and blood pressure control

The patient was hospitalized for 1 month. The right hemiplegia resolved, but the ocular motility signs persisted. Early in April, he was discharged to rehabilitation with the plan to readmit him in 3 months for cerebral angiography to rule out a thalamic arteriovenous malformation (AVM). He was noncompliant.

In January 1995, 10 years after the thalamic bleed, he was readmitted for a left vertebral arteriogram. The study showed a small tortuous artery feeding a small thalamic AVM lateral to the third ventricle. A stereotactic craniotomy was performed with resection of the AVM. Postoperatively, the patient had a transient right hemiplegia, which resolved over 4–5 days.

Special Explanatory Note

Thalamic lesions are characterized by disturbance of both horizontal and vertical gaze.[92,93] Hemorrhage affecting the medial thalamus may result in conjugate deviation of the eyes contralateral to the side of the lesion (wrong-way deviation[94] (wrong-way eyes)–a phenomenon yet to be explained). Tonic downward deviation of the eyes with convergence and miosis (affected patients appear to be peering at the tip of their nose),[95] is regarded as a unique sign of thalamic hemorrhage that is usually the result of intraventricular hemorrhage compressing the pretectum. Downward deviation of the eyes typically resolves following treatment of raised intracranial pressure.[96]

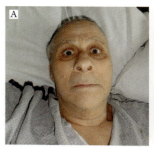
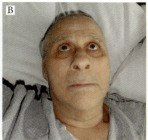
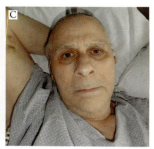

FIGURE 7-21 A sixty-two-year-old man with the pretectal syndrome due to hydrocephalus and malfunction of a ventriculoperitoneal shunt. He had light-near dissociation of the pupils and (A) Collier's "tucked lid" sign and (B) Supranuclear upgaze paresis. (C) Normal examination 12 hours post-shunt revision.

Acute *thalamic esotropia* (stupor and impaired upward gaze) is a phenomenon associated with thalamic hemorrhage and infarction.[97] The pupils are normal. It is characterized by monocular tonic adduction with the eye remaining adducted despite oculocephalic and caloric stimulation, while at the same time the contralateral eye is fully mobile. Magnetic resonance imaging has shown infarction at the interface of the posterior thalamus and the midbrain in the territory of penetrating branches of the basilar-communicating (mesencephalic) artery, with embolism to the top of the basilar artery the presumed precipitating event.

Cautionary note: upward gaze palsy and light-near dissociation of the pupils are reliable signs of increased intracranial pressure and a sensitive indicator of shunt failure in patients treated for hydrocephalus with a ventriculoperitoneal shunt.[98] Shunt revision typically restores pupil reflexes and vertical upgaze to normal. A personal case is illustrated in Figure 7-21A–C. The patient had cancer of the prostate metastasizing to the cerebellum and causing obstructive hydrocephalus. He was admitted for revision of a malfunctioning ventriculoperitoneal shunt.

CASE 7-4 Supranuclear Downgaze Palsy and Paralysis of Convergence

Video Display

This case, published in 1980,[99] is one of the earliest reports localizing selective supranuclear paralysis of downgaze to pathological lesions in the midbrain. It is of particular interest because an examination 11 weeks post stroke documented full recovery of downgaze (Figure 7-22) and only mild convergence insufficiency prior to the patient's death years later.

The patient is a 58-year-old man who was admitted in 1975 with dyspnea and a heart murmur. Cardiac catheterization revealed moderately severe mitral regurgitation. After the procedure, the patient was somnolent and unable to read the menu to order his meals. Seven days later, the cardiologist requested a neurovisual consultation.

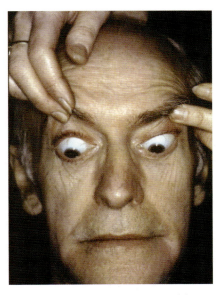

FIGURE 7-22 A fifty-eight-year-old patient 11 weeks post stroke with full recovery of downgaze palsy.

Analysis of the History

- What are the major presenting symptoms?
- Where are the CNS lesion(s) likely to be?

CASE 7-4 SYMPTOMS

Symptoms	Location Correlation
Somnolent	Mesencephalic reticular formation
Unable to read	Vergence system, paralysis of convergence

The analysis guides the clinical examination.

Examination

Neuro-ophthalmological

- Visual acuity 20/30 OU, Reads J2
- Confrontation visual fields and fundus examination normal
- Pupils 3 mm, equal, sluggish to light and near
- Global paralysis of downgaze (saccades and pursuit)
- Absent convergence
- Slow saccades on upgaze
- Horizontal gaze-evoked nystagmus to the right

- A left ocular tilt reaction (OTR)
- Optokinetic nystagmus absent with vertical rotation of the drum
- Normal vertical oculocephalic reflex (Doll's head maneuver)
- Bell's reflex normal (upward deviation of the eyes under closed lids)

The neurological examination was normal.

Localization and Differential Diagnosis

Supranuclear paralysis of downgaze is due to bilateral lesions of the riMLF and skew deviation to a lesion of the INC. Convergence is invariably absent in the presence of a supranuclear downgaze palsy.

What Diagnostic Tests Should Follow?

- Brain MRI (unavailable at the time)
- Brain CT

Test Results

Brain CT showed no abnormality.

Diagnosis: Midbrain Infarction

Treatment

The patient's blood pressure was stable and he received no medical treatment. Cardiac surgery was performed 6 weeks later, and a Starr-Edwards ball valve implanted. By 11 weeks post stroke, he had regained full downgaze.

Five years later, the patient entered the hospital with fever and right hip pain. Despite extensive evaluation and antibiotic therapy, he developed septic shock and died on the 10th hospital day.

Prior to his death, he had shown only mild convergence insufficiency. A general autopsy (sparing the brain) revealed a psoas abscess and perforation of the duodenum.

Special Explanatory Note

In preparing this case for publication as a clinicopathological case,[100] John Trojanowski reviewed the patient's record and found a drawing of the midbrain that I had placed in the chart at the time of my consultation (Figure 7-23). The drawing indicated the probable location of bilateral midbrain infarcts causing the patient's downgaze paralysis, and it prompted Trojanowski to retrieve the patient's brain and to step-section the brainstem in the horizontal plane.

At the level of the rostral midbrain, the autopsy showed two old irregularly shaped, slit-like, "butterfly" cavitary infarcts on either side of the cerebral aqueduct where it originates from the third ventricle (matching very closely the drawing in the chart) (Figure 7-24A). The infarcts extended from the dorsomedial surface of the red

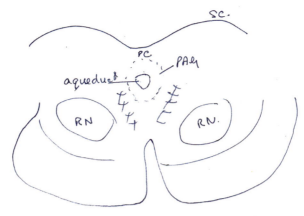

FIGURE 7-23 Drawing, placed in the patient's record, of a transverse section of the midbrain at the level of the superior colliculus indicating the probable location of "butterfly" infarcts (*marked xxx*) of the rostral interstitial nucleus of the medial longitudinal fasciculi. SC: superior colliculus; PC: posterior commissure; PAG: periaqueductal gray; RN: red nucleus.

Reproduced with permission.[99]

nucleus dorsolaterally into the ventral portion of the tegmentum. In the dorsoventral plane, the infarct extended from the most ventral portion of the pretectum to the most ventral limit of the cerebral aqueduct. A transverse section through the meso-diencephalic junction showed the extent of the bilateral infarcts (Figure 7-24B).

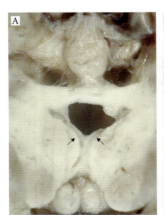
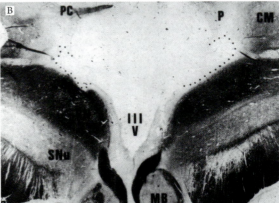

FIGURE 7-24 (A) Cut surface of bilateral rostral midbrain infarct. (B) Transverse section of the mesodiencephalic junction demonstrating bilateral infarcts (outlined with stippled lines). This section demonstrates the largest extent of the lesions. (Hematoxylin and eosin plus Luxol fast blue), CM: centromedianum MB: mammillary body P: pretectum PC: posterior commissure and nuclei SNu: subthalamic nucleus III V: third ventricle.

Reproduced with permission.[99]

TABLE 7-3: Intrinsic Disorders of the Midbrain Affecting Vertical Gaze

---

Primary brainstem tumor (glioma, ependymoma)
Metastatic brainstem tumor
Third ventricular tumors
Stroke
   Infarction
   Hemorrhage (thalamic)
   Trauma (surgery, head injury)
Multiple sclerosis
Infection (syphilis, encephalitis)
Lipid storage disease
Transtentorial herniation
Wernicke's syndrome
Bassen-Kornzweig's syndrome
Vitamin B$_{12}$ deficiency
Gastric bypass

Modified and reproduced with permission.[43]

Only four autopsy cases[101–104] were available when the findings in Case 7-4 were published, but destruction of fiber tracts and neurons in the region bordering the dorsomedial portion of the red nucleus was a feature common to all four. In 1982, Büttner-Ennever et al.[105] reconstructed autopsy findings in six cases (including the one in Case 7-4) and showed that the riMLF was the common area destroyed in every case.

The recovery of the downgaze palsy in the Trojanowski/Wray patient suggests that some of the fibers originating from neurons generating downgaze were intact and it may also suggest that the neuronal population itself was only partially involved.

Intrinsic disorders of the midbrain that affect vertical gaze are shown in Table 7-3.

Vertical Supranuclear Syndrome

Supranuclear vertical gaze palsy affecting all classes of eye movements is the hallmark sign of cerebral Whipple's disease in advance of dementia. The disease itself is a rare relapsing systemic illness presenting most often with symptoms of gastrointestinal malabsorption, chronic diarrhea, weight loss, migratory polyarthralgias, and fever of unknown origin.[106–108] It is caused by a gram-positive bacillus, *Tropheryma whippelii*, which resides predominantly in the gut, but the CNS, retina, liver, spleen, and heart are all vulnerable. Whipple's disease may present solely with CNS involvement.[109–114]

The case of Whipple's disease presented here is a cautionary one. It draws attention to the risk of misdiagnosis because of failure to reexamine previous tissue biopsies and/or failure to take into account the significance of a vertical supranuclear gaze palsy.

CASE 7-5 Supranuclear Vertical Gaze Palsy and Dementia

Video Display

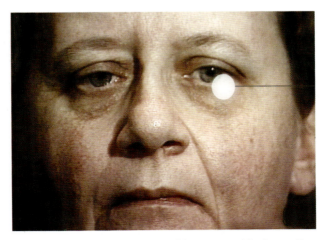

FIGURE 7-25 A fourty-four-year-old woman with dementia.

The patient is a 44-year-old woman with a past history of alcohol abuse. She had three hospital admissions for evaluation of memory impairment over a period of 13 months prior to transfer to the Massachusetts General Hospital in March 1993.

In February 1992, she had developed marked impairment of short-term memory, difficulty recalling where she placed objects, what she had just eaten, or what she had just read. These symptoms took her to the hospital for her first admission, and it appeared that, at that time, her care team focused on her history of alcohol abuse and treated her with intravenous (IV) thiamine.

In June 1992 (9 months prior to admission [PTA] to the Massachusetts General Hospital), she experienced an episode of excruciating abdominal pain and hematuria; investigations included a negative IV pyelogram and a negative CT of the abdomen.

In September 1992 (6 months PTA,) a brain MRI, without gadolinium, was normal. A spinal tap showed a mildly elevated CSF protein of 78 mg/dL and 10 lymphocytes. An ESR of 57 in I hour, and a low serum sodium of 123 were due to the syndrome of inappropriate antidiuretic hormone secretion (SIADH). A small bowel biopsy was done and read as normal. No diagnosis was made.

In November 1992, at the time of her third hospital admission, she had on examination a supranuclear vertical upgaze palsy and tests showed hypothalamic dysfunction with a normal prolactin level.

In March 1993, she was transferred and admitted to the Massachusetts General Hospital with a diagnosis of CNS vasculitis for consideration of a brain biopsy (Figure 7-25).

Her Past history: She had formerly been a heavy drinker (1 liter of rum/day) and a heavy smoker (over 100 (five packs of cigarettes/day)). Her father had died of Alzheimer's disease.

Analysis of the History

· What are the major presenting symptoms?
· Where are the CNS lesion(s) likely to be?

CASE 7-5 SYMPTOMS

Symptoms	Location Correlation
Memory impairment	Mammillary bodies (frequently involved in Korsakoff's pyschosis)
	Ventromedial hypothalamus
Dementia	Cerebral cortex
Supranuclear vertical gaze palsy	Pretectum-Midbrain

The analysis guides the clinical examination.

Examination

Neurological

· Disinhibited, emotionally labile, and euphoric
· Poor attention span
· Speech normal
· Oriented to person only
· 0/3 recall in 1 minute
· Unable to subtract 3 from 100
· Motor strength 4/5 throughout
· Reflexes symmetric 2+ plantar flexor
· Jaw jerk and facial jerks 1+
· No abnormal facial movements

Neuro-ophthalmological

· Visual acuity 20/30 OU
· Fundus examination normal
· Pupils 3 mm OU, sluggishly reactive to light and near
· Constant convergent pendular oscillations in primary gaze
· Supranuclear paralysis up and downgaze
· Absent convergence
· Horizontal gaze (saccades and pursuit) normal
· Preserved oculocephalic reflex
· Bell's reflex intact

Localization and Differential Diagnosis

This patient, at age 44, presented with impaired memory and a history of alcohol abuse. Over the next year, she became slowly demented, and a diagnosis of primary vasculitis of the CNS was made. A brain biopsy was recommended. When she developed a supranuclear vertical gaze palsy and hypothalamic dysfunction, a diagnosis of Whipple's disease became likely.

What Diagnostic Tests Should Follow?

Prompt diagnosis of CNS Whipple's disease is imperative because the disease is treatable, and the dementia potentially reversible.[115] Guidelines for diagnosing Whipple's disease include tissue biopsy of the small bowel, brain, lymph node, or vitreous fluid; polymerase chain reaction (PCR) analysis of intestinal tissue, blood,[116] and CSF;[117] and MRI neuroimaging.[118]

Special Explanatory Note

The classic method for diagnosing Whipple's disease is periodic acid Schiff (PAS) staining of small-bowel biopsy specimens, which on light microscopical examination show magenta-stained inclusions within the macrophages of the lamina propria. Several biopsy samples should be studied because the lesions are often focal and sparse.

Immunohistochemical staining with polyclonal rabbit anti-T Ripley antibody has also been used to detect the organism in various tissues and bodily fluids, such as the aqueous humor and blood monocytes, providing direct visualization of the bacilli.

In addition, PCR assays can be used to detect *T. whippelii*. The bacterial 16S ribosomal RNA sequence can be amplified directly from a variety of tissue(s) and body fluids including CSF, first with broad-range primers and then with specific primers.

On the basis of genome analysis, a new quantitative real-time PCR assay has been developed that targets repeated sequences of *T. whippelii* with substantially greater sensitivity than the earlier PCR assays and with the same specificity. As with all PCR assays, it is critical to avoid contamination of the DNA sample and to include positive and negative controls to validate the test.

It is specially important to pay attention to a positive PCR assay even when a duodenal biopsy specimen is negative on PAS staining.

Test Results

The patient had an extremely extensive workup with consultations from rheumatology, infectious disease, oncology, and neurosurgery.

Blood Studies

The results of blood studies showed an ESR of 88 mm/hr, abnormal serum protein electrophoresis IgM 560 (56–352), IgA 479 (7–312), and negative urine Bence-Jones. The test for porphyria was negative.

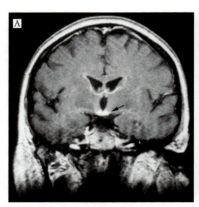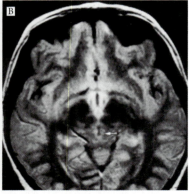

FIGURE 7-26 Brain magnetic resonance imaging (MRI). (A) Coronal T1 postcontrast image shows marked enhancement of the hypothalamus (*arrow*). (B) Axial T2 fluid-attenuated inversion recovery (FLAIR) image shows hyperintensity of the hypothalamus, mammillary bodies and periaqueductal gray (*arrow*).

A spinal tap showed CSF protein at 45 mg/dL, eight white blood cells (WBC) (92% lymphocytes and 8% monocytes), absent oligoclonal bands, and a negative cytology.

Brain MRI postcontrast showed marked enhancement of the hypothalamus, mammillary bodies, and periaqueductal gray (Figure 7-26A–B).

Treatment

The patient was treated for CNS vasculitis and received an empiric course of high-dose IV methylprednisolone (1 g IV q.d.× 3 days, 500 mg × 3 days, 250 mg × 3 days), followed by cyclophosphamide 100 mg p.o. q.d. with prednisolone 25 mg p.o. q.d. with no improvement of her clinical signs.

Three months later, a repeat MRI showed prominent enhancement of the hypothalamus and mammillary bodies and abnormal signals in the pons and periaqueductal region. At this time, a neurovisual consultation was requested.

Examination

Neuro-ophthalmological

- Pupils equal and reactive to light and near
- Constant pendular vergence oscillations
- A global supranuclear paralysis of vertical gaze (i.e., absent vertical saccadic and pursuit eye movements)
- Normal horizontal eye movements
- Convergence absent
- Normal vestibular oculocephalic reflexes
- Normal Bell's reflex

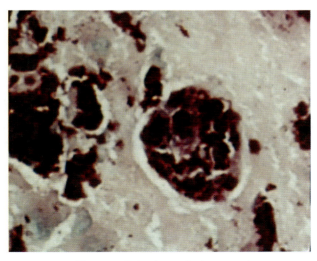

FIGURE 7-27 Biopsy of the hypothalamus shows parenchymal infiltration with foamy macrophages laden with periodic acid Schiff-positive material.

What Tests Should Follow?

Brain biopsy[119,120] is warranted as a diagnostic method in cases of high suspicion, but it needs to be noted that the lesions are often inaccessible and the focal nature of the disease leads to a moderately high rate of false negatives. As imaging techniques improve, the biopsy may be more accurately directed, and the yield from this procedure should improve.

In August 1993 brain biopsy of the hypothalamus showed perivascular and parenchymal infiltration with foamy macrophages laden with periodic acid Schiff-positive material consistent with a diagnosis of CNS Whipple's disease due to the bacillus T. whippelii (Figure 7-27). Unfortunately, neither electromicroscopy nor PCR could be satisfactorily performed on the biopsy tissue.

Subsequent reevaluation of the jejunal tissue from the original biopsy performed at the outside hospital in September 1992 was confirmatory for Whipple's disease.

Diagnosis: Whipple's Disease

Special Explanatory Note

A major manifestation of Whipple's disease in this case was hypothalamic dysfunction—an area crucial for the storage of new items of information (recent memory). Lesions in the ventromedial hypothalamus causing bilateral interruption of the mammillothalamic tract may also produce memory loss.

The inflammatory process of CNS Whipple's has a predilection for the gray matter of the hypothalamus, cingulate gyrus, basal ganglia, insular cortex, and cerebellum. It is not yet clear why these tissues are preferentially involved and why they appear to be resistant to therapy designed to cross both the disrupted and intact blood–brain barrier.

Treatment

Chloramphenicol and trimethoprim-sulfamethoxazole may arrest the course of CNS Whipple's—gaze palsies and nystagmus are signs most responsive to treatment.

Therapy with trimethoprim-sulfamethoxazole is usually preceded by streptomycin together with penicillin G or ceftriaxone for 2 weeks.

The patient was treated for 2 weeks with IV penicillin (following PCN desensitization) and intramuscular streptomycin and started on a course of IV trimethoprim/sulfamethoxazole for 2 weeks followed by oral trimethoprim/sulfamethoxazole twice daily for 1 year.

She was discharged in December 16, 1993, 10 months after admission, to a chronic nursing facility.

Special Explanatory Note

Pendular nystagmus with a vergence component, present in this case, is a unique form of nystagmus that may be due to either a phase difference between the conjugate oscillatory drive reaching the eye or to oscillations of the vergence system—hence the term "pendular vergence oscillations" (PVO).[121] In cerebral Whipple's, the oscillations are smooth, pendular, convergent movements with a velocity characteristic of normal convergence/divergence eye movements; with a frequency of about I.0 Hz. The movements are present under closed eyelids and during sleep. The continuous nature of PVOs distinguishes them from the nystagmus of the pretectal syndrome (convergence retraction nystagmus), which is episodic and provoked by voluntary saccadic eye movements, especially attempted upgaze.

The pathogenesis of PVOs is unknown. In Whipple's disease, the ocular oscillations are frequently associated with lesions in the rostral midbrain and cerebellum, with a predilection for the periaqueductal gray and tegmentum. The complex waveforms observed may reflect several sources contributing to the oscillation, or one source influencing different oculomotor subsystems—for example, instability within the brainstem–cerebellar connections of the vergence system, such as those between the nucleus reticularis tegmenti pontis and the cerebellar posterior interposed nuclei (Chapter 9).

Slow PVOs synchronized with concurrent contractions of the masticatory muscles suggest a diagnosis of *oculomasticatory myorhythmia*.[122,123]

Oculomasticatory myorhythmia is pathognomonic of Whipple's. It is thought to be a form of segmental rhythmic myoclonus of the brainstem involving the vergence system, masticatory segments of the midbrain and upper pons,' and less apparently, segments of the lower pons and medulla.

The leading causes of supranuclear gaze palsies associated with dementia are shown in Table 7-4.

TABLE 7-4: Supranuclear Gaze Palsies Associated with Dementia

Progressive supranuclear palsy

Parkinson's disease

Huntington's disease

Corticobasal degeneration

Neuroacanthocytosis

Wilson's disease

Creutzfeldt-Jakob disease

Gerstmann-Straussler-Scheinker disease

Lipid storage diseases (including adult dystonic lipidosis)

Spinocerebellar degenerations

Ataxia telangiectasia

Whipple's disease

Progressive multifocal leukoencephalopathy

Neoplasms involving mesodiencephalic junction

Reproduced with permission.[124]

SELECTED REFERENCES

1. Blumenfeld H. *Neuroanatomy Through Clinical Cases.* 2nd ed. Sunderland, MA: Sinauer Associates; 2010.

2. Horn AKE, Leigh RJ. The anatomy and physiology of the ocular motor system. In: Kennard C, Leigh RJ, eds. *Neuro-ophthalmology.* Vol 102, 3rd series: Handbook of Clinical Neurology. Amsterdam: Elsevier B.V.; 2011;Ch 2:21–69.

3. Büttner-Ennever JA, Büttner U. The reticular formation. In: Büttner-Ennever JA, ed. *Neuroanatomy of the Oculomotor System.* New York: Elsevier; 1988:119–176.

4. Meissner I. Sapir S, Kokmen E, Stein SD. The paramedian diencephalic syndrome: a dynamic phenomenon. *Stroke.* 1987;*18*:380–385.

5. Segarra JM. Cerebral vascular disease and behavior: I. The syndrome of the mesencephalic artery. *Arch Neurol.* 1970;*22*:408–418.

6. Caplan LR. Top of the basilar syndrome: selected clinical aspects. *Neurology.* 1980;*30*:72–79.

7. Mehler MF. A novel basilar artery syndrome with acute confusion and benign outcome. *Neurology.* 1984;*34*:203.

8. Mehler MF. The neuro-ophthalmic spectrum of the rostral basilar artery syndrome. *Arch Neurol.* 1988;*45*:966–971.

9. Castaigne P, Lhermitte F, Buge A, Escourolle R, Hauw JJ, Lyon-Caen O. Paramedian thalamic and midbrain infarcts: clinical and neuropathological study. *Ann Neurol.* 1981;*10*:127–148.

10. Hommel M, Bogousslavsky J. The spectrum of vertical gaze palsy following unilateral brainstem stroke. *Neurology.* 1991;*41*:1229–1234.

11. Helmchen C, Rambold H, Kempermann U, Büttner-Ennever JA, Büttner U. Localizing value of torsional nystagmus in small midbrain lesions. *Neurology.* 2002;*59*:1956–1964.

12. Suzuki Y, Büttner-Ennever JA, Straumann D, Hepp K, Hess BJ, Henn V. Deficits in torsional and vertical rapid eye movements and shift of Listing's plane after uni- and bilateral lesions of the rostral interstitial nucleus of the medial longitudinal fasciculus. *Exp Brain Res.* 1995;*106*:215–232.

13. Alemdar M, Kamaci MD, Budak F. Unilateral midbrain infarction causing upward and downward gaze palsy. *J Neuro-ophthalmol.* 2006;*26*:173–176.

14. Ranalli PJ, Sharpe JA, Fletcher WA. Palsy of upward and downward saccadic, pursuit, and vestibular movements with a unilateral midbrain lesion: pathophysiologic correlations. *Neurology.* 1988;38(1):114–122.

15. Wall M, Slamovits TL, Weisberg LA, Trufant SA. Vertical gaze ophthalmoplegia from infarction in the area of the posterior thalamo-subthalamic paramedian artery. *Stroke.* 1986;17:546–555.

16. Percheron G. Les artères du thalamus humain. II. Artères et territoires thalamiques paramédians de l'artère basilaire communicante. *Rev Neurol.* 1976;132:309–324.

17. Percheron G. The anatomy of the arterial supply of the human thalamus and its use for the interpretation of the thalamic vascular pathology. *Z Neurol.* 1973;205:1–13.

18. Miller RN. The pretectal region of the human brain. *J Comp Neurol.* 1949;91:369–407.

19. Hutchins B, Weber JT. The pretectal complex of the monkey: a reinvestigation of the morphology and retinal terminations. *J Comp Neurol.* 1985;232:425–442.

20. Gamlin PDR. The pretectum: connections and oculomotor-related roles. *Prog Brain Res.* 2006;151:379–405.

21. Das VE, Economides JR, Ono S, Mustari MJ. Information processing by parafoveal cells in the primate nucleus of the optic tract. *Exp Brain Res.* 2001;140:301–310.

22. Horn AKE, Büttner-Ennever JA, Gayde M, Messoudi A. Neuroanatomical identification of mesencephalic premotor neurons coordinating eyelid with upgaze in monkey and man. *J Comp Neurol.* 2000;420:19–34.

23. Christoff N. A clinicopathological study of vertical eye movements. *Arch Neurol.* 1974;31:1–8.

24. Pasik P, Pasik T, Bender MB. The pretectal syndrome in monkeys. I. Disturbances of gaze and posture. *Brain.* 1969;92:521–534.

25. Daroff RB, Hoyt WF. Supranuclear disorders of ocular control systems in man: Clinical, anatomical and physiological correlations. In: Bach-y-Rita P, Collins CC, Hyde JE, eds. *The Control of Eye Movements.* New York: Academic Press; 1971:175–235.

26. Parinaud H. Paralysie des mouvements associés des yeux. *Arch Neurologie.* 1883; 5:145–172.

27. Parinaud H. Paralysis of the movement of convergence of the eyes. *Brain.* 1886; 9:330–341.

28. Koerber HL. Üeber drei Fälle von Retraktionsbewegung des Bulbus. *Ophthalmol Klin.* 1903;7:65–67.

29. Salus R. Über erworbene Retraktionsbewegungen der Augen. *Arch Kinderkeilk.* 1910;47:61–76.

30. Elschnig A. Nystagmus retractorius, ein cerebrales Herdsymptom. *Med Klin.* 1913; 9:8–11.

31. Keane JR, Davis RL. Pretectal syndrome with metastatic malignant melanoma to the posterior commissure. *Am J Ophthalmol.* 1976;82:910–914.

32. Keane JR. The pretectal syndrome: 206 patients. *Neurology.* 1990;40:684–690.

33. Wong AMF. *Eye Movement Disorders.* New York: Oxford University Press; 2008.

34. Graybiel AM. Organization of oculomotor pathways in the case and rhesus monkey. In: Baker R, Berthoz A, eds. *Control of Gaze by Brain Stem Neurons.* Amsterdam: Elsevier/North Holland; 1977:79–88.

35. Büttner-Ennever JA, Büttner U, Cohen B, Baumgartner G. Vertical gaze paralysis and the rostral interstitial nucleus of the medial longitudinal fasciculus. *Brain.* 1982;105:125–149.

36. Pierrot-Deseilligny CH, Chain F, Gray F, Serdaru M, Escourolle R, Lhermitte F. Parinaud's syndrome: electro-oculographic and anatomical analyses of six vascular cases with deductions about vertical gaze organization in the premotor structures. *Brain.* 1982;105:667–696.

37. Bogousslavsky J, Miklossy J, Regli F, Janzer R. Vertical gaze palsy and selective unilateral infarction of rostral interstitial nucleus of the medial longitudinal fasciculus (riMLF). *J Neurol Neurosurg Psychiatr.* 1990;53:67–71.

38. Seifert T, Enzinger C, Ropele S, Storch MK, Fazekas F. Midbrain ischemia presenting as vertical gaze palsy: value of diffusion-weighted magnetic resonance imaging. *Cerebrovasc Dis.* 2004;18:3–7.

39. Büttner U, Büttner-Ennever JA. Present concepts of oculomotor organization. *Prog in Brain Res.* 2006;151:1–42.

40. Helmchen C, Glasauer S, Bartl K, Büttner U. Contralesionally beating torsional nystagmus in a unilateral rostral midbrain lesion. *Neurology.* 1996;47:482–486.

41. Suzuki Y, Büttner-Ennever JA, Straumann D, Hepp K, Hess BJ, Henn V. Deficits in torsional and vertical rapid eye movements and shift of Listing's plane after uni- and bilateral lesions of the rostral interstitial nucleus of the medial longitudinal fasciculus. *Exp Brain Res.* 1995;106:215–232.

42. Helmchen C, Rambold H, Kempermann U, Büttner-Ennever JA, Büttner U. Localizing value of torsional nystagmus in small midbrain lesions. *Neurology.* 2002;59L:1956–1964.

43. Lavin PJM, Donahue SP. Disorders of supranuclear control of ocular motility. In: Yanoff M, Duker JS, eds. *Ophthalmology*. 2nd ed. St. Louis: Mosby; 2004:1305–1314.

44. Jampel RS, Fells P. Monocular elevation paresis caused by a central nervous system lesion. *Arch Ophthalmol*. 1968;*80*:45–57.

45. Kirkham TH, Kline LB. Monocular elevator paresis. Argyll Robertson pupils and sarcoidosis. *Can J Ophthalmol*. 1976;*11*:330–335.

46. Thomke F, Hopf HC. Acquired monocular elevation paresis: an asymmetric upgaze palsy. *Brain*. 1992;*115*:1901–1910.

47. Lessell S. Supranuclear paralysis of monocular elevation. *Neurology*. 1975;*25*:1134–1136.

48. Hriso E, Masdeu JC, Miller A. Monocular elevation weakness and ptosis: an oculomotor fascicular syndrome? *J Clin Neuroophthalmol*. 1991;*11*:111–113.

49. Gauntt CD, Kashii S, Nagata I. Monocular elevation paresis caused by an oculomotor fascicular impairment. *J Neuroophthalmol*. 1995;*15*:11–14.

50. Castro O, Johnson LN, Mamourian AC. Isolated inferior oblique paresis from brain-stem infarction: Perspective on oculomotor fascicular organization in the ventral midbrain tegmentum. *Arch Neurol*. 1990;*47*:235–237.

51. Carpenter MB, Pierson RJ. Pretectal region and the pupillary light reflex. An anatomical analysis in the monkey. *J Comp Neurol*. 1973;*149*:271–300.

52. Seybold ME, Yoss RE, Hollenhorst RW, Moyer NJ. Pupillary abnormalities associated with tumors of the pineal region. *Neurology*. 1971;*21*:232–237.

53. Wray SH. The neuro-ophthalmic and neurologic manifestations of pinealomas. In: Schmidek H, ed. *Pineal Tumors*. New York: Masson Publishing; 1977:21–59.

54. Wilson SA. Ectopia pupillae in certain mesencephalic lesions. *Brain*. 1906; *29*:524–536.

55. Selhorst JB, Hoyt WF, Feinsod M, Hosobuchi Y. Midbrain corectopia. *Arch Neurol*. 1976;*33*:193–195.

56. Collier J. Nuclear ophthalmoplegia with especial reference to retraction of the lids and ptosis and to lesions of the posterior commissure. *Brain*. 1927;*50*:488–498.

57. Büttner-Ennever JA, Acheson JF, Büttner U, Graham EM, Leonard TJK, Sanders MD, Russell RR. Ptosis and supranuclear downgaze paralysis. *Neurology*. 1989; *39*(3):385–389.

58. Büttner-Ennever JA Jenkins C, Armin-Parsa H, Horn AKE, Elston JS. A neuroanatomical analysis of lid-eye coordination in ptosis and downgaze paralysis. *Clin Neuropathol*. 1996;*15*:313–318.

59. Maranhao-Filho P, Campos JC, Lima MA. Bilateral ptosis and supranuclear downgaze paralysis. *Arq Neuropsiquiatr*. 2007;*65*(4A):1007–1009.

60. Growdon JH, Winkler GF, Wray SH. Midbrain ptosis: A case with clincopathologic correlation. *Arch Neurol*. 1974;*30*:179–181.

61. Ohtsuka K, Maeda S, Oguri N. Accommodation and convergence palsy caused by lesions in the bilateral rostral superior colliculus. *Am J Ophthalmol*. 2002;*133*:425–427.

62. Kirkham TH, Bird AC, Sanders MD. Divergence paralysis with raised intracranial pressure. *Br J Ophthalmol*. 1972;*56*:776–782.

63. Jacobson DM. Divergence insufficiency revisited. Natural history of idiopathic cases and neurologic associations. *Arch Ophthalmol*. 2000;*118*:1237–1241.

64. deManchy SJR. Rhythmical convergence spasm of the eyes in a case of tumor of the pineal gland. *Brain*. 1923;*46*:176–188.

65. Cogan DG. Convergence nystagmus. *Arch Ophthalmol*. 1959;*62*:295–298.

66. Segarra JM, Ojemann RJ. Convergence nystagmus. *Neurology*. 1961;*11*:883–893.

67. Rambold H, Kompf D, Helmchen C. Convergence retraction nystagmus: A disorder of vergence? *Ann Neurol*. 2001;*50*:677–681.

68. Ochs AL, Stark L, Hoyt WF, D'Amico D. Opposed adducting saccades in convergence-retraction nystagmus. A patient with sylvian aqueduct syndrome. *Brain*. 1979;*102*:497–508.

69. Atkin A, Bender MB. "Lightning eye movements" (ocular myoclonus). *J Neurol Sci*. 1964;*1*:2–12.

70. Pasik T, Pasik P, Bender MB. The pretectal syndrome in monkeys: spontaneous and induced nystagmus and "lightning" eye movements. *Brain*. 1969;*92*:871–884.

71. Fisher CM. Acute hypertensive cerebellar hemorrhage. *J Nerv Ment Dis*. 1965; *140*:38–57.

72. Masdeu J, Brannegan R, Rosenberg M, Dobben G. Pseudo abducens palsy with midbrain lesions. *Ann Neurol.* 1980;*10*:103 (Abstract).

73. Truax BT, Shin I, Soumekh F, Chutkow JG. Bilateral pseudo-sixth nerve palsies in midbrain infarction. *Neurology.* 1988;38:421 (Abstract).

74. Keane JR. Pretectal pseudobobbing. Five patients with 'V'-pattern convergence nystagmus. *Arch Neurol.* 1985;*42*:592–594.

75. McCowan PK, Cook LC, Cantab BA. Oculogyric crises in chronic epidemic encephalitis. *Brain.* 1928;*51*:285–309.

76. Onuaguluchi G. Crises in post-encephalitic parkinsonism. *Brain.* 1961;*84*:395–414.

77. Nasrallah HA, Pappas NJ, Crowe RR. Oculogyric dystonia in tardive dyskinesia. *Am J Psychiatry.* 1980;*137*:850–852.

78. FitzGerald PM, Jankovic J. Tardive oculogyric crises. *Neurology.* 1989;39:1434–1437.

79. Berchou RC. Carbamazepine-induced oculogyric crisis. *Arch Neurol.* 1979;36:522–523.

80. Burstein AH, Fullerton T. Oculogyric crisis possibly related to pentazocine. *Ann Pharmacother.* 1993;*27*:874–876.

81. Fraunfelder FW, Fraunfelder FT. Oculogyric crisis in patients taking cetirizine. *Am J Ophthalmol.* 2004;*137*:355–357.

82. Jhee SS, Zarotsky V, Mohaupt SM, Yones CL, Sims SJ. Delayed onset of oculogyric crisis and torticollis with intramuscular haloperidol. *Ann Pharmacother.* 2003; 37:1434–1437.

83. Ramos AE, Shytle RD, Silver AA, Sanberg PR. Ziprasidone-indued oculogyric crisis. *J Am Acad Child Adolesc Psychiat.* 2003;*42*:1013–1014.

84. Leigh RJ, Foley JM, Remler BF, Civil RH. Oculogyric crisis: a syndrome of thought disorder and ocular deviation. *Ann Neurol.* 1987;*22*:13–17.

85. FitzGerald PM, Jankovic J, Glaze DG, Schultz R. Percy AK. Extrapyramidal involvement in Rett's syndrome. *Neurology.* 1990;*40*:293–295.

86. Jinnah HA, Lewis RF, Visser JE, Eddey GE, Barabas G, Harris JC. Ocular motor abnormalities in Lesch-Nyhan disease. *Pediatr Neurol.* 2001;*24*:200–204.

87. Shimpo T, Fuse S, Yoshizawa A. Retrocollis and oculogyric crisis in association with bilateral putaminal hemorrhages. *Rinsho Shinkeigaku.* 1993;*33*:40–44.

88. Ringertz N, Nordenstam H, Flyger G. Tumors of the pineal region. *J Neuropathol Exp Neurol.* 1954;*13*:540–561.

89. Apuzzo MLJ, Davey LM, Manuelidis EE. Pineal apoplexy associated with anticoagulant therapy. Case report. *J Neurosurg.* 1976;*45*:223–226.

90. Swash M. Periaqueductal dysfunction (the Sylvian aqueduct syndrome): A sign of hydrocephalus? *J Neurol Neurosurg Psychiat.* 1974;*37*:21–26.

91. Chattha AS, DeLong GR. Sylvian aqueduct syndrome as a sign of acute obstructive hydrocephalus in children. *J Neurol Neurosurg Psychiat.* 1975;*38*:288–296.

92. Fisher A, Knezevic W. Ocular and ocular motor aspects of primary thalamic hemorrhage. *Clin Exp Neurol.* 1985;*21*:129–139.

93. Fisher CM. Some neuro-ophthalmological observations. *J Neurol Neurosurg Psychiat.* 1967;*30*:383–392.

94. Keane JR. Contralateral gaze deviation with supratentorial hemorrhage. Three pathologically verified cases. *Arch Neurol.* 1975;*32*:119–122.

95. Choi KD, Jung DS, Kim JS. Specificity of 'peering at the tip of the nose' for a diagnosis of thalamic hemorrhage. *Arch Neurol.* 2004;*61*:417–422.

96. Waga S, Okada M, Yamamoto Y. Reversibility of Parinaud's syndrome in thalamic hemorrhage. *Neurology.* 1979;*29*:407–409.

97. Gomez CR, Gomez SM, Selhorst JB. Acute thalamic esotropia. *Neurology.* 1988; 38:1759–1762.

98. Shallat RF, Paul RP, Jerva MJ. Significance of upward gaze palsy (Parinaud's syndrome) in hydrocephalus due to shunt malfunction. *J Neurosurg.* 1973; 38:717–721.

99. Trojanowski JQ, Wray SH. Vertical gaze ophthalmoplegia—Selective paralysis of downgaze. *Neurology.* 1980;*30*:605–610.

100. Case Records of the Massachusetts General Hospital. *N Engl J Med.* 1979;301:370–377.

101. André-Thomas J, Shaeffer H, Bertrand I. Paralysis of downgaze, paralysis of the depressors, hypertonia of the elevators and of the levators. *Rev Neurol.* 1933; 40:535–542.

102. Jacobs L, Anderson PJ, Bender MB. The lesions producing paralysis of downward but not upward gaze. *Arch Neurol.* 1973;28:319–323.

103. Cogan D. Paralysis of downgaze. *Arch Ophthalmol.* 1974;91:192–199.

104. Shuster P. Zur Pathologie der vertikalen Blicklähmung. *Dtsch Z Nervenheilk.* 1921; 70:97–115.

105. Büttner-Ennever JA, Büttner U, Cohen B, Baumgartner G. Vertical gaze paralysis and the rostral interstitial nucleus of the medial longitudinal fasciculus. *Brain.* 1982;105:125–149.

106. Whipple GH. A hitherto undescribed disease characterized anatomically by deposits of fat and fatty acids in the intestinal and mesenteric lymphatic tissues. *Johns Hopkins Hosp Bull.* 1907;18:382–391.

107. Dvorak A, Monahan R. Weight loss, fatigue, diarrhea, fever and lymphadenopathy in a 48-year-old male industrial engineer. *Electron Optics Report.* 1984;31:10–21.

108. Kitamura T. Brain involvement in Whipple's disease: a case report. *Acta Neuropathol.* 1975;33:275–278.

109. Pollock S, Lewis PD, Kendall B. Whipple's disease confined to the nervous system. *J Neurol Neurosurg Psychiat.* 1981;44:1104–1109.

110. Romanul FC, Radvany J, Rosales RK. Whipple's disease confined to the brain: a case studied clinically and pathologically. *J Neuro Neurosurg Psychiat.* 1977; 40:901–909.

111. Halperin J, Landis DMD, Kleinman GM. Whipple's disease of the nervous system. *Neurology.* 1982;32:612–617.

112. Adams M, Rhyner PA, Day J, DeArmond S, Smuckler EA. Whipple's disease confined to the central nervous system. *Ann Neurol.* 1987;21:104–108.

113. Finelli PF, McEntee WJ, Lessell S, Morgan TF, Copetto J. Whipple's disease with predominantly neuro-ophthalmic manifestations. *Ann Neurol.* 1977;1:247–252.

114. Knox DL, Green WR, Troncoso JC, Yardley JH, Hsu J, Zee DS. Cerebral ocular Whipple's disease: A 62-year odyssey from death to diagnosis. *Neurology.* 1995; 45:617–625.

115. Ryser RJ, Locksley RM, Eng SC, et al. Reversible dementia associated with Whipple's disease by trimethoprim-sulfamethoxazole, drugs that penetrate the blood-brain barrier. *Gastroenterology.* 1984;86:745–751.

116. Relman DA, Schmidt TM, MacDermott RP, Falkow S. Identification of the uncultured bacillus of Whipple's disease. *N Engl J Med.* 1992;327:293–301.

117. Cohen L, Berthet K, Dauga C, Thivart L, Deseilligny C. Polymerase chain reaction of cerebrospinal fluid to diagnose Whipple's disease. *Lancet.* 1996;347:329.

118. Davion T, Rosat P, Sevestre H, Desablens B, Debussche C, Delamarre J, Capron JP. MR imaging of CNS relapse of Whipple's disease. *J Comput Assist Tomgr.* 1990; 14:815–817.

119. Johnson L, Diamond I. Cerebral Whipple's disease. Diagnosis by brain biopsy. *Am J Clin Pathol.* 1980;74:486–490.

120. Warren JD, Schott JM, Fox NC, Thom M, Revesz T, Holton JL, Scaraville F, Thomas DG, Plant GT, Rudge P, Rossor MN. Brain biopsy in dementia. *Brain.* 2005;128:2016–2025.

121. Averbuch-Heller L, Zivotofsky AZ, Remler BF, Das VE, Dell'Osso LF, Leigh RJ. Convergent-divergent pendular nystagmus: Possible role of the vergence system. *Neurology.* 1995;45:509–515.

122. Schwartz MA, Selhorst JB, Ochs AL, Beck RW, Campbell WW, Harris JK, Waters B, Velasco ME. Oculomasticatory myorhythmia: A unique movement disorder occurring in Whipple's disease. *Ann Neurol.* 1986;20:677–683.

123. VanBogaert L, Lafon R, Pages P, Lahauge R. Sur une encéphalite subaiguë on classable, principalement charactérisée par des myoythmies oculo-facio-cervicales. *Rev Neurol (Paris).* 1963;109:443–453.

124. Mendez MF, Cummings JL. Parkinsonian disorders with dementia. In: Mendez MF, Cummings JL eds. *Dementia: A Clinical Approach.* Butterworth Heinemann; 3rd edition Philadelphia. 2003;Ch 7:235–290.

| 8 |
DIZZINESS, VERTIGO, AND SYNDROMES OF THE MEDULLA

THE MEDULLA

The medulla is the most caudal portion of the brainstem, extending from the pons to a level just rostral to the point of emergence of the first spinal nerve root. The transition between the medulla and spinal cord is marked by the pyramidal decussation.

The medulla is home to the motor and sensory nuclei of the vestibular and cochlear nerve (CN VIII), the vagus (CN X), the glossopharyngeal nerve (CN IX), the nucleus ambiguus (CN IX and X), the hypoglossal nerve (CN XII), and an important sensory nucleus, the nucleus solitarius whose caudal cardiorespiratory segment receives input from CNs IX and X.

The medulla is also home to critically important structures for eye movement control: the vestibular nuclei, the perihypoglossal nuclei, and the inferior olivary nuclear complex.

The Vestibular Nuclei

The vestibular nuclei lie within the medulla and the pons in four major nuclear groups: the superior, medial, lateral, and inferior nuclei. The inferior vestibular nucleus connects with the superior, lateral, and medial nuclei. Major projections run to and from the cerebellum, particularly to the so-called vestibulocerebellum (the inferior vermis and flocculonodular lobes).

Motion receptors in the membranous labyrinth transmit signals to the vestibular nuclei through the vestibular nerve (CN VIII), which enters the brainstem at the pontomedullary level. The superior portion of the nerve carries information from the anterior and horizontal (lateral) semicircular canals and from the utricle. The inferior portion of the nerve carries information from the posterior semicircular canal and the saccule. The semicircular canals project preferentially to the superior and medial vestibular nuclei (MVN) in what is called the *rostral vestibular complex.* The utricular and saccular macular fibers (the otolith pathway) project mainly to the medial and inferior vestibular nuclei—the *caudal vestibular complex.* Still other afferent projections from the vestibular nerve enter the cerebellum by way of the inferior cerebellar peduncle (the restiform body) and terminate in the vestibulocerebellum.

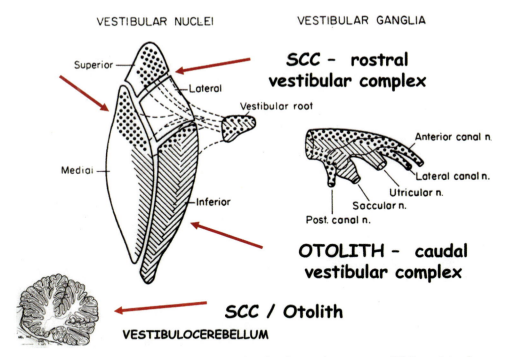

FIGURE 8-1 The vestibular nuclei and peripheral and central projections. SCC, semicircular canals; n, nerve.

Reproduced with permission.[1]

The vestibular nuclei and peripheral cerebral connections are shown in Figure 8-1.[1]

Connections between the vestibular nuclei and the cerebellum are important not simply for the vestibular-ocular reflexes (VORs) but for their closely associated importance in the control of balance and equilibrium. These connections—which are concerned with integration and feedback of information from the cerebellum, spinal cord, and brainstem—include:

- The medial longitudinal fasciculus (MLF)
- The medial vestibulospinal tract
- The lateral vestibulospinal tract

All the vestibular nuclei project to the MLF, with the difference that the superior vestibular nucleus projects only to the ipsilateral MLF whereas the other nuclei project to the contralateral MLF.

Through its cerebellar projections, the vestibular nuclei influence the reticular formation (especially the lateral reticular nucleus and the nucleus reticularis pontis chordalis).

The Perihypoglossal Nuclei

The perihypoglossal nuclei consist of:

- The nucleus prepositus hypoglossi (NPH), which lies in the floor of the fourth ventricle
- The nucleus of Roller
- The nucleus intercalatus

The NPH is an important component of the pontine network involved in gaze control. Adjacent to it in the medulla is the MVN and the MVN with the NPH form the NPH/MVN region, the neural integrator for horizontal saccades. Together with the interstitial nucleus of Cajal (INC), the neural integrator for vertical gaze the NPH/MVN region, play an extremely important role in holding steady all positions of gaze.

Lesions of the perihypoglossal nuclei, the nucleus intercalatus, and the nucleus of Roller have upbeat nystagmus as a prominent sign.[2–4] Medullary lesions causing upbeat nystagmus may also affect the nucleus pararaphales, which lies approximately halfway between the abducens nucleus and the hypoglossal nucleus and receives inputs from the INC with projections to the cerebellum. More rostral medullary lesions cause upbeat nystagmus by affecting projections from the superior vestibular nucleus.

The Inferior Olivary Nuclear Complex

The inferior olivary nuclear complex lies in the ventral medulla and gives rise to olivocerebellar fibers that cross the medulla to enter the contralateral cerebellum. These fibers run in the inferior cerebellar peduncle (restiform body) and terminate as climbing fibers throughout the cerebellum. The dentate nucleus projects to the inferior olivary nucleus via the contralateral parvocellular division of the red nucleus (there is no synapse in the red nucleus) and then via the central tegmental tract. The pathway completes a loop running from cerebellum, to dentate nucleus, to contralateral parvocellular red nucleus, to inferior olive via the central tegmental tract, and then crosses back to the original cerebellar hemisphere, forming the Guillain-Mollaret triangle[5–7] (Figure 8-2).

A lesion of the central tegmental tract results in pseudohypertrophy of the olive and the syndrome of oculopalatal tremor[8] (Case 8-1).

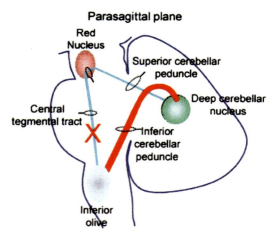

FIGURE 8-2 Schematic representation of the Guillain-Mollaret triangle formed by connections between the deep cerebellar nuclei and contralateral inferior olive, which pass near the red nucleus shows a lesion (red X) in the central tegmental tract resulting in hypertrophy of inferior olive neurons.

Reproduced with permission.[7]

CASE 8-1 Oculopalatal Tremor: Acquired Pendular Nystagmus

Video Display

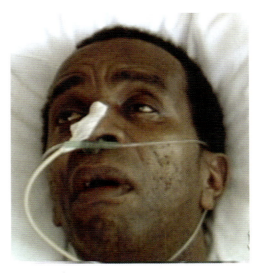

FIGURE 8-3 A fourty-four-year-old hypertensive man with an acute pontine hemorrhage.

The patient is a 44-year-old left-handed man with uncontrolled hypertension and a history of intravenous (IV) drug abuse (heroin and cocaine), alcoholism, and rheumatic fever. At 3 A.M. on the day of admission, he had headache, acute dizziness, slurred speech, left-sided weakness, and difficulty walking. He was admitted to a local hospital, intubated for airway protection, and transferred to the Massachusetts General Hospital (Figure 8-3).

Analysis of the History

· What are the major presenting symptoms?
· Where are the central nervous system (CNS) lesion(s) likely to be?

CASE 8-1 SYMPTOMS

Symptoms	Lesion Correlation
Headache	Increased intracranial pressure
Acute dizziness	Vestibular system
Slurred speech (dysarthria)	
Left hemiplegia	Corticospinal tracts

The analysis guides the clinical examination.

Examination

Neurological

- Intubated
- Alert and cooperative
- Obeyed simple one-step commands
- Pinpoint pupils reactive to light
- Left lower motor neuron facial weakness (Bell's palsy)
- Left hemiplegia with hyperreflexia

Ocular Motility

- Esotropia at rest OS > OD
- Bilateral horizontal gaze palsy involving saccades, pursuit, and vestibular eye movements
- Normal convergence
- Patient converged his eyes when attempting to look right or left
- Full vertical gaze
- Upbeat nystagmus on upgaze
- Torsional (rotary) nystagmus (unsustained) on downgaze
- Horizontal and vertical oculocephalic reflexes absent
- Ice water caloric response absent

Localization and Differential

Bilateral horizontal gaze palsies involving saccades, pursuit, and vestibular eye movements, no response to ice water stimulation, and a Bell's palsy localize precisely to a lesion involving the paramedian pontine reticular formation and the abducens nucleus. The left hemiplegia, due to involvement of the corticospinal tracts, extends the lesion into the basis pontis. The differential diagnosis rests between hemorrhage versus infarction and favors hemorrhage in a patient with headache and hypertension (Chapter 6).

What Diagnostic Tests Should Follow?

Brain neuroimaging

Test Results

Axial head CT showed an intraparenchymal hemorrhage in the central pons and blood in the ventricles (Figure 8-4).

Treatment

The patient was placed on antihypertensive medication and, when stable, transferred to rehab. During the next 2 months, his hemiplegia and gait improved considerably.

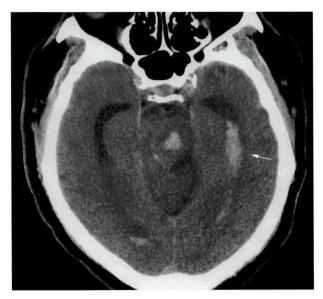

FIGURE 8-4 Axial head computed tomography (CT) shows intraparenchymal pontine hemorrhage in the central pons and blood in the lateral ventricle (*arrow*).

Two years later, the patient developed palatal tremor and rhythmic movements of the facial muscles and neck. Periodic myoclonic discharges were recorded in the orbicularis oculi muscle bilaterally, and a palatal needle electrode recorded rhythmic 2–3 Hz palatal movement bilaterally, synchronous with myoclonus of the orbicularis oculi muscle.

Special Explanatory Note

Oculopalatal tremor is among the rarest of movement disorders, and palatal oscillations (formerly termed myoclonus) typically develop first. The oscillations meet all the criteria for a tremor: they are rhythmic, involuntary, jerking movements of the soft palate (that persist during sleep), often accompanied by movements of adjacent structures derived from the brachial arch—the face, neck, larynx, and diaphragm. The tremor is generated by rhythmic contractions of the levator veli palatini muscle innervated from the nucleus ambiguus by the facial or glossopharyngeal nerve, and it varies from 40 to 200 beats per minute. A click can usually be heard by placing a stethoscope on the neck just below the ramus of the mandible.

An axial FLAIR magnetic resonance (MR) image showed a hyperintense signal in the right hypertrophied olive (Figure 8-5).

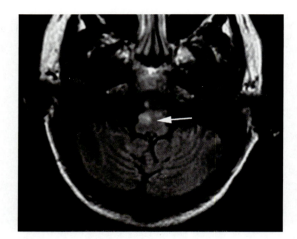

FIGURE 8-5 Magnetic resonance axial fluid-attenuated (FLAIR) image shows hyperintensity of the right inferior olivary nucleus in the medulla (*arrow*).

Special Explanatory Note

Hypertrophic degeneration (pseudohypertrophy) of the inferior olive is the characteristic pathological finding in oculopalatal tremor, and pseudohypertrophy of the contralateral right olive was visualized in this case by neuroimaging of the brainstem.[9] Functional MRI has also demonstrated increased glucose metabolism in the medulla of patients with palatal tremor, possibly reflecting increased metabolic activity in the nucleus.

Seven months later, the patient developed blurred vision and oscillopsia and was readmitted.

Examination

Ocular Mobility

- Constant pendular nystagmus increasing in amplitude on upgaze
- Lid nystagmus with accentuation of nystagmus on lid closure
- Bilateral horizontal gaze palsy
- Normal convergence
- Converged his eyes to attempt to look laterally
- Full vertical gaze with saccadic pursuit
- Torsional nystagmus rotating toward the left shoulder on downgaze

Acquired pendular nystagmus (APN) in oculopalatal tremor is predominantly vertical with smaller torsional and horizontal components and is distinct from the pendular vergence oscillations seen in Whipple's disease (Chapter 7, Case 7-5). APN may be synchronous with palatal tremor, brought out or increased by eyelid closure, and may disappear with sleep. In cases where the tremor is unilateral, the ocular oscillations can have a see-saw pattern, with the ipsilateral eye intorting as it rises and extorting as it falls, while the contralateral eye extorts as it rises and intorts as it falls (Chapter 10).

Diagnosis: Oculopalatal Tremor Post Pontine Hemorrhage with Bilateral Horizontal Gaze Palsy

Treatment

Memantine and gabapentin have been reported to partially suppress the pendular nystagmus but, in some patients with oculopalatal tremor the nystagmus is often less affected by these drugs than is the APN associated with multiple sclerosis. Neither drug suppresses the palatal tremor, which is usually asymptomatic.

No medications to suppress nystagmus were available to the patient at this time.

Special Explanatory Note

The oculopalatal syndrome is due to disruption of the pathway passing from the deep cerebellar nuclei to the inferior olivary nucleus in the medulla via the superior cerebellar peduncle, red nucleus, and central tegmental tract. Climbing fibers from olivary neurons cross to the contralateral cerebellar cortex via a pathway in the inferior cerebellar peduncle (see Figure 8-2).

Normally, inferior olivary neurons share subthreshold membrane oscillations because they are electronically coupled via dendrodendritic gap junctions formed by pre- and postsynaptic connexons. Lesions that disrupt the pathway from the deep cerebellar nuclei to the olive remove gamma aminobutyric acid (GABA)-mediated inhibitory modulation of these junctions which leads, over time, to abnormal electronic coupling of inferior olivary neurons, the development of synchronous discharges, and maladaptive learning in the cerebellum, expressed as ocular oscillations.[7]

This suggests that drugs designed to reduce electronic coupling within the inferior olivary nuclear complex (such as the antimalarial agent mefloquine) might be the drug of choice to treat APN in oculopalatal tremor.

THE VESTIBULAR LABYRINTH

Understanding how the receptors in the labyrinth function to detect motion is essential to correctly evaluating a patient with vestibular signs. Two VORs—the rotational and the translation reflexes—act together to generate eye movements that compensate for head movements. When the head is still, the tonic activity in the two labyrinths (specifically in the coplanar semicircular canals) must be perfectly balanced (Figure 8-6).[10]

When the head moves, the VORs are activated depending on the type of head movement. If the head rotates, the semicircular canals (anterior, posterior, and lateral), oriented at 90 degrees to

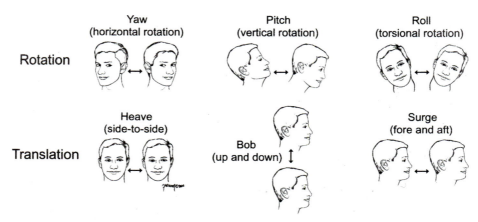

FIGURE 8-6 The Vestibulo-ocular reflex; rotation, translation.

Reproduced with permission.[10]

one another, sense angular acceleration of the head by movement of endolymph within the canal, which activates the vestibular nerve in three directions: horizontal (yaw), vertical (pitch), and torsional (roll), around the naso-occipital axis. Once integrated, this information provides the brain with a head-velocity signal.

The Semicircular Canals

The semicircular canals are arranged so that each canal on one side of the head is paired with the other on the opposite side, both lying in nearly the same plane. Stimulation of a single canal produces slow phase movements of both eyes in a plane parallel to the plane in which the canal lies (Figure 8-7A–B).[11]

Table 8-1 shows the connections of the semicircular canals with the extraocular muscles of the eyes.[12] For example, stimulation of the left posterior canal causes excitation of the ipsilateral superior oblique and the contralateral inferior rectus muscles while inhibiting the ipsilateral inferior oblique and the contralateral superior rectus. An oblique downward movement in the plane of the left posterior canal is the final result.

The semicircular canal ocular reflex (the rotational/angular VOR) produces eye movements to compensate for head movements by counter-rotating the eyes at the same speed as the head but in the opposite direction. Together with the optokinetic and smooth pursuit systems, the rotational VOR acts to maintain steady fixation and prevent nystagmus, which results when any part of the system fails or is out of balance. Examples of the eye movements elicited by stimulation of the semicircular canals are shown in Figure 8-8.[13]

Otolith Receptors: Utricle and Saccule

The ocular-otolith reflex (the translation/linear VOR) originates in the hair cells on the maculae of the otolith organs, the utricle and saccule. The utricular hair cells are oriented in the horizontal

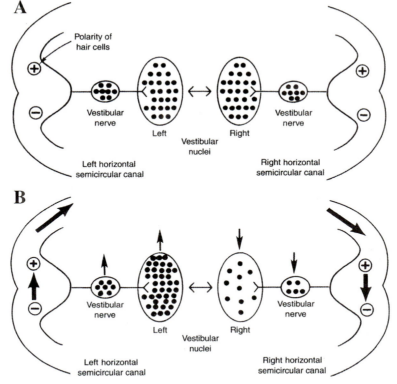

FIGURE 8-7 Push-pull action of the horizontal vestibulo-ocular reflex. (A) With no head movement, left and right vestibular influences are balanced. (B) With head movement to the left, endolymph flow produces an excitatory stimulus in the left horizontal semicircular canal and an inhibitory stimulus in the right horizontal semicircular canal. The excitatory stimulus increases neural activity in the vestibular nerve and vestibular nuclei, and the inhibitory stimulus decreases such activity. The brain interprets the difference in neural activity between the vestibular nuclei as a head movement to the left and generates appropriate vestibulo-ocular and postural responses.

Reproduced with permission.[11]

TABLE 8-1: Connections of the Semicircular Canals with the Extraocular Muscles of the Eyes

	Excitation	Inhibition
Anterior Canal	i—superior rectus	i—inferior rectus
	c—inferior oblique	c—superior oblique
Posterior Canal	i—superior oblique	i—inferior oblique
	c—inferior rectus	c—superior rectus
Horizontal Canal	i—medial rectus	i—lateral rectus
	c—lateral rectus	c—medial rectus

(i, ipsilateral; c, contralateral)

Modified and reproduced with permission.[12]

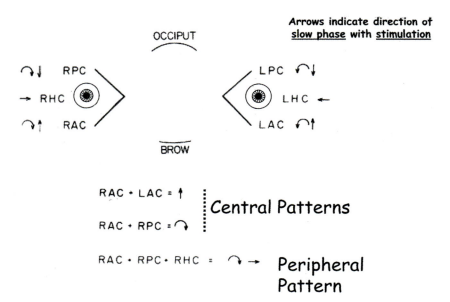

FIGURE 8-8 Central and peripheral patterns of eye movement with stimulation of the semicircular canals. Arrows indicate direction of the slow phase of nystagmus.

Reproduced with permission.[1]

plane and detect horizontal translation and head tilt. The utricular neurons have a strong projection to the eye muscles. The saccular neurons project to the neck muscles.

The translation VOR produces eye movements that compensate for linear displacement of the head (analogous to the role of the rotational VOR during angular displacement of the head). For example, the translation VOR responds to side-to-side (heave), up and down (bob), and fore and aft (surge) head movements, as well as to static lateral head tilt (ocular counterroll) (see Figure 8-6).

Skew Deviation and Ocular Tilt Reaction

A lesion of the otolith pathway results in skew deviation with ocular counter-roll and a tilt of the subjective visual vertical (SVV), a most sensitive sign of vestibular tone imbalance in the roll plane[14,15] that can be very simply assessed using the bucket test.[16]

The bucket test measures both the monocular and binocular visual vertical. Patients sit upright, looking straight ahead into a translucent plastic bucket placed so that the bucket's rim prevents any gravitational orientation clues (Figure 8-9A). On the bottom inside the bucket there is a dark, straight, diametric line that should be positioned vertically (Figure 8-9B). On the bottom outside, there is a perpendicular, horizontal line centered on the vertical inside line. When level, the horizontal line indicates the true vertical and it is the center line, marked zero, of a quadrant divided into degrees. To measure the SVV, the examiner rotates the bucket clockwise or counterclockwise to a quadrant end position and then slowly rotates it back toward the zero degree position. Patients signal stop when they estimate the inside line to be truly vertical, and the examiner reads the degree of tilt on the outside scale. A total of 10 repetitions should be

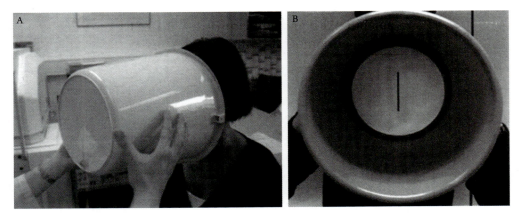

FIGURE 8-9 The bucket test for determining the subjective visual vertical.

Reproduced with permission.[16]

performed, and an eye patch used for monocular testing. It is important to remember that pontomedullary brainstem lesions cause *ipsilateral* SVV tilts, whereas pontomesencephalic lesions cause *contralateral* SVV tilts.

Skew deviation and a tilt of the SVV are reported with lesions of the labyrinth, vestibular nerve, the vestibular nuclei (as part of Wallenberg's syndrome), the midbrain, and the cerebellum. The localizing value of skew, particularly in infarction of the brainstem, has been established by clinical observation and neuroimaging and *it is a bedside predictor of central brainstem causes of acute vertigo.*

The key to bedside diagnosis of skew is the ocular tilt reaction (OTR)—the combination of a lateral head tilt of varying degree *and* vertical divergence of the eyes with hypotropia of the eye on the side of the lesion (the undermost eye). In persistent tonic OTR, there is a deviation of the internal representation of the subjective vertical and a significant compensatory deviation in the direction of the head tilt. However, there is no close correlation between net tilt angles of the eyes and the subjective visual vertical, and, surprisingly, most patients do not complain of a perceptual tilt of the visual world[17–20] (Figure 8-10).

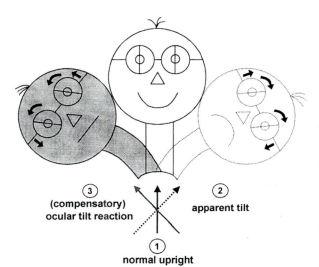

FIGURE 8-10 Ocular tilt reaction represented as a "motor compensation" of a lesion-induced apparent eye-head tilt (*dashed line*), which would be opposite in direction to the apparent tilt. The eyes and head are continuously adjusted to what the lesioned brain computes as being vertical.

Reproduced with permission.[20]

The OTR is attributed to an imbalance in otolith-ocular and otolith-collic reflexes. A case of OTR was reported in 1979 by Halmagyi et al.[21] in a patient who had selective loss of vestibular function as a complication of stapedectomy (the surgical treatment for conductive hearing loss associated with otosclerosis) in the ear subject to the procedure. (Post left-sided stapedectomy, she had (Figure 8-11) unopposed activity of the intact right labyrinth resulting in:

- A leftward head tilt (approximately 10 degrees)
- Vertical misalignment of the eyes, a right-over-left hypertropia in primary gaze, and a left skew deviation
- Twenty-five degrees of leftward counter-rolling of the 12 o'clock ocular meridians—each optic nerve rotated clockwise by approximately 25 degrees relative to the macula
- First-degree horizontal nystagmus beating to the right

The ocular-otolith pathway crosses the midline of the brainstem at pontine level and gives rise to two types of OTR: the "ascending" unilateral pontomedullary VOR-OTR that causes an *ipsilateral*

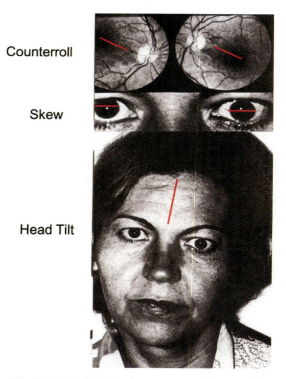

FIGURE 8-11 Head and eye posture of the seated patient during the first postoperative week following a left stapedectomy. There is leftward tilting of the head (about 10 degrees) and right-over-left skew deviation of the eyes. Note the leftward counter-rolling of the 12 o'clock meridian in the fundus photographs.

Reproduced with permission.[21]

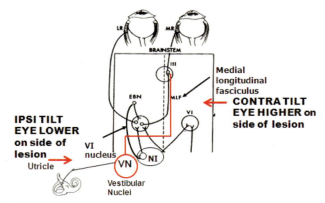

Vertical deviation, Comitant, Lower eye on side of lower ear
Head tilt toward side of lower eye (and ear)
Ocular counterroll (torsion), Top poles toward the lower eye (and ear)

FIGURE 8-12 Ocular tilt reaction (OTR) pathway. Utricle → Vestibular Nuclei → MLF → III, IV → INC. MLF: medial longitudinal fasciculus; III: oculomotor nerve; IV: trochlear nerve; INC: interstitial nucleus of Cajal; VN, vestibular nuclei.

Reproduced with permission.[1]

skew deviation and the "descending" mesencephalic integrator—OTR that causes a *contralateral* skew deviation, with the OTR probably due to involvement of the INC.[22]

The typical ocular pattern of OTR in Wallenberg's syndrome (skew deviation with monocular excyclotropia of the ipsilateral hypotropic eye) can be explained by a circumscribed lesion of the ascending pathways of the ipsilateral posterior semicircular canal (Figure 8-12).

DIAGNOSTIC SYMPTOMS AND SIGNS

Dizziness and Vertigo

Dizziness has its ultimate root in the medulla through its causal linkage with the vestibular nuclei. It ranks high among the symptoms patients commonly complain of when they seek emergency medical care but, as common a symptom as it is, it is also a nonspecific one.

Dizziness is a term patients use to refer to some sort of ill-feeling—light-headedness, near faint, unsteadiness standing or walking, confusion, or even anxiety. Vertigo, on the other hand, is an illusion of movement, an erroneous perception of motion (usually rotation) of either the sufferer or the environment and is strongly suggestive of an imbalance within the vestibular system. This sensation of motion differentiates vertigo from other causes of dizziness, although it does not indicate where in the system the imbalance originates.

A pathological lesion of the vestibular system causes classic symptoms: vertigo, nystagmus, gait unsteadiness, nausea, and vomiting, and these symptoms correlate with different aspects of vestibular function and arise from different sources.

Vertigo results from a disturbance of cortical spatial orientation—an imbalance within the vestibular system. Nystagmus is secondary to semicircular canal imbalance, which activates neural circuits in the brainstem. Postural unsteadiness of gait (postural vestibular ataxia) is due to inappropriate or abnormal activation of the vestibulospinal pathways that link the labyrinth receptors with antigravity motor neurons in the spinal cord to maintain head and body posture. Nausea and vomiting, frequently associated with vertigo, are triggered by chemical activation of the medullary vomiting center.

The Dizziness-Vertigo History

Taking the history is of paramount importance in patients presenting with vestibular symptoms. The patient should always be asked to describe what he feels as clearly as he possibly can in order to establish whether he is actually experiencing a sensation of motion. A diagnosis of vertigo rests on this, and these key questions help.

- Is the feeling of divzziness you have one of light-headedness, or a feeling that you might faint?
- Is the sensation you are experiencing a feeling of spinning—of yourself or the world around you?
- Do you feel at all unsteady or off balance walking?

Asking patients specifically about the direction of self-rotation they experience with their eyes closed helps to evaluate vestibular involvement: a rotational, spinning feeling suggests disturbance of the semicircular canals, whereas sensations of body tilt and unsteadiness imply disturbance of the otolith receptors. Asking about the direction in which the images seem to move with the eyes open helps identify the direction of nystagmus because the direction of apparent motion of the visual world is usually opposite to the direction of the slow phase of nystagmus.

Patients with acute dizziness are often unable to reliably describe the type of dizziness they are experiencing. Is it rotary (spinning), or to and fro, or light-headedness?[23]

In these cases, it is the *triggers* of dizziness that become a key source of diagnostic information. The patient should be asked:

- What were you doing when the dizziness started?
- Can you make your dizziness worse by moving your head?
- Do you get dizzy doing anything in particular—turning over in bed, extending your head back at the hairdresser or the dentist, reversing your car out of the garage?

These questions begin to differentiate dizziness brought on by change in head position, which is usually a benign peripheral problem, from existing and sustained vertigo made worse by movement that changes the position of the head and/or body. However, symptoms of both benign peripheral and central vertigo are worsened by sudden changes of position that cause a rush of disordered stimuli to the CNS, and these two conditions, benign or sustained, must be distinguished from each other. Onset and duration are important in doing so.

Questions to ask:

- Have you had a blow to your head recently or in the past?
- Is this the first time an episode of dizziness has occurred, or have you had similar episodes before?
- Did the feeling of dizziness come on gradually or acutely?
- How long does the attack of dizziness last?

With trauma and vascular occlusion, vertigo is long-lasting but usually episodic and abrupt in onset. It is typically more gradual in onset (over hours) with viral vestibular neuritis. Episodes lasting seconds only, suggest a diagnosis of benign paroxysmal positional vertigo. An episode lasting minutes suggests a transient vascular ischemic attack—it is the typical duration of vertigo with transient vertebro-basilar ischemia.[24] Migraine, which is very variable, and Ménière's disease can be accompanied by vertigo lasting for hours.[25]

TABLE 8-2: Duration of Episodes in Common Causes of Vertigo

Seconds	Benign positional vertigo
Minutes	Vertebrobasilar insufficiency
Hours	Mèniére's syndrome, Migraine
Days	Vestibular neuritis
	Infarction of the labyrinth

Modified and reproduced with permission.[26]

The duration of episodes in common causes of vertigo is shown in Table 8-2.[26] And once timing is clarified, it is particularly important to ask about associated visual symptoms:

- Do you have blurred vision?
- Do you see the visual world moving (oscillopsia)?
- Do you have double vision?

Blurred vision is nonspecific but may be due to oscillopsia, which suggests that the patient has spontaneous nystagmus (Chapter 10). Diplopia is an uncommon symptom in vertiginous patients and when vertical diplopia is present it suggests vertical misalignment of the eyes—a feature of skew deviation (Chapter 4).

There may also be associated auditory symptoms:

- Is your hearing normal?
- Do you have any noise in your ears (tinnitus)?
- Do loud noises make you dizzy?

Auditory symptoms point to Ménière's syndrome,[27] which typically begins with a sensation of fullness and pressure in the ear along with decreased hearing and tinnitus. Vertigo rapidly follows, is usually at its maximum intensity within minutes and then slowly resolves.

Some Ménière's patients may experience abrupt episodes of falling to the ground without loss of consciousness or associated neurological symptoms,[28,29] and they may report a feeling of being pushed to the ground. These episodes can be confused with, and easily misdiagnosed as, drop attacks seen with vertebrobasilar insufficiency.

Sudden congruent deafness suggests infarction of the labyrinth in the territory of the anterior-inferior cerebellar artery.

Vertigo caused by a loud noise or even by the patient humming—the Tullio phenomenon—can occur in several clinical syndromes including dehiscence of the superior semicircular canal.[30]

Important associated neurological symptoms may need to be elicited:

- Have you any headache or neck pain?
- Do you have a history of migraine or excessive motion sickness as a child?

Headache and neck pain are common symptoms of dissection of the vertebral artery,[31,32] and young patients are particularly at risk of receiving a misdiagnosis of migraine when they present with these symptoms.[33] Bear in mind that craniocervical pain caused by dissection of the vertebral artery is often sudden, severe, and sustained. *In these patients, emergency brain MRI is mandatory to establish the diagnosis of vertebral artery dissection.*

In contrast, headache pain characteristic of migraine develops gradually over hours and usually disappears within 24–48 hours. The headache of vestibular migraine with vertigo will vary in severity.[34–37]

There are other questions that should always be asked:

- Are you having difficulty walking or sitting upright?
- Do you get dizzy or light-headed if you suddenly stand up?

Severe truncal ataxia (inability to sit with arms crossed unaided) is a red flag because *ataxia may be the only neurological sign of stroke.*

Dizziness on suddenly sitting up and/or standing is suggestive of *orthostatic hypotension,* a condition that should be routinely checked in all dizzy patients. Diagnosis is based on a drop in systolic blood pressure by 20 mm Hg or more when the dizzy patient stands up. Antihypertensive drugs, some antidepressants, and long-term bed rest predispose a patient to orthostatic hypotension.[38]

By this stage of taking the history, patients complaining of dizziness, light-headedness and/or imbalance and unsteadiness of gait but with no erroneous perception of motion will be identified, and it is this nonvertiginous "dizzy" patient who needs to be asked:

- Have you ever had symptoms associated with imbalance or light-headedness as a side effect of medication?
- Do you have a history of alcohol or drug abuse?
- Do you think your symptoms could be related to stress, anxiety, or depression?

Medications, Drugs, Alcohol

A detailed history of medications is critical to accurate evaluation. Antihypertensive and antidepressant medications are common causes of light-headedness. Ototoxic drugs, such as aminoglycosides and cisplatin, can cause bilateral loss of vestibular function and produce disequilibrium and oscillopsia when moving the head and walking.[39,40] A light-headed swimming sensation is typically associated with chronic alcohol use.

Anxiety and Depression

Taking a social history helps to evaluate a dysfunctional lifestyle, stress, and anxiety. A useful question is:

- What do you yourself think your symptoms are due to?

Dizziness and vertigo not fully explained by an identifiable medical illness can be related to phobic, panic, anxiety, and/or depressive disorders, and the patient may reveal this. A final diagnosis of psychophysiological dizziness rests on a history of acute and chronic anxiety, in many cases side by side with symptoms of chronic depression.[41–43]

Concurrent Illness and Gait Unsteadiness

Keep in mind that there are also groups of patients who may be symptomatic because of concurrent illnesses such as diabetes mellitus, hypertension, and hyperlipidemia (all stroke risk factors);[44] multiple sclerosis; HIV/AIDS; metastatic cancer; severe malnutrition or post stroke complications. There is as well the causal possibility of Lyme disease, syphilis, or zoster (Ramsey Hunt, so look in the patient's ears.)

In the elderly, dizziness is common,[45] and unsteadiness of gait may be an early symptom of Parkinson's disease or of progressive supranuclear palsy, and it may be accompanied by a fear of falling.[46]

To sum up: of these two classes of dizzy patients—the unsteady, light-headed patient and the vertiginous patient afflicted with an erroneous perception of motion of herself and/or the world around her—it is the latter who presents the greater clinical challenge, and the characteristics of her "dizziness" are the key to diagnosis.

LOCALIZING NYSTAGMUS

Nystagmus is discussed in detail in Chapter 10. Its principal relevance here is as a localizing sign of the vestibular lesion causing vertigo. It is the key to understanding vertigo's "dizziness."

Lesions of the vestibular labyrinth or CN VIII typically interrupt tonic afferent signals originating from the motion receptors in the labyrinth. Nystagmus results, with combined torsional, horizontal, and vertical components but with the horizontal component dominant because the tonic activity from the intact vertical canals and otolith partially cancel each other out.

Nystagmus, in the form of peripheral vestibular nystagmus, is *unidirectional,* meaning that the primary direction of the fast phase does not change. If the nystagmus is right-beating, for example, it will not change to left-beating even on left gaze. Based on its presence during visual fixation in different positions of horizontal gaze, peripheral vestibular nystagmus is graded as *first-degree, second-degree, or third-degree vestibular nystagmus (Figure 8-13).*

- *First-degree* nystagmus refers to nystagmus that is present only on gaze in the direction of the fast phase.
- *Second-degree* nystagmus is present in the primary position and on gaze in the direction of the fast phase.
- *Third-degree* nystagmus is present even on gaze away from the direction of the fast phase.

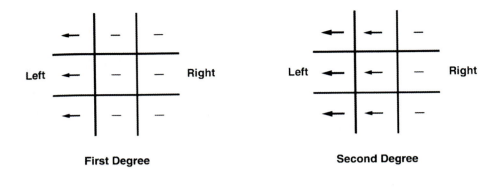

First Degree　　　　　　　　　Second Degree

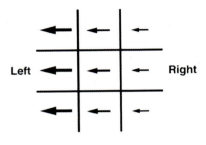

Third Degree

FIGURE 8-13 Alexander's system of grading vestibular nystagmus. Note that only the horizontal quick components of nystagmus are illustrated for the nine standard positions of gaze with the head motionless. The length and thickness of the arrows signify the intensity of the nystagmus. The patient had a first-degree left-beating vestibular nystagmus as a result of a right-sided peripheral vestibular loss.

Reproduced with permission.[11]

Peripheral vestibular nystagmus is strongly inhibited by fixation. Usually it subsides within a few days due to central rebalancing in the vestibular nuclei.

Central vestibular nystagmus is present with and without fixation and may be purely vertical, horizontal, or torsional or have some combination of torsional and horizontal components (Chapter 10). As with peripheral vestibular nystagmus, gaze in the direction of the fast component usually increases nystagmus frequency and amplitude, but, unlike peripheral nystagmus, gaze away from the direction of the fast component will often change the direction of the nystagmus.

Differentiation between vestibular nystagmus of peripheral versus central origin is shown in Table 8-3.[12]

Direction-changing horizontal nystagmus on lateral gaze is a highly important clinical sign whose presence identifies a central cause of acute vertigo. Direction-changing horizontal nystagmus presents as right-beating nystagmus in right gaze and left-beating nystagmus in left gaze. Nystagmus may be absent or present when the patient looks straight ahead. This type of nystagmus is gaze-evoked and reflects dysfunction of gaze-holding mechanisms located in the pons and cerebellum.

TABLE 8-3: Differentiation Between Vestibular Nystagmus of Peripheral and Central Origin

	Appearance	Fixation	Gaze	Mechanism	Localization
Peripheral	Combined horizontal, torsional	Inhibited	Unidirectional (Alexander's law)	Asymmetric loss of peripheral vestibular tone	Labyrinthine or vestibular nerve
Central	Often pure vertical, horizontal, or torsional	Usually little effect	May change direction	Imbalance in central oculomotor tone; usually central vestibular, may be pursuit or OKN	CNS, usually brainstem or cerebellum

CNS, central nervous system; OKN, optokinetic nystagmus

Reproduced with permission.[12]

Positional Nystagmus

Positional nystagmus (nystagmus evoked by head or body movements) can be either paroxysmal or persistent.

Paroxysmal Positional Nystagmus

The most common type of paroxysmal positional nystagmus is induced by a rapid change from erect sitting to the supine head-hanging left or right position (Dix-Hallpike test). A key feature is that the patient experiences severe vertigo with the initial positioning, but with repeated positioning, it fatigues and disappears. This type of paroxysmal positional nystagmus is specific for the posterior canal variant (posterior benign paroxysmal positional vertigo [P-BPPV]) of canalithiasis. A personal case illustrates the condition.

CASE 8-2 Benign Paroxsysmal Positional Vertigo

No Video Display

The patient is an elderly physician in excellent health and on no medication. One week prior to an acute episode of positional vertigo, she noticed on getting out of bed in the morning a sense of mild disequilibrium and unsteadiness walking. These symptoms persisted for 7 days and then, one night, when lying down in bed she experienced an acute rapid spinning sensation to the right without nausea, or vomiting. The episode lasted minutes only. The same sensation could be easily reproduced by staying in the supine position and turning her head to the left, with the left ear down. The sensation of spinning to the right was identical each time she did this. Sitting up was accompanied by a feeling of disequilibrium but no rotation.

The patient diagnosed her condition as benign paroxysmal positional vertigo and she consulted a neuro-otologist for treatment. This physician repeated the Dix-Hallpike maneuver from erect sitting to supine head-hanging left (approximately 45 degrees from the body) while viewing the patient's eyes with Frenzel lenses. The rapid movement produced acute vertigo, a sensation of rotating to the right. It elicited a mixed vertical torsional nystagmus, slow phase down. The latency before nystagmus and vertigo developed was very short, of the order of 30 seconds, and the nystagmus was transient, lasting less than 15 seconds. The nystagmus reversed direction on sitting up.

The response to this maneuver is illustrated in Figure 8-14.[47]

Diagnosis of BPPV rests on provoking vertigo with the characteristic nystagmus. The typical nystagmus induced by the upright to supine Dix-Hallpike test has combined torsional (fast component toward the undermost ear) and vertical fast components.[48] The eyes beat upward (toward the forehead) with the upper poles beating toward the ground producing an upbeat torsional nystagmus. Reverse nystagmus (downbeat and torsional) usually occurs if the patient is brought directly back up from the head-hanging position to the sitting position.[49,50] Treatment with the Epley maneuver is often successful.

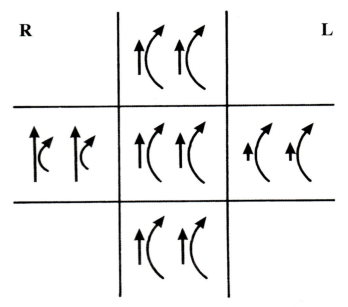

FIGURE 8-14 Benign paroxysmal positional vertigo. Drawing shows jerk nystagmus—a combination of vertical and torsional vectors. Nystagmus plane and direction (*curved arrow*) approximate that produced by stimulation of the left posterior semicircular canal. Lines with arrowhead indicate trajectory and direction of quick phases for each eye. Lengths of lines depict relative intensity of vertical and torsional components in each gaze position.

Reproduced with permission.[47]

An illustration of the modified Epley maneuver is shown in Figure 8-15.[12]

The treatment of BPPV using the Epley repositioning procedure is based on specific knowledge of the vertigo's cause. For BPPV to occur, otoconia (calcium carbonate crystallites) must be free floating in the utricle and when they enter a canal, usually the posterior canal symptoms occur. Rapid repositioning movements of the head unplug the canal, and positional vertigo and nystagmus stop. Spontaneous resolution of symptoms can take up to 10 weeks.[51,52]

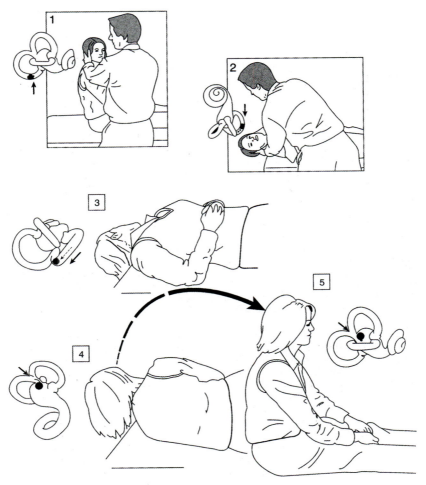

FIGURE 8-15 Modified Epley maneuver for treating the posterior canal variant of benign positional vertigo. After turning the head toward the affected side (right side in this case), the patient moves from a sitting to head hanging position (the Dix-Hallpike test, 1–2); once the nystagmus and vertigo have subsided, the patient rolls across to the opposite side, nose facing the ground, all in one motion (2–4); finally, after about 30 seconds, the patient returns to the sitting position (4–5).

Reproduced with permission.[12]

Benign paroxysmal positional vertigo is reported in migraine-related dizziness.[53] but true rotational vertigo, alone or associated with nausea and vomiting, often constitutes a migraine aura.[54] Attacks lasting for days or weeks in a milder form may produce a sensitivity to motion resulting in imbalance.[55] In some individuals, headache and vertigo accompanied by dysarthria, diplopia, and ataxia suggest basilar migraine.[56,57]

Persistent Positional Nystagmus

Persistent positional nystagmus persists as long as the head or body position is held, although it may fluctuate in frequency and amplitude. An unusual form of persistent positional nystagmus (direction-changing and *apogeotropic* or beating away from the ground), was one of the most important signs in Case 8-3.

CASE 8-3 Upbeat and Apogeotropic Nystagmus

Video Display

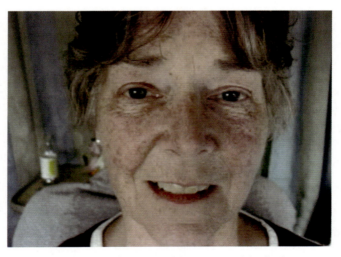

FIGURE 8-16 A sixty-five-year-old woman with dizziness and vertical oscillopsia.

The patient is a 65-year-old woman who, developed dizziness and an "inability to sense myself in space" during a transcontinental flight in August 2009. Her feeling of imbalance intensified, and she had difficulty standing. She was unable to walk off the plane without support. When fully upright, she felt "a sensation of being pulled backward with someone trying to push me off my heels."

She also had a 2-month history of impairment of short-term memory, recent intermittent blurring of vision ("eyes bobbing up and down"), and a 20-pound weight loss. She had smoked 1–2 packs of cigarettes a day, but quit at age 60. She currently drank two or more glasses of wine a night. Vestibular neuritis was diagnosed, and prednisone prescribed, but her symptoms progressed. She was admitted to the Massachusetts General Hospital.

Analysis of the History

- What are the major presenting symptoms?
- Where are the CNS lesion(s) likely to be?

CASE 8-2 SYMPTOMS

Symptoms	Location Correlation
Impaired memory	Medial temporal lobes
	Hippocampi
Dizziness	Vestibular system
Unsteady walking	Cerebellar vermis or cerebellar pathways
Sensation of being pulled backwards	Otolith pathway
Vertical oscillopsia	Vestibular pathways

The analysis guides the clinical examination.

Examination

Neurological

- Alert and appropriately interactive, but depressed
- Registered three items but failed to recall any at 5 minutes
- Unable to name the month of the year or the name of the hospital
- Followed complex commands
- Speech normal
- Able to spell WORLD backwards
- Marked truncal ataxia, fell backwards sitiing
- Bilateral lower limb ataxia
- Gait ataxic unable to walk and tandem
  Motor strength 5/5, normal reflexes
  Sensation intact

Ocular Motility

- Blurred vision (vertical oscillopsia) reading
- Spontaneous upbeat nystagmus
- Lid nystagmus
- Saccadic intrusions
- Upbeat nystagmus suppressed during convergence
- Persistent nystagmus, changing direction with changes in head/body position:
  Upbeat when erect
  Absent when supine
  Reduced when prone
  Beating away from the ground—apogeotropic—when lying on either side
  Horizontal and vertical saccades dysmetric
- Saccadic pursuit in all directions

Localization and Differential Diagnosis

Upbeat nystagmus with concomitant oscillopsia and postural instability reflec an imbalance of the vestibulo-ocular reflexes (the rotational and translation VORs, which generate eye movements that compensate for head movements) mediated by pathways from the vertical semicircular canals and the otoliths. Defects in cognition suggest that the medial temporal lobes and adjacent limbic areas are involved. Taken together, these signs are evidence of an underlying encephalitic process, possibly a "remote effect" of cancer.[58]

The differential diagnosis includes other encephalitic syndromes. These syndromes typically present with an acute febrile illness, meningeal involvement (sometimes only headache), and various combinations of symptoms and signs—convulsions, delirium, coma, aphasia, hemiparesis, ataxic, and myoclonic jerks. The spinal fluid in these cases invariably shows a cellular reaction and elevated protein. Early imaging studies are often normal.

What Diagnostic Tests Should Follow?

- A lumbar puncture for analysis of the cerebrospinal fluid (CSF).
- Blood tests including paraneoplastic markers.
- A search for an occult malignancy.
  Chest x-ray
  Brain MRI
  Mammogram
  Computerised (CT) scan abdomen/pelvis

Test Results

The spinal fluid showed elevated CSF protein at 69 mg/dL, sugar 60 mg/dL, and 7 leukocytes/mm^3 (97% lymphocytes, 3% monocytes and no malignant cells, oligoclonal bands, malignant or viral titers.Blood tests: Immunoglobulin was 22.5 mg/dL (elevated), albumin 33.2 mg/dL (normal).

Paraneoplastic antibody testing (anti-Ri, anti-Yo, anti-Hu, anti-MA1, anti-MA2, anti-ZiC4, and anti-CV2) was positive for anti-Hu antibodies at a titer of 1/15,360. Brain MRI (early in the admission) showed no signs of inflammation of the brain or

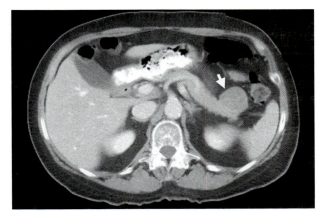

FIGURE 8-17 Computed tomography scan of abdomen and pelvis with intravenous contrast: solid appearing 3.8 cm well-defined heterogeneous mass (*arrows*) arising from the tail of the pancreas.

Reproduced with permission.[59]

cerebellum, only small vessel ischemia. Chest x-ray and scan were normal (ruling out coexisting cancer of the lung associated with positive anti-Hu antibodies).

The brain MRI and mammogram were normal.

Computed tomography (CT) of the abdomen/pelvis with contrast revealed a heterogeneous mass (arrow) arising from the tail of the pancreas (Figure 8-17).

A CT-guided core biopsy of the mass revealed a pancreatic endocrine neoplasm.

Diagnosis: Paraneoplastic Encephalitic Upbeat Nystagmus with Endocrine Carcinoma of the Pancreas

A spleen-sparing distal pancreatectomy was performed on day 8, and a well-differentiated endocrine carcinoma with metastases to one of 23 regional lymph nodes was excised.

Treatment

The patient was treated with cyclophosphamide, one dose IV 1,100 mg (600 mg/m²), followed by oral 75 mg/day (1 mg/kg/day), and a course of IV immunoglobulin (0.5 g/kg/day for 5 days). A 4-month trial of memantine 10 mg b.i.d. did not suppress the nystagmus. She was last seen in May 2013, wheelchair bound, but independent, cooking doing crosswords and able to take care of herself. Although in remission from her cancer, her husband had noted progressive short term memory loss and further cognitive decline.

Special Explanatory Note

There was clinical evidence for a paraneoplastic pathogenesis of this patient's upbeat nystagmus.[59] An immune attack, on either neuronal channels in the nodulus and ventral uvula of the cerebellum that govern otolith responses, or on acetylcholine receptors in brainstem pathways subserving the otolithic-ocular responses, might have been the mechanism, although antibodies against surface neuronal antigens, including receptors and channels, seemed more likely to account for the clinical findings.[60,61]

PROVOCATIVE TESTS TO ELICIT NYSTAGMUS BY SUPPRESSING FIXATION

Preventing visual fixation by occlusive ophthalmoscopy or head shaking can elicit nystagmus in cases where it has been so suppressed by visual fixation as to be invisible clinically. For example, in some stroke patients with acute vestibular syndrome nystagmus is only apparent when fixation is prevented.

Horizontal head shaking may elicit nystagmus in peripheral, as well as in central vestibular lesions.[62,63] In unilateral labyrinthine hypofunction, head shaking rapidly back and forth and from side to side for approximately 10–15 seconds, immediately induces a vigorous horizontal nystagmus (usually with a torsional component) with slow phases directed initially toward the affected labyrinth[64] and then toward the unaffected labyrinthduring the compensatory recovery phase.[65] With central vestibular lesions, the direction of the nystagmus is nonlocalizing. In some cases of cerebellar infarction, vertical nystagmus is induced by head shaking.[66]

Hyperventilation-induced nystagmus, with slow phases directed away from the side of the lesion (often with a torsional component prominent) can be induced in a number of disorders, including compression of the vestibular nerve by a vestibular schwannoma or demyelination of central pathways in multiple sclerosis. Hyperventilation enhances downbeat nystagmus in patients with cerebellar lesions (attributed to metabolic effects in the calcium channels of Purkinje cells).

The Valsalva maneuver can induce nystagmus by increasing intracranial pressure (as with weight-lifting). Blowing out against pinched nostrils increases pressure in the middle ear and may produce symptoms and signs in patients with hydrocephalus.

The cold caloric test (often valuable in determining the side of a peripheral lesion) has largely been replaced by the head impulse test as a test of the horizontal VOR. However, it can be performed at the bedside using only 2 mL of ice water and its usefulness should not be overlooked[67] (see Chapter 6, Case 6-5).

DIAGNOSTIC GUIDELINES FOR THE BEDSIDE EXAMINATION

The clinician's first task is to assess the function of the VOR. And there are two tests of VOR function that should be performed: the *dynamic visual acuity* (DVA) test and the *horizontal head impulse* test (h-HIT).

The DVA test requires the patient to read the letters of a Snellen visual acuity chart at standard distance, first with his head still and then while shaking his head rapidly, first horizontally, then vertically, and then in the roll plane from ear to shoulder, at a relatively high frequency of about 2 cycles/sec. Loss of three or more lines of visual acuity (head moving versus head stationary) indicates some degree of failure of vestibular function. DVA testing does not localize the lesion but it clearly identifies patients with bilateral vestibular loss from vestibular drug-induced ototoxicity.[68–70]

The h-HIT is a simple way to identify a complete unilateral or bilateral loss of vestibular function.[71] The test is best performed by sitting opposite the patient, grasping her head, and applying brief, small-amplitude, *high-acceleration* head rotation, first to one side and then to the other. Before starting, the examiner must warn the patient that the head will be rotated very rapidly (and it is advisable to start by rotating the head slowly several times before conducting the higher speed maneuver). The test must be performed with the patient fixating either on the examiner's nose or on a distant object and with the head positioned about 20 degrees away from the side to which it is to be thrust (Figure 8-18).

The normal VOR to rapid rotation of the head with fixation is an equal and opposite eye movement that leaves the eyes stationary in primary gaze when the head stops moving.

A *normal response* in a patient with an acute vestibular syndrome is a strong indicator that the labyrinth and vestibular nerve are intact, thus increasing the likelihood of a central brainstem or cerebellar lesion.[72,73]

An *abnormal response,* due to loss of vestibular input, results in the inability to maintain fixation on the examiner's nose, and, when the head stops moving, a corrective gaze shift (refixation saccade) directly opposite to the direction of the head movement is made to bring the eyes back to primary gaze. Corrective refixation saccades indicate the h-HIT is positive, a very strong indicator of a peripheral lesion of the labyrinth or vestibular nerve.

An equally important bedside test is the alternate cover test (Chapter 4) for vertical ocular misalignment indicative of skew. Its importance needs to be underlined: *skew deviation with vertigo points to a central lesion.*

In a study of 101 patients with acute vertigo, the authors found that the presence of *any one* of the three danger signs—negative head impulse test, direction-changing horizontal nystagmus on lateral gaze, and vertical misalignment due to skew—had a sensitivity of 100% ($n = 76/76$) and a specificity of 96% ($n = 24/25$) for stroke.

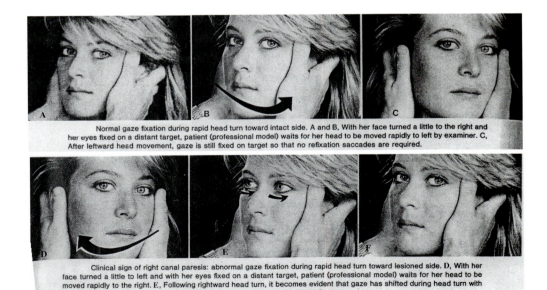

Normal gaze fixation during rapid head turn toward intact side. A and B, With her face turned a little to the right and her eyes fixed on a distant target, patient (professional model) waits for her head to be moved rapidly to left by examiner. C, After leftward head movement, gaze is still fixed on target so that no refixation saccades are required.

Clinical sign of right canal paresis: abnormal gaze fixation during rapid head turn toward lesioned side. D, With her face turned a little to left and with her eyes fixed on a distant target, patient (professional model) waits for her head to be moved rapidly to the right. E, Following rightward head turn, it becomes evident that gaze has shifted during head turn with head to right. F, Leftward or compensatory saccade is now required to refix gaze.

FIGURE 8-18 The head impulse test. A–C, Normal test, D–F, Right canal paresis—positive head impulse test.

Modified and reproduced with permission.[71]

These three components of bedside testing (the head impulse test [HI], direction-changing horizontal nystagmus on lateral gaze [N], and test of skew [TS], originally given the acronym HINTS), appear to rule stroke in or out with more accuracy than urgent MRI with diffusion-weighted imaging.[74]

VASCULAR SYNDROMES OF THE MEDULLA

Wallenberg's syndrome, due to infarction of the lateral medulla, is the most recognized syndrome of the medulla. It presents acutely with severe vertigo, nausea, vomiting, and unsteadiness—to which diplopia and headache can often be added. Fisher's comment that vomiting is out of proportion to dizziness in ischemic strokes of the brainstem is worth remembering.[75]

CASE 8-4 Wallenberg's Syndrome: The Lateral Medullary Syndrome

No Video Display

The patient is a 46-year-old left-handed man with a history of hypertension, hyperlipidemia, depression, and attention deficit disorder.

Having gone to bed at 11 P.M., he woke at 1:30 A.M. with a dull frontal headache, extreme dizziness/light-headedness, and diplopia. His voice was hoarse (dysphonia) and he complained of numbness involving his left side. He was brought to the ER at 3 A.M. and at that time the NIH stroke scale was noted to be 3 (right arm drift, right hand ataxia). The patient denied any recent head/neck trauma, chiropractor visits, loud coughing or sneezing, and no recent episodes of chest pain or palpitations.

A dizziness history confirmed he had vertigo.

Analysis of the History

- What are the major presenting symptoms?
- Where are the CNS lesion(s) likely to be?

CASE 8-3 SYMPTOMS

Symptoms	Location Correlation
Dizziness	Vestibular system
Dysarthria and hoarseness	Nucleus ambiguus in the medulla
Left hemisensory loss	Spinothalamic tract
Right facial numbness	Trigeminal nucleus/fasiculus CN V

The analysis guides the clinical examination.

Examination

Neurological

- Fatigued and drowsy, requiring frequent redirection
- Oriented ×3
- Obeyed three-step commands
- Dysarthric with a hoarse quality to his voice

Ipsilateral signs
- Facial hypalgesia and thermoanesthesia due to involvement of the trigeminal nucleus and descending tract
- No ipsilateral facial pain
- Palatal, pharyngeal, and vocal cord paralysis with dysphagia and dysarthria due to involvement of the nucleus ambiguus
- Right limb cerebellar ataxia due to involvement of the inferior cerebellar peduncle and cerebellum

Contralateral signs
- Crossed hemisensory loss with left extremity hypalgesia and thermoanesthesia due to involvement of the spinothalamic tract

Ocular Motility

- Right Horner's syndrome (ptosis and miosis) due to involvement of the descending sympathetic pathway
- Full vertical and horizontal saccadic eye movements
- Horizontal gaze-evoked, direction changing, torsional nystagmus gaze right and left most pronounced looking right
- OTR with ipsilateral hypotropia and head tilt to the right
- Saccadic pursuit in all directions
- Normal oculocephalic reflex
- Lateropulsion of horizontal saccades to the right under closed lids

Localization and Differential Diagnosis

The classic constellation of ipsilateral and contralateral signs characteristic of Wallenberg's syndrome results from infarction of a wedge-shaped area of the lateral medulla and inferior cerebellum (Figure 8-19).[12]

Involvement of the nucleus ambiguus results in paralysis of the ipsilateral palate, pharynx, and larynx producing dysphagia, dysarthria, and hoarseness. Dysarthria and hoarseness are often combined and are present in 30–60% of patients.

Headache, especially unilateral headache localized to the upper posterior cervical region, is particularly common when the syndrome is due to vertebral artery dissection.

The motor system, tongue movements, and vibration and position sense are spared because the corresponding anatomic structures are located in the medial medulla.

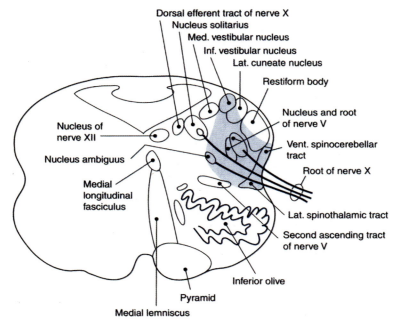

FIGURE 8-19 Cross-section of the medulla illustrating the zone of infarction with Wallenberg's syndrome (red area).

Reproduced with permission.[12]

What Diagnostic Tests Should Follow?

· Brain MRI
· Brain magnetic resonance angiography (MRA) or
· CT angiography (CTA) of the posterior circulation[76–78]

Test Results

Brain MRI showed an acute DWI bright/ADC dark right lateral medullary infarct. The study was not retained. MRI images of a similar case are shown in Figure 8-20. An MRA was not done. A CT/CTA of the head and neck showed irregular narrowing of a segment of the distal right cervical vertebral artery just proximal to dural penetration. Opacification of intradural segment, on delayed images, was attributed to critical narrowing rather than complete occlusion, suggesting a right vertebral artery dissection.

Diagnosis: Right Lateral Medullary Infarction with Dissection of the Right Vertebral Artery

The patient was told that he had a dissection of the right vertebral artery. He then recalled that he had had minor trauma to his neck a few days prior to admission. He was washing laundry at the time and threw a large bag of dirty laundry over his shoulder hitting his neck. Trauma, as in this case, or neck manipulation, are the leading causes of vertebral artery dissection, particularly in young patients.[79]

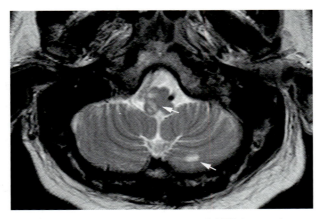

FIGURE 8-20 Magnetic resonance axial T2 image in a patient with a classic Wallenberg syndrome shows hyperintensity in the right lateral medulla involving the olivary nucleus (*arrow*). There is also hyperintensity in the right vertebral artery representing thrombus in contrast to the intact flow void in the left vertebral artery. A small old infarct is also present in the left cerebellar hemisphere (*arrow*).

Courtesy of Anne Osborn, M.D.

Treatment

· Anticoagulation

The patient received IV heparin and transitioned to Coumadin prior to discharge. He was instructed to stay on Coumadin for 6 months and return for a repeat CTA.

Special Explanatory Note

Disordered perceptions of verticality can be quite bizarre in Wallenberg's syndrome.[80] For example, a transient visual illusion with a 180-degree reversal of vision—the "floor on ceiling" upside-down phenomenon[81]—is attributed to ischemia of the central vestibulo-ocular integrative control system.

More often, patients experience a prominent motor disturbance that causes the body to deviate toward the side of the lesion as if being pulled by a strong external force.[82,83] This so-called *lateropulsion* affects the oculomotor system, causing excessively large voluntary and involuntary saccades directed toward the side of the lesion, whereas saccades away from the lesion side are abnormally small.[84,85]

Lateropulsion is prominent when the patient blinks. Typically, the eyes deviate horizontally under closed lids to the side of the lesion (ipsipulsion) and, on eye opening, they make a spontaneous corrective saccade to place the eye in primary gaze. Ipsipulsion, in Wallenberg's syndrome is attributed to interuption

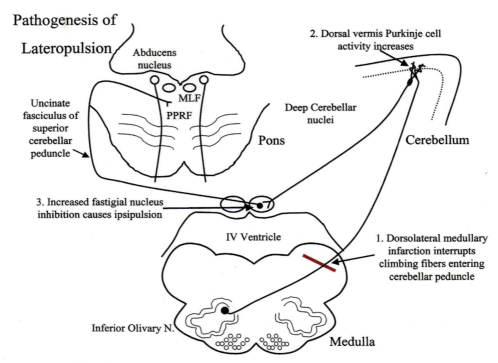

FIGURE 8-21 Hypothetical scheme to account for lateropulsion of saccades. Interruption of climbing fibers originating from the inferior olivary nucleus may occur prior to their crossing in the medulla (1) or as they enter the inferior cerebellar peduncle (in Wallenberg's syndrome. (2) Loss of climbing fiber inputs to Purkinje cells in the dorsal vermis causes the latter to inhibit the fastigial nucleus (4), which causes ipsipulsion of saccades. Pharmacological inactivation of the dorsal vermis (3) causes contrapulsion (although clinical lesions produce bilateral hypometria). Interruption of crossed fastigial nucleus outputs in the superior cerebellar peduncle (uncinate fasciculus, 5) causes contrapulsion. Thus, contrapulsion arises at sites 1, 3 and 5, and ipsipulsion at sites 2–4.

Reproduced with permission.[13]

of inputs (climbing fibres) from the contraleteral inferior olive in the medulla to the cerebellar vermis in the inferior cerebellar peduncle that is thought to increase activity of Purkinje cells and cause a unilateral (functional) fastigial nucleus "lesion". Interuption of the crossed output of the fastigeal nucleus in the superior cerebellar peduncle causes contrapulsion of saccades character-ised by overshooting contralaterally, undershooting ipsilaterally (Figure 8-21).[21]

Patients with Wallenberg's syndrome may develop hiccups several days after stroke onset and the hiccups usually subside within a few days but can persist for weeks. Intractable hiccups is a rare syndrome of the medulla and a unique case is presented here.

CASE 8-5 Intractable Hiccups

Video Display

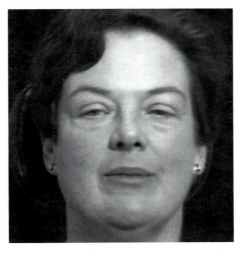

FIGURE 8-22 A fifty-year-old woman with intractable hiccups.

The patient is a 50-year-old woman who presented in November 1977 with vertigo, a transient facial droop, nystagmus, diplopia, and dysarthria (Figure 8-22). She had an extensive workup, including CT brain scan, angiogram, and spinal tap. A brainstem lesion was detected. She received a brief course of steroids, with complete resolution of her symptoms in 6 weeks.

Fourteen years later, in August 1991, she developed sinusitis and bilateral headache. She was seen by an otorhinologist and a brain MRI was scheduled. Five days prior to her appointment, she developed intractable hiccup (Figure 8-22).

Analysis of the History

- What are the major presenting symptoms?
- Where are the CNS lesion(s) likely to be?

CASE 8-4 SYMPTOMS

Symptoms	Location Correlation
Headache	Intracranial
Intractable hiccup	Medullary nuclei

The analysis guides the clinical examination.

Examination

Ocular Motility

- Upbeat nystagmus in primary gaze
- Lid nystagmus
- Vertical gaze full with upbeat nystagmus
- Horizontal gaze full
- Convergence normal
- Vertical and horizontal saccadic pursuit
- Vertical and horizontal saccadic hypermetria
- Horizontal vestibular ocular reflex suppressed (tested by rotating the patient in the chair and asking her to fix on her thumb held up on her outstretched arm moving with her)

The neurological examination was normal.

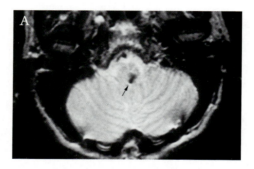

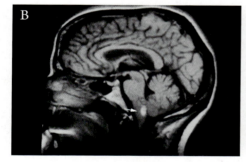 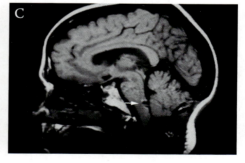

FIGURE 8-23 Brain magnetic resonance imaging (MRI). (A) An axial susceptibility sequence shows focal hemorrhage in the medulla (*arrow*). (B) Sagittal T1 image shows a cavernous malformation at the pontomedullary junction with adjacent hyperintense hemorrhage in the medulla (*arrow*). (C) Sagittal paramedian T1 image shows a cavernous malformation in the dorsal pontomedullary junction (*arrow*).

Localization and Differential Diagnosis

Vertigo, nystagmus, and dysarthria localizes to the nuclei in the medulla. Headache—the initial symptom—was highly important.

What Diagnostic Tests Should Follow?

· Review of the 1977 imaging studies (not available)
· Brain MRI, noncontrast

Axial Brain MRI susceptibility study showed a low signal rim (hemosiderin) around a hemorrhage in the dorsal pontomedullary junction (Figure 8-23A). Saggital brain T1 images showed a cavernous malformation at the pontomedullary junction with adjacent hemorrhage in the medulla (Figure 8-23B–C).

Diagnosis: Left Medullary Hemorrhage with Cavernous Angioma

Treatment

· Surgical resection

The patient underwent suboccipital craniotomy and resection of a medullary cavernous angioma, confirmed histopathologically. Postoperatively, the hiccups stopped but vertical oscillopsia and extreme sensitivity to motion required her to move extremely slowly so as not to trigger vertigo.

Examination

Neurological

· Extremely sensitive to motion, which provoked vertigo
· Marked gait ataxia and truncal ataxia with difficulty standing
· Motor strength 5/5 throughout, normal reflexes

Ocular Motility

· Upbeat nystagmus
· Lid nystagmus (synkinetic lid twitches in conjunction with the fast phase up)
· Full horizontal and vertical eye movements
· Normal convergence
· Saccadic pursuit in all directions of gaze
· Saccadic hypermetria vertically and horizontally

What Further Diagnostic Studies Should Follow?

· Brain MRI

Test Results

@ Brain MRI showed an area of decreased signal on T1 measuring 6 mm in diameter at the level of the pontomedullary junction and no hemorrhage.

Treatment

· Medication to suppress upbeat nystagmus

The patient received Klonopin 0.5 mg t.i.d. and steadily improved.

Special Explanatory Note

Hiccups consist of brief bursts of intense inspiratory activity with abrupt involuntary contraction of the diaphragm and inspiratory intercostal muscles, with sudden closure of the glottis 35 msec after onset, generating the characteristic sound and sense of discomfort.[86,87] The term "intractable" refers to hiccups with a duration ranging from 24 hours to several years—other terms include chronic, persistent, and obstinate. Hiccups continuing for longer than 24 hours are rare and may indicate serious underlying disease, in particular structural or functional disturbances of the medulla affecting the dorsal motor nucleus of the vagus (CN X), the nucleus tractus solitarius, and, more likely, the neurons related to expiration and inspiration in the reticular formation near the nucleus ambiguus, the vagal nuclei, and the nucleus tractus solitarius associated with respiratory control, or afferent or efferent nerves to the respiratory muscles.

Although hiccups are particularly associated with infarction in the territory of the posterior inferior cerebellar artery or a bleed into a cavernous angioma (as in this case), tumor,[88] and multiple sclerosis are also possible.[89,90] Hiccup occurrence may anticipate the onset of irregularities of the respiratory rhythm, culminating in respiratory arrest.

The Medial Medullary Syndrome

The medial medullary syndrome, also known as Dejerine's anterior bulbar syndrome, is caused by occlusion of the anterior spinal artery (ASA) or its parent vertebral artery.[91] The ASA supplies a medial segment of the medulla containing the pyramid, medial lemniscus, and hypoglossal nucleus.

Occlusion of the ASA produces a classic clinical triad of signs:

- *Contralateral* hemiplegia due to involvement of the pyramid with sparing of the face.
- *Contralateral* loss of joint position and vibratory sensation in the limbs due to involvement of the medial lemniscus, sparing pain and temperature sensitivity.
- *Ipsilateral* paresis, atrophy, and fibrillation of the tongue due to involvement of the hypoglossal nucleus. The protruded tongue deviates toward the side of the lesion and away from the hemiplegia.

Notably, ipsilateral paresis of the tongue is the most topographically localizing sign of the medial medullary syndrome.[92]

Several types of eye movement disorders (most often upbeat nystagmus) have been reported in medial medullary infarction. They include bow-tie and hemi-see-saw nystagmus, the OTR, and saccadic lateropulsion or contrapulsion.

Before the advent of MRI, infarction of the medial medulla was verifiable only at autopsy. MRI reports have expanded clinical knowledge of the medullary syndromes, and they suggest that the

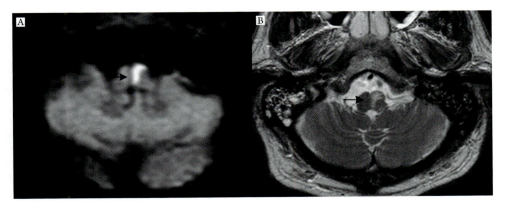

FIGURE 8-24 Brain magnetic resonance imaging (MRI). (A) Axial diffuse-weighted image shows hyperintensity in the left medial medulla consistent with infarction. (B) Axial T2 image demonstrates hyperintensity in the left medial medulla corresponding to the area of restricted diffusion, consistent with a lesion of greater than a few hours duration.

frequency of medial medullary infarction has previously been underestimated.[93] A brain MRI in a patient with a medial medullary infarction is shown in Figure 8-24A–B.

Occlusion of the anterior inferior cerebellar artery (AICA) results in infarction of the dorsolateral pontomedullary region and the middle cerebellar peduncle. Pofound unilateral or bilateral hearing loss and vertigo can be the initial or sole manifestation of occlusion of the AICA[94,95] due to infarction of the labyrinth, CN VIII or the CN VIII nerve root entry zone in the brainstem. Suspicion of a cerebellar infarction is increased if truncal ataxia and direction-changing gaze-evoked nystagmus are present.

SELECTED REFERENCES

1. Leigh JR, Zee DS. With permission 2013.
2. Pierrot-Deseilligny C, Milea D. Vertical nystagmus: clinical facts and hypotheses. *Brain.* 2005;128:1237–1246.
3. Munro NA, Gaymard B, Rivaud S, Majdalani A, Pierrot-Deseilligny C. Upbeat nystagmus in a patient with a small medullary infarct. *J Neurol Neurosurg Psychiat.* 1993;56:1126–1128.
4. Nakamagoe K, Iwamoto Y, Yoshida K. Evidence for brainstem structures participating in oculomotor integration. *Science.* 2000;288:857–859.
5. Guillain G, Mollaret P. Deux cas myoclonies synchrones et rhythmees velo-pharyngo-laryngo-oculodiaphragmatiques: Le problem anatomique et physiolopathologique de ce syndrome. *Rev Neurol (Paris).* 1931;2:545–566.
6. Barmack NH. Central vestibular system: vestibular nuclei and posterior cerebellum 2. *Brain Res Bul.* 2003;60:511–541.
7. Shaikh AG, Hong S, Liao K, Tian J, Solomon D, Zee DS, Leigh RJ, Optican LM. Oculopalatal tremor explained by a model of inferior olivary hypertrophy and cerebellar plasticity. *Brain.* 2010;133:923–940.
8. Leigh RJ, Hong S, Zee DS, Optican LM. Oculopalatal tremor: clinical and computational study of a disorder of the inferior olive. *Soc Neurosci Abstr.* 2005; 933.8.
9. Kim JS, Moon SY, Choi KD, Kim JH, Sharpe JA. Patterns of ocular oscillation in oculopalatal tremor: imaging correlations. *Neurology.* 2007;68(14):1128–1135.
10. Wong AMF. *Eye Movement Disorders.* New York: Oxford University Press; 2008.
11. Furman JM, Cass SP, Whitney SL. *Vestibular Disorders: A Case-study Approach to Diagnosis and Treatment.* 3rd ed. Oxford: Oxford University Press; 2010.

12. Baloh RW, Kerber KA. *Clinical Neurophysiology of the Vestibular System.* 4th ed. Philadelphia, PA: Oxford University Press; 2011.

13. Leigh JR, Zee DS. *The Neurology of Eye Movements.* 4th ed. New York: Oxford University Press; 2006.

14. Dieterich M, Brandt T. Ocular torsion and tilt of subjective visual vertical are sensitive brainstem signs. *Ann Neurol.* 1993;33:292–299.

15. Zwergal ACC, Arbusow V, Glaser M, Fesl G, Brandt T, Strupp M. Unilateral INO is associated with ocular tilt reaction in pontomesencephalic lesions: INO plus. *Neurology.* 2008;71:590–593.

16. Zwergal A, Rettinger N, Frenzel C, Dieterich M, Brandt T, Strupp M. A bucket of static vestibular function. *Neurology.* 2009;72:1689–1692.

17. Brandt T, Dieterich M. Skew deviation with ocular torsion: a vestibular brainstem sign of topographic diagnostic value. *Ann Neurol.* 1993;33:528–534.

18. Brandt T, Dieterich M. Central vestibular syndromes in roll, pitch, and jaw planes: topographic diagnosis of brainstem disorders. *Neuro-ophthalmology.* 1995; 15(6):291–303.

19. Brandt T, Dieterich M. Different types of skew deviation. *J Neurol Neurosurg Psychiat.* 1991;54:549–550.

20. Brandt T, Dieterich M. Pathological eye-head coordination in roll: tonic ocular tilt reaction in mesencephalic and medullary lesions. *Brain.* 1987;110:649–666.

21. Halmagyi GM, Gresty MA, Gibson WPR. Ocular tilt reaction with peripheral vestibular lesion. *Ann Neurol.* 1979;6:80–83.

22. Brandt T, Dieterich M. Two types of ocular tilt reaction: the "ascending" pontomedullary VOR-OTR and the "descending" mesencephalic integrator-OTR. *Neuro-ophthalmology.* 1998;19(2):83–92.

23. Newman-Toker DE, Cannon LM, Stofferahn ME, Rothman RE, Hsieh YH, Zee DS. Imprecision in patient reports of dizziness symptom quality: a cross-sectional study conducted in an acute care setting. *Mayo Clin Proc.* 2007;82(11):1329–1340.

24. Grad A, Baloh RW. Vertigo of vascular origin. Clinical and oculographic features. *Arch Neurol.* 1989;46:281–284.

25. Cheung CS, Mak PS, Manley KV, Lam JMY, Tsang AYL, Chan HMS, Rainer TH, Graham CA. Predictors of important neurological causes of dizziness among patients presenting to the emergency department. *Emerg Med J.* 2010;27(7):517–521.

26. Baloh RW, Honrubia V. *Clinical Neurophysiology of the Vestibular System.* 2nd ed. Philadelphia, PA: FA Davis; 1990.

27. Havia M, Kentala E. Progression of symptoms of dizziness in Meniere's disease. *Arch Otolaryngol Head Neck Surg.* 2004;130(4):431–435.

28. Baloh RW, Jacobson K, Winder AT. Drop attacks with Meniere's syndrome. *Ann Neurol.* 1990;28:384–387.

29. Ishiyama G, Ishiyama A, Jacobson K, Baloh RW. Drop attacks in older patients secondary to an otologic cause. *Neurology.* 2001;57(6):1103–1106.

30. Watson SRD, Halmagyi GM, Colebatch JG. Vestibular hypersensitivity to sound (Tulio phenomenon). *Neurology.* 2000;54:722–728.

31. Silbert PL, Mokri B, Schievink WI. Headache and neck pain in spontaneous internal carotid and vertebral artery dissections. *Neurology.* 1995;45(8):1517–1522.

32. de Sousa JE, Halfon MJ, Bonardo P, Reisin RC, Fernandez Pardal MM. Different pain patterns in patients with vertebral artery dissections. *Neurology.* 2005; 64(5):925–926.

33. Yen JC, Chan L, Lai YJ. Vertebral artery dissection presented as lateral medullary syndrome in a patient with migraine: a case report. *Acta Neurol Taiwan.* 2010; 19(4):275–280.

34. Lee H, Jen JC, Cha YH, Nelson SF, Baloh RW. Phenotypic and genetic analysis of a large family with migraine-associated vertigo. *Headache.* 2008;48(10):1460–1467.

35. Vuković V, Plavec D, Galinović I, Lovrencić-Huzjan A, Budisić M, Demarin V. Prevalence of vertigo, dizziness, and migrainous vertigo in patients with migraine. *Headache.* 2007;47(10):1427–1435.

36. Neuhauser H, Leopold M, von Brevern M, Arnold G, Lempert T. The interrelations of migraine, vertigo, and migrainous vertigo. *Neurology.* 2001;56(4):436–441.

37. Furman JM, Marcus DA, Balaban CD. Migrainous vertigo: development of a pathogenetic model and structured diagnostic interview. *Curr Opin Neurol.* 2003; 16(1):5–13.

38. Freeman R. Current pharmacologic treatment for orthostatic hypotension. *Clin Auton Res.* 2008;18(suppl 1):14–18.

39. Halmagyi GM, Fattore CM, Curthoys IS, Wade S. Gentamicin vestibulotoxicity. *Otolaryngol Head Neck Surg.* 1994;111:571–574.
40. Ishiyama G, Ishiyama A, Kerber K, Baloh RW. Gentamicin ototoxicity: clinical features and the effect on the human vestibulo-ocular reflex. *Acta Otolaryngol.* 2006;126(10):1057–1061.
41. Yardley L, Owen N. Nazareth I, Luxon L. Panic disorder with agoraphobia associated with dizziness: characteristic symptoms and psychosocial sequelae. *J Nerv Ment Dis.* 2001;189(5):321–327.
42. Clark MR, Sullivan MD, Fischl M, Katon WJ, Russo JE, Doble RA, Voorhees R. Symptoms as a clue to otologic and psychiatric diagnosis in patients with dizziness. *J Psychosom Res.* 1994;38(5):461–470.
43. Lahmann C, Henningsen P, Dieterich M, Feuerecker R, Cyran CA, Schmid G. The Munich diagnostic and predictor study of dizziness: objectives, design, and methods. *J Neurol.* 2012;259:702–711.
44. Hsu LC. Isolated dizziness/vertigo, vascular risk factors and stroke. *Acta Neurol Taiwan.* 2011;20(2):75–76.
45. Tinetti ME, Williams CS, Gill TM. Dizziness among older adults: a possible geriatric syndrome. *Ann Intern Med.* 2000;132(5):337–344.
46. Masdeu JC, Wolfson L. White matter lesions predispose to falls in older people. *Stroke.* 2009;40(9):e546.
47. Fletcher WA. Nystagmus: An overview. In: Sharpe JA, Barber HO, eds. *Vestibulo-ocular Reflex, Nystagmus and Vertigo.* New York: Raven Press; 1993;Ch 16:195–215.
48. Dix MR, Hallpike CS. The pathology, symptomatology and diagnosis of certain common disorders of the vestibular system. Section of Otology. *Proc R Soc Med.* 1952;45:341–354.
49. Harbert F. Benign paroxysmal positional nystagmus. *Arch Ophthalmol.* 1970; 84(3):298–302.
50. Baloh RW, Sakala SM, Honrubia V. Benign paroxysmal positional nystagmus. *Am J Otolaryngol.* 1979;1(1):1–6.
51. Imai T, Ito M, Takeda N, Uno A, Matsunaga T, Sekine K, Kubo T. Natural course of the remission of vertigo in patients with benign paroxysmal positional vertigo. *Neurology.* 2005;64:920–921.
52. Lopez-Escamez JA, Gamiz MJ, Fernandez-Perez A, Gomez-Finana M. Long-term outcome and health-related quality of life in benign paroxysmal positional vertigo. *Eur Arch Otorhinolaryngol.* 2005;262:507–511.
53. Ishiyama A, Jacobson KM, Baloh RW. Migraine and benign positional vertigo. *Ann Otol Rhinol Laryngol.* 2000;109:377–380.
54. Selby G, Lance JW. Observations on 500 cases of migraine and allied vascular headache. *J Neurol Neurosurg Psychiat.* 1960;23(1):23–32.
55. Cutrer FM, Baloh RW. Migraine-associated dizziness. *Headache* 1992; 32:300–304.
56. Bickerstall ER. Basilar artery migraine. *Lancet.* 1961;1:15–17.
57. Harker LA. Migraine-associated vertigo. In: Baloh RW, Halmagyi GM, eds. *Disorders of the Vestibular System.* New York: Oxford University Press; 1996:407–417.
58. Ko MW, Dalmau JO, Galetta SL. Neuro-ophthalmologic manifestations of paraneoplastic syndromes. *J Neuro-ophthalmol.* 2008;28:58–68.
59. Wray SH, Dalmau J, Chen A, King S, Leigh RJ. Paraneoplastic disorders of eye movements. *Ann NY Acad Sci.* 2011;1233:279–284.
60. Wray SH, Martinez-Hernandes E, Dalmau J, Maheshwari A, Chen A, King S, Bishop-Pitman M, Leigh RJ. Paraneoplastic upbeat nystagmus. *Neurology.* 2011; 77:691–693.
61. Graus E, Saiz A, Dalmau J. Antibodies and neuronal autoimmune disorders of the CNS. *J Neurol.* 2010;257:509–517.
62. Hain TC, Spindler J. Head-shaking nystagmus. In: Sharpe JA, Barber HO, eds. *The Vestibulo-ocular Reflex and Vertigo.* New York: Raven Press; 1993:217–228.
63. Takahashi S, Fetter M, Koenig E, Dichgans J. The clinical significance of head-shaking nystagmus in the dizzy patient. *Acta Otolaryngol.* 1990;109:8–14.
64. Strupp M. Perverted head-shaking nystagmus: two possible mechanisms. *J Neurol.* 2002;249(1):118–119.
65. Choi K-D, Oh SY, Kim HJ, Kim JS. The vestibulo-ocular reflexes during head impulse in Wernicke's encephalopathy. *J Neurol Neurosurg Psychiat.* 2007; 78(10):1161–1162.
66. Huh YE, Kim JS. Patterns of spontaneous and head-shaking nystagmus in cerebellar infarction: imaging correlations. *Brain.* 2011;134:3662–3671.
67. Schmal F, Lubben B, Weiberg K, Stoll W. The minimal ice water caloric test compared with established vestibular caloric test procedures. *J Vestib Res.* 2005; 15(4):215–224.
68. Longridge NS, Mallinson AI. The dynamic illegible E (DIE) test: a simple technique for assessing the vestibulo-ocular reflex to overcome vestibular pathology. *Can J Otolaryngol.* 1987;16:97–103.

69. Burgio DL, Blakely BW, Myers SE. The high frequency oscillopsia test. *J Vestib Res.* 1992;2:221–226.

70. Kaeser PF, Borruat FX. Altered vision during motion: an unusual symptom of cerebellar dysfunction, quantifiable by a simple clinical test. *Acta Ophthalmol.* 2010;88(7):791–796.

71. Halmagyi GM, Curthoys IS. A clinical sign of canal paresis. *Arch Neurol.* 1988;45:737–739.

72. Newman-Toker DE, Kattah JC, Alvernia JE, Wang DZ. Normal head impulse test differentiates acute cerebellar strokes from vestibular neuritis. *Neurology.* 2008;70:2378–2385.

73. Tarnutzer AA, Berkowitz AL, Robinson KA, Hsieh Y-H, Newman-Toker DE. Does my dizzy patient have a stroke? A systematic review of bedside diagnosis in acute vestibular syndrome. *CMAJ.* 2011;183(9):1–22.

74. Kattah JC, Talkad AV, Wang DZ, Hsieh Y-H, Newman-Toker DE. HINTS to diagnose stroke in the acute vestibular syndrome: three-step bedside oculomotor examination more sensitive than early MRI diffusion-weighted imaging. *Stroke.* 2009;40:3504–3510.

75. Fisher CM. Vomiting out of proportion to dizziness in ischemic brainstem strokes. *Neurology.* 1996;46(1):267–268.

76. Fisher CM, Karnes WE, Kubik CS. Lateral medullary infarction—the pattern of vascular occlusion. *J Neuropathol Exp Neurol.* 1961;20:323–379.

77. Bartels E. Dissection of the extracranial vertebral artery: clinical findings and early noninvasive diagnosis in 24 patients. *J Neuroimaging.* 2006;16(1):24–33.

78. Arnold M, Bousser MG, Fahrni G, Fischer U, Georgiadis D, Gandjour J, Benninger D. Vertebral artery dissection presenting findings and predictors of outcome. *Stroke.* 2006;37:2499–2503.

79. Frumkin LR, Baloh RW. Wallenberg's syndrome following neck manipulation. *Neurology.* 1990;40:611–615.

80. Dieterich DM, Brandt T. Wallenberg's syndrome: lateropulsion, cyclorotation, and subjective visual vertical in thirty-six patients. *Ann Neurol.* 1992;31:399–408.

81. Steiner I, Shahin R, Melamed E. Acute "upside down" reversal of vision in transient vertebrobasilar ischemia. *Neurology.* 1987;37:1685–1686.

82. Bjerner K, Silfverskold BJ. Lateropulsion and imbalance in Wallenberg's syndrome. *Acta Neurol Scand.* 1968;44:91–100.

83. Nowak DA, Topka HR. The clinical variability of Wallenberg's syndrome. The anatomical correlate of ipsilateral axial lateropulsion. *J Neurol.* 2006;253(4):507–511.

84. Kommerell G, Hoyt WF. Lateropulsion of saccadic eye movements: electro-oculographic studies in a patient with Wallenberg's syndrome. *Arch Neurol.* 1973;28:313–318.

85. Choi KD, Kim HJ, Cho BM, Kim JS. Saccadic adaptation in lateral medullary and cerebellar infarction. *Exp Brain Res.* 2008;188(3):475–482.

86. Newsom-Davis J. An experimental study of hiccup. *Brain.* 1970;93:851–872.

87. Newsom-Davis J. Pathological interoperative responses in respiratory muscles and the mechanism of hiccup. In: Desmedt J, ed. *New Developments in EMG and Clinical Neurophysiology.* Vol 3. Basel: Karger; 1973:751–760.

88. Slotka VL, Barcay SJ, Bell HS, Clare FB. Intractable hiccough as the primary manifestation of brain stem tumor. *Am J Med.* 1962;32:13–15.

89. McFarling DA, Susac JO. Hoquet diabolique: intractable hiccups as a manifestation of multiple sclerosis. *Neurology.* 1979;29:797–801.

90. Howard RS, Wiles CM, Hirsch NP, Loh L, Spencer GT, Newsom-Davis J. Respiratory involvement in multiple sclerosis. *Brain.* 1992;115:479–494.

91. Davison C. Syndrome of the anterior spinal artery of the medullar oblongata. *Arch Neurol Psychiat.* 1937;37:91–107.

92. Ho KL, Meyer KR. The medial medullary syndrome. *Arch Neurol.* 1981;38:385–387.

93. Kameda W, Kawanami T, Kurita K, Daimon M, Kayama T, Hosoya T, Kato T. Lateral and medial medullary infarction: a comparative analysis of 214 patients. *Stroke.* 2004;35:694–699.

94. Lee H, Ahn BH, Baloh RW. Sudden deafness with vertigo as a sole manifestation of anterior inferior cerebellar artery infarction. *J Neurol Sci.* 2004;222(1–2):105

95. Lee H, Yi HA, Baloh RW. Sudden bilateral simultaneous deafness with vertigo as a sole manifestation of vertebrobasilar insufficiency. *J Neurol Neurosurg Psychiat.* 2003;74(4):539.

| 9 |

THE CEREBELLUM AND ITS SYNDROMES

THE CEREBELLUM

The cerebellum is responsible for optimizing movement of the eyes to provide the clearest possible vision. It makes the minute adjustments needed for visual accuracy and stability and, equally important, it also maintains the body's equilibrium and muscle tone.

The cerebellum is located in the posterior fossa, which is formed by the occipital bones and clivus inferiorly and by the dura of the tentorium cerebelli superiorly. It lies dorsal to the pons and medulla (Figure 9-1).[1]

The cerebellum consists of a central portion, the vermis, and two lateral portions, the cerebellar hemispheres. It is connected to the brainstem by three large cerebellar peduncles: the inferior (restiform body), the middle (brachium pontis), and the superior (brachium conjunctivum) peduncles. The inferior peduncle connects the cerebellum to the medulla, the middle peduncle connects the cerebellum to the pons, and the superior peduncle connects the cerebellum to the midbrain.

There are three functional regions of the cerebellum contributing to the control of gaze: the dorsal oculomotor vermis (the OMV, lobules VI and VII), which is essential for the accuracy of saccades; the flocculus plus ventral paraflocculus, which are concerned with optokinetic movements, gaze-holding, and smooth pursuit; and the nodulus and ventral uvula, which play an important role in control of the vestibulo-ocular reflex (VOR).

A schematic drawing of the cerebellum showing the three separate regions involved in different eye movement functions is shown in Figure 9-2.[2]

The cerebellum constantly monitors and recalibrates oculomotor reflexes and eye movements, using not only cues from the cerebral cortical areas that process visual motion, but information from every source available, including proprioceptive information from the extraocular muscles. In this way, it determines the best relation of the eyes and the body to the outside world, particularly when normal inputs become defective and incongruent due to disease. This adaptive control of eye movements by the cerebellum—for this is what it is—largely depends on the dorsal vermis of the posterior lobe and the underlying posterior portion of the fastigial nucleus and the vestibulocerebellum.

All outputs from the cerebellum are carried by Purkinje cells to the deep cerebellar nuclei or vestibular nuclei.

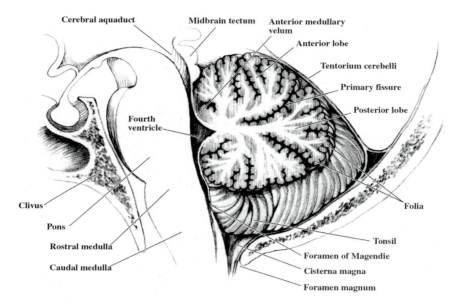

FIGURE 9-1 Sagittal view in situ: The cerebellum and brainstem lie within the posterior fossa formed by the occipital bones and clivus inferiorly and by the dura of the tentorium cerebelli superiorly.

Reproduced with permission.[1]

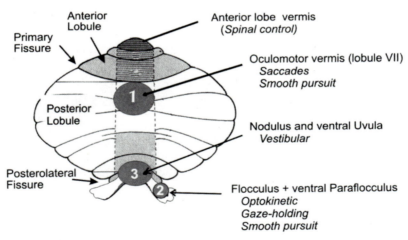

FIGURE 9-2 Schematic drawing of the cerebellum to show the three separate regions involved in different eye movement functions. (1) Dorsal vermis of lobule VI and VII. (2) Flocculus and ventral paraflocculus. (3) Nodulus and ventral uvula.

Reproduced with permission.[2]

TOPOGRAPHIC SYNDROMES

The Dorsal Vermis (Lobules VI and VII)

The dorsal vermis, lobules VI and VII, which comprise the OMV, are particularly important for controlling the speed and accuracy of saccades—a role they share with the fastigial nuclei, which comprise the fastigial oculomotor region (FOR).[3]

The dorsal vermis facilitates ipsilateral saccades and contributes to the termination of contralateral saccades. As a result, unilateral OMV lesions lead to hypometric ipsilateral and hypermetric contralateral saccades, whereas bilateral OMV lesions cause hypometric saccades in both horizontal directions; vertical saccades show ipsipulsion (an oblique trajectory toward the side of the lesion) but vertical pursuit is little affected. Unilateral lesions of the OMV also cause horizontal pursuit deficits in both directions.[4]

The dorsal vermis receives mossy fiber inputs from the paramedian pontine reticular formation (PPRF), from the nucleus reticularis tegmenti pontis (NRTP), the dorsolateral and dorsomedial pontine nuclei, and the vestibular nuclei and prepositus hypoglossi nuclei, as well as from climbing fiber input from the inferior olivary nucleus.[5,6] Signals from the frontal eye fields and superior colliculus to the cerebellum are relayed through the NRTP and provide the cerebellum with the information necessary for planning saccades. Signals from the dorsolateral pontine nuclei are concerned with smooth pursuit. Outputs from the dorsal vermis reach the fastigial nucleus and are then carried out of the cerebellum via the superior cerebellar peduncle in a crossed pathway to reach the thalamus (ventral lateral nucleus).

Purkinje cells in the dorsal vermis discharge before saccades,[7] and a topographic organization is evident: upward saccades are evoked from the anterior part of the vermis, downward saccades from the posterior part, and ipsilateral horizontal saccades from the lateral part.[8]

Lesions of the dorsal vermis and fastigial nucleus cause *saccadic dysmetria*.[9] In which a saccade to a visual target that is either too small and undershoots (hypometria), or too large and overshoots (hypermetria), has to be followed by a corrective saccade. The difference is that lesions of the OMV[10] cause ipsilateral hypometria and contralateral hypermetria of saccades, and lesions of the FOR[11] cause ipsilateral hypermetria and contralateral hypometria of saccades. Patients with lesions involving the dorsal vermis may also have impaired smooth pursuit, predominantly toward the side of the lesion.[12]

■ **Clinical Points to Remember About Lesions of the OMV (Dorsal Vermis Lobules VI, VII)**

Lesions of the OMV cause:
- Ipsilateral saccadic hypometria and contralateral hypermetria.
- Impaired initiation of smooth pursuit (first 100 ms) of a target moving toward the side of the lesion.
- Tonic conjugate gaze deviation away from the side of the lesion.   ■

The Flocculus and Paraflocculus

The flocculonodular lobes and inferior vermis are referred to as the *vestibulocerebellum* because they project mainly to the vestibular nuclei and are particularly important in the control of smooth pursuit, vestibular eye movements, and holding positions of gaze.

The flocculi are paired structures that lie adjacent to the cerebellar tonsils (paraflocculi) and ventral to the inferior cerebellar peduncle. Both the flocculi and paraflocculi receive climbing fiber inputs from the contralateral inferior olivary nucleus, which may provide information important for adaptive oculomotor control. The main projections of the flocculus and paraflocculus are to the ipsilateral vestibular nuclei and the y-group, a small group of cells that cap the inferior cerebellar peduncle. The y-group receives input from Purkinje cells in the flocculus and may contribute, with the flocculus, in the adaptive control of both the VOR and smooth pursuit.[13] The paraflocculus contributes mainly to smooth pursuit. The y-group projects to the oculomotor and trochlear nuclei in the midbrain via the brachium conjunctivum and the crossing ventral tegmental tract. Most fibers leaving the vestibulocerebellum project to the vestibular nuclei located in the medulla, rather than to the cerebellum, and the vestibular nuclei function in some ways like additional deep cerebellar nuclei.

Unilateral lesions of the flocculus impair ipsilateral smooth pursuit, and severe damage to the flocculus and paraflocculus produces a characteristic syndrome similar to the syndrome encountered clinically in patients with the Chiari malformation (see Case 9-3). This syndrome includes downbeat nystagmus, impaired smooth pursuit, and eye–head tracking, as well as impaired gaze-holding.[14,15]

■ **Clinical Points to Remember About Lesions of the Flocculus and Paraflocculus**

The following functions are impaired:
- Smooth pursuit eye movements
- Suppression of the VOR
- Suppression of caloric nystagmus by fixating a stationary target
- Nystagmus may be present
- Downbeat nystagmus, often greatest on looking laterally
- Gaze-evoked nystagmus, centripetal and rebound nystagmus ■

The Nodulus and Ventral Uvula

The nodulus is the midline portion of the flocculonodular lobe adjacent to the uvula, and, together with the flocculus and paraflocculus (cerebellar tonsils), it is part of the vestibulocerebellum. It receives input from the vestibular nuclei, nucleus prepositus hypoglossi, and inferior olivary nucleus.[16-18] The nodulus and uvula project to the vestibular nuclei and control the velocity-storage mechanism of the horizontal VOR and can enhance the response of the VOR to low-frequency stimuli.[19,20] When this process is interrupted, periodic alternating nystagmus (PAN) can result.

Periodic alternating nystagmus is the most important cerebellar sign produced by lesions affecting the nodulus and ventral uvula. The oscillations PAN produces would ordinarily be blocked by visual fixation mechanisms that tend to suppress nystagmus, but disease of the cerebellum causing PAN also impairs these mechanisms.[21,22]

In typical cases of PAN, the nystagmus reverses direction every 2–4 minutes. The nystagmus finishes one-half cycle (e.g., right-beating nystagmus) and a brief transition period occurs during which there may be upbeating or downbeating nystagmus or square-wave jerks before the next half cycle (e.g., left-beating nystagmus) begins. The congenital form of PAN is usually much less regular in the timing of reversal of direction, and slow-phase waveforms are typical.[23,24]

Lesions of the nodulus and uvula typically cause PAN in the dark, and lesions of the flocculus and ventral paraflocculus cause PAN during visual fixation in the light.

Table 9-1: Disorders Associated with Periodic Alternating Nystagmus

---

Ataxia telangiectasia
Brainstem infarction
Cerebellar degeneration
Cerebellar tumor, abscess, cyst, and other mass lesion
Chiari type I malformation
Congenital nystagmus—periodic form especially in albinos
Creutzfeldt-Jakob disease
Hepatic encephalopathy
Infections affecting the cerebellum, including syphilis
Lithium and anticonvulsant medications
Multiple sclerosis
Severe visual loss (due to vitreous hemorrhage or cataract)
Trauma

Reproduced with permission.[33]

Periodic alternating nystagmus was the first form of nystagmus for which an effective treatment was identified. The gamma aminobutyric acid (GABA)-ergic drug baclofen abolishes acquired PAN in most patients[25] but helps only occasionally in cases of congenital PAN.[26]

Periodic alternating nystagmus is reported in association with a number of conditions that affect the cerebellum (Table 9-1). The commonest are cerebellar degeneration, cerebellar mass lesions (tumor, abcess or cyst), multiple sclerosis, trauma, Chiari malformation and ataxia telangiectasia. Other unusual etiologies are hepatic encephalopathy, Creutfeldt-Jakob disease and drug toxicity due to lithium or anticonvulsant medications.

■ Clinical Points to Remember About Lesions of the Nodulus and Ventral Uvula

The signs are:
- Periodic alternating nystagmus in darkness
- Periodic alternating nystagmus present in light indicates that the floccular and paraflocculus are also lesioned, thus impairing visual fixation.
- Periodic alternating nystagmus may be associated with positional nystagmus and downbeat nystagmus.
- Convergence may be preserved and can be used to suppress PAN in some patients.[27]
- Impaired smooth pursuit and optokinetic nystagmus.
- Inability to suppress postrotational nystagmus. ■

The Fastigial Nucleus and Deep Cerebellar Nuclei

The dentate nucleus, emboliform nucleus, globose nucleus, and fastigial nucleus are the deep cerebellar or roof nuclei (running from lateral to medial) (Figure 9-3).[28]

The *dentate nuclei* are the largest of these four nuclei. They receive projections from Purkinje cells in the lateral cerebellum, and their output fibers project to the contralateral red nucleus in the midbrain, where some fibers terminate in the rostral parvocellular division of the red nucleus.

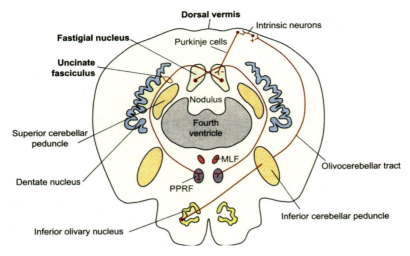

FIGURE 9-3 Lesions in the dorsal vermis, fastigial nucleus, and uncinate fasciculus.

Reproduced with permission.[28]

Projections from the dentate nucleus pass through the red nucleus (without a synapse) and connect to the ipsilateral inferior olive by way of the central tegmental tract—the triangle of Guillain and Mollaret (see Chapter 8, Figure 8-2, Case 8-1).

The emboliform and globose nuclei are together called *the interposed nuclei*. They receive projections from the intermediate cerebellar hemisphere, which is involved in control of movements of the limbs. They project via the superior cerebellar peduncle, contralaterally to the thalamus and to the magnocellular division of the red nucleus. They are active during movement of the limbs and a lesion of the left cerebellar hemisphere (intermediate portion or interposed nuclei) causes ataxia of the left (ipsilateral) extremities.

The *fastigial nucleus* (FN), the most medial of the deep cerebellar nuclei, plays a major role in the control of both saccades[29] and smooth pursuit.[30] The caudal region of the fastigial nucleus, the FOR, receives input from Purkinje cells of the dorsal vermis, from the inferior olivary nucleus, and from axon collaterals from mossy fibers projecting to the dorsal vermis from pontine nuclei, and in particular from the NRTP.[31,32] This wide range of connections allows the FOR to receive a copy of saccadic command signals relayed by the NRTP from the frontal eye fields and superior colliculus.

■ **Clinical Points to Remember About Lesions of the Fastigial Nucleus**

- Clinical lesions of the FN are invariable bilateral (because their axons cross to the opposite nucleus) and cause bilateral saccadic hypermetria and macrosaccadic oscillations (Chapter 10)
- Unilateral lesion of the FN cause:
  - Ipsilateral hypometria and mild contralateral hypermetria of saccades—"ipsipulsion" (Chapter 8)
  - Gaze is tonically deviated towards the side of the lesion
  - Smooth pursuit is impaired for targets moving *away* from side of lesion
- All ocular motility signs seen in Wallenberg's syndrome (Chapter 8). ■

Periodic alternating nystagmus is a rare form of nystagmus characterized by a horizontal jerk nystagmus whose slow component velocity changes in amplitude and direction periodically. The periodicity is often about 4 mm, with 2 mm of right-beating and 2 mm of left-beating nystagmus. The acquired form of PAN occurs in a number of disorders, including spinocerebellar degenerative and posterior fossa neoplasm. Periodic alternating nystagmus is caused by an instability in the velocity-storage mechanism, a neural circuit that perseverates (loss of habituation to repetitive vestibular stimulation), the eye movement response to both vestibular and optokinetic stimulation. Clinical lesions of the nodulus and ventral uvula can result in an increase in the duration of vestibular responses that may predispose the patient to the development of PAN (Case 9-4).

Saccadic Dysmetria

Saccadic dysmetria is a very specific cerebellar eye sign that the examiner should look for in all patients with a history of unsteadiness and mild incoordination, keeping in mind the probability of a cerebellar syndrome. Saccadic dysmetria (analogous to overshoot on finger-nose-finger test with upper limb ataxia) is diagnostic of a lesion of the OMV or the FOR.

Saccadic dysmetria is most easily demonstrated by asking the patient to look from an eccentric point back to the midline. Normally, the saccade is executed with remarkable precision and accuracy, but, with a cerebellar lesion, there is a characteristic overshoot (*hypermetria*) if the deep nuclei are involved or undershoot (*hypometria*) if the vermis alone is involved. With saccadic hypermetria, pendular excursions of the eyes—referred to as macrosaccadic oscillations—occur when the eyes overshoot prior to final stable fixation.

Saccadic Pursuit

Saccadic pursuit is often seen in patients with cerebellar disease who partially compensate for pursuit impairment with frequent catch-upsaccades (saccadic pursuit) to hold the object of interest on the fovea. Both the OMV and FOR participate in the generation of smooth pursuit eye movements. The OMV facilitates ipsilateral pursuit and contributes to the termination of contralateral pursuit. The flocculus and paraflocculus also contribute to smooth pursuit, and one possible division of labor is that the OMV/FOR is more concerned with the initiation and termination of pursuit, whereas the flocculus and paraflocculus—the vestibulocerebellum—are more concerned with pursuit during sustained tracking. Neurons in the FOR discharge early during contralateral pursuit and late for ipsilateral pursuit, analogous to activity associated with saccades.

■ **Clinical Points to Remember About Smooth Pursuit Eye Movements**

- Lesions of the OMV and FOR mainly affect eye acceleration during the initial period of smooth pursuit (the first 100 ms of tracking after a target has started moving or has changed its speed) and have a smaller effect during the sustained tracking period.
- A lesion in the OMV impairs ipsilateral pursuit.
- A lesion in the FOR impairs contralateral pursuit.
- Vertical pursuit is little affected following OMV lesions, but FOR lesions impair downward pursuit to a greater degree than upward pursuit. ■

Ataxia

Cerebellar incoordination or ataxia is the most prominent manifestation of cerebellar disease affecting intended (volitional) movement. The terms *dyssynergia, dysmetria,* and *dysdiadochokinesis* are all used to describe cerebellar abnormalities in movements requiring alternation or rapid change in direction.[35] The abnormalities are brought out by finger-to-nose or heel-to-shin movement (running the heel down the opposite shin) or tracing a square in the air with a hand or foot.

The examiner should ask the patient to move the limb to the target accurately and rapidly. There is usually an irregularity, with slowing of the movement in both acceleration and deceleration.[36] The limb may overshoot the target (hypermetria) due to delayed activation and diminished contraction of antagonist muscles, then the error is corrected by a series of secondary movements in which the finger or toe sways away from the target before coming to rest, or moves from side to side a few times (intention tremor) when it is actually on the target.

A simple test for dysmetria is to ask the patient to rest the arms extended with the hands on the knees and on command "go" raise them straight up as quickly as possible to the level of your outstretched hand held 12 or more inches above the resting position. A dysmetric ataxic arm typically overshoots the target while the unaffected arm stops abruptly and accurately at the level of the outstretched hand.

All the foregoing defects together impart a highly characteristic clumsiness to the cerebellar syndrome. Acts that require coordination of rapid smooth and accurate movements, such as screwing in a light bulb, are impaired. Babinski called this abnormality adiadochokinesis. Patients with the cerebellar syndrome also have variable degrees of difficulty in standing and walking. Gait ataxia may be quite mild and not detected unless the examiner asks the patient to tandem (i.e., walk heel to toe). When severe, standing with feet together may be impossible or maintained only briefly before the patient pitches to one side or backward. When the cerebellar disturbance is limited to one of stance and gait, the pathological changes are restricted to anterior parts of the superior vermis (Case 9-2). A rhythmic tremor of the head or upper trunk (3–4 per second) is called titubation and implies midline cerebellar disease. When truncal ataxia is severe, patients are unable to sit up without support (Chapter 8, Case 8-3).

Dysarthria

Dysarthria in cerebellar lesions may take one of two forms: either a slow, *slurred* dysarthria, similar to that following interruption of the corticobulbar tract, or a *scanning* dysarthria with variable intonation. In addition to its scanning quality, speech is slow and, after an involuntary interruption, each syllable may be uttered with less or more force than is natural (explosive speech). Functional magnetic resonance imaging (fMRI) in patients with cerebellar dysarthria has localized the area involved to the upper paravermal area of the right cerebellar hemisphere, the site of coordination of articulatory movements of the tongue and orofacial muscles.[37]

Hypotonia

Hypotonia refers to a decrease in the normal resistance muscles offer to passive manipulation— for example flexion and extension of the limb. It is the least evident of the cerebellar signs and much more apparent with acute than with chronic lesions. Hypotonia is attributed to a depression of gamma and alpha motor neuron activity, and it may produce mild flabbiness of the muscles on the affected side. With time, fusimotor activity is restored as hypotonia disappears. A simple test for hypotonia is to tap firmly the dorsum of both wrists of the outstretched arms, in which case the affected limb (or both limbs in diffuse cerebellar disease) will be displaced downwards through a wider range of motion than normal and may rebound due to a failure of hypotonic muscles to fixate the arm at the shoulder

ATAXIC SYNDROMES OF THE CEREBELLUM

Autosomal Dominant Ataxia

Hereditary ataxias are the major congenital syndromes of the cerebellum, and the majority of the ocular motor abnormalities they produce can be attributed to degenerative changes within the cerebellar system. Spinocerebellar ataxias (SCA), SCA-1 (SCA type 1), SCA-2, and SCA-3, represent autosomal, dominantly inherited, untreatable, and ultimately fatal ataxic diseases. They belong to the group of CAG repeat or polyglutamine diseases with expanded CAG triplets at disease-specific gene loci.[38,39] Machado-Joseph disease,[40] SCA-3, is the most common dominantly inherited ataxia in the world, and six additional SCA diseases are recognized—SCA-1, SCA-2, SCA-6, SCA-7, SCA-8, and SCA-20.

Ocular motility abnormalities are shared across the spectrum of autosomal dominant spinocerebellar ataxias. They include intrusions that disrupt fixation: square-wave jerks, macrosaccadic oscillations, nystagmus or flutter, and impaired pursuit and saccadic dysmetria.[41–43]

> ■ **Clinical Points to Remember About Eye Movements in Dominant SCA**
>
> - SCA1: slow saccades, gaze-evoked and rebound nystagmus
> - SCA2: very slow saccades [44]
> - SCA3: hypometria, impaired smooth pursuit [45, 46]
> - SCA6: downbeat, gaze-evoked, rebound nystagmus
> - SCA7: slow saccades, pigmentary maculopathy and visual loss
> - SCA8: gaze-evoked nystagmus, saccadic dysmetria ■

Autosomal Recessive Ataxia

Friedreich's ataxia is the most common recessive form of hereditary ataxia. It was identified by Nikolaus Friedreich in 1863 as a degenerative disease with sclerosis of the spinal cord. The syndrome is characterized by ataxia, hyporeflexia, an axonal sensory neuropathy, cardiomyopathy, diabetes, and scoliosis.[47] Fixation instability, accompanied by saccadic intrusions, square-wave jerks, ocular flutter, and PAN,[48] yet with relatively preserved smooth pursuit, are frequent findings in this disorder.[49]

Ataxia telangiectasia—the Louis-Bar syndrome—is also an autosomal recessive ataxic degenerative disease characterized by impaired initiation of horizontal saccades (indicative of ocular

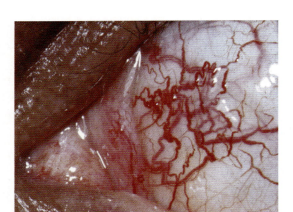

FIGURE 9-5 Telangiectasia of the conjunctival blood vessels in a patient with ataxia telangiectasia.

Courtesy of Nicholas Hogan, M.D., Ph.D.

motor apraxia [OMA]—or Cogan's congenital OMA with head thrusts). The disorder presents with cerebellar ataxia (with onset at approximately 4 years of age) followed by progressive ataxia, athetoid movements, slow dysarthric speech, telangiectasia of the bulbar conjunctiva (Figure 9-5), and recurrent respiratory infections, with mental retardation in 50% of cases. This syndrome affects both sexes equally, and death usually occurs in early childhood or adolescence from pulmonary infection or a lymphoreticular malignant tumor.[50–52] The ocular motor signs in ataxic telangiectasia are OMA, saccadic hypometria, saccadic pursuit, gaze-evoked nystagmus, square-wave jerks, and PAN.

Spastic Ataxia of Charlevoix-Saguenay

A Canadian study of the most common recessive ataxia, Friedreich's ataxia,[53] pointed the way to diagnosis of the patient presented in Case 9-1. The study reported a new syndrome of autosomal recessive spastic ataxia in patients isolated in the Charlevoix-Saguenay region of Quebec, a mountainous area east of Quebec City where, between 1665 and 1725, some 40 families settled and propagated with very high fertility.

The study, conducted by Bouchard et al. in 1978, investigated 14 of 42 patients drawn from 24 sibships in the region.[54] Many of these patients were found to have biochemical changes that included impaired pyruvate oxidation, hyperbilirubinemia, low serum beta-lipoproteins, and HDL apoproteins. Clinically they typically showed spasticity, dysarthria, distal muscle wasting, foot deformities, truncal ataxia, absence of sensory evoked potentials in the lower limbs, retinal striation reminiscent of early Leber's hereditary optic atrophy, and, in 57% of cases, prolapse of the mitral valve.

More recent genetic studies link autosomal recessive spastic ataxia of Charlevoix-Saguenay to nonsense mutations of the SACS gene.[55]

The case presented here shares many of the Quebec abnormalities.

CASE 9-1 Spastic Ataxia of Charlevoix-Saguenay

Video Display

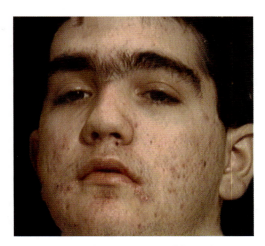

FIGURE 9-6 A nineteen-year-old student with progressive ataxia.

The patient is a 19-year-old high school student who was born at term, walked at 9 months, and developed well with normal milestones. At age 10, he began to have difficulty speaking, occasional involuntary movements of the head, and progressive clumsiness playing baseball, falling when running, and unsteadiness on his feet. Despite these difficulties, he attended normal classes up to the 8th grade, when he fell behind and had to attend special classes. He worked occasionally as a bagger at a supermarket, but, by age 17, he needed to use a walker.

In March 1988, at age 19, he was admitted under a neuropediatrician at the Massachusetts General Hospital for evaluation of progressive ataxia, mental retardation, memory loss, increased drooling, and inability to care for himself (Figure 9-6).

His past history was notable for seizure disorder since childhood. Nerve conduction studies and visual evoked potentials performed in 1987 were normal. In 1989, he was treated for reactive psychosis, which resolved with antipsychotic medication.

His family history was notable for the following:

- Negative for neurological disease
- Brother, age 24, normal
- Both parents came from the Nova Scotia region of Canada.
- Father, French-Canadian with five siblings and no known neurological disease
- Mother had an Italian father and German mother, five siblings, and no known neurological disease.

Analysis of the History

- What are the major presenting symptoms?
- Where are the central nervous system (CNS) lesion(s) likely to be?

CASE 9-1 SYMPTOMS

Symptoms	Location Correlation
Progressive retardation	Cerebral cortex
Ataxia	Cerebellum
Spasticity	Corticospinal tracts

The analysis guides the clinical examination.

Examination

Neurological

- Wheelchair bound
- Severe spastic ataxic dysarthria
- Able to show two fingers, unable to subtract 7 from 100
- Slow obeying one-step commands
- Spastic tongue only minimal movement
- Brisk jaw and facial jerks

Motor System
- Dystonic posture of the hands
- Axial extensor rigidity, particularly in the neck
- Occasional spontaneous extensor movements of the legs
- Marked increase in tone in the limbs
- Movement of arms and legs produces a rubral tremor and pronounced ataxia
- Strength good allowing for limited extent testable
- Hyperreflexia bilaterally, sustained ankle clonus, plantar responses extensor
- No pes cavus
- Marked ataxia finger-nose-finger, heel-knee-shin, and foot tapping
- Bilateral dysdiadochokinesis
- Truncal ataxia, wide-based ataxic gait, only able to take a few steps

Sensory System
- Limited—normal light touch and vibration sense

Neuro-ophthalmological

- Visual acuity: J2 OU, visual fields, color vision and pupils normal
- Fundus: normal optic discs, granularity of the macular area, and no striations of the retinal nerve fiber layer

Ocular Motility

- Supranuclear global vertical gaze palsy—saccades and pursuit
- Slow to initiate horizontal saccades—used head thrust to initiate looking right and left consistent with ocular motor apraxia
- Slow horizontal hypometric saccades
- Saccadic smooth pursuit in all directions
- Saccadic dysmetria—hypermetric horizontally and vertically
- No nystagmus or square-wave jerks
- Convergence absent
- Optokinetic nystagmus not elicited
- Normal Bell's reflex—eyes deviated up under closed lids
- Vertical oculocephalic reflex normal

Localization and Differential Diagnosis

The extent of the neurological and ocular signs:

- Mental deficiency
- Spastic and ataxic dysarthria
- Marked gait, trunk, and limb ataxia
- Spastic quadriparesis with hyperreflexia
- Global supranuclear paralysis of vertical gaze
- Slow horizontal hypometric saccades
- Oculomotor apraxia with head thrust
- Saccadic pursuit
- Saccadic hypermetria

Indicates the range of diagnostic differentials that need to be considered for this patient. They include Niemann-Pick type C or a mitochondrial disorder.

Niemann-Pick type C is an autosomal recessive lysosomal storage disease in which the gene *NPC1* maps to chromosome 18q11-12 and a variety of lipids, including GM2 and GM3 ganglioside, in addition to cholesterol, accumulate in the brain. The classic patient with Niemann-Pick disease type C appears normal at birth, and it may take as long as 7 years for neurologic signs to become apparent. Impairment of upgaze may be the first clinical finding, downgaze may also be impaired, and, on examination, the key finding is vertical supranuclear ophthalmoplegia. Ophthalmoplegia may ultimately be complete. Speech is dysarthric, and the patient may have ataxia and abnormal behavior progressing to dementia or psychosis.

Diagnosis is made by examination of cultured fibroblasts, which show both impaired cholesterol esterification and the accumulation of free cholesterol.[56]

The mitochondrial differential leans toward a maternally inherited neurodegenerative *mitochondrial disorder* characterized by **n**eurogenic muscle weakness, **a**taxia, pigmentary **r**etinopathy, and **p**eripheral neuropathy that has been given the acronym NARP. The NARP mutation T8993G of mitochondrial DNA (mtDNA) correlates closely with the severity of the NARP syndrome. The clinical features of the syndrome include progressive unsteadiness walking and absent ankle jerks. Nerve conduction velocity is reduced in a pattern of axonal sensory neuropathy. Night blindness (often the first symptom in these patients) is followed by loss of peripheral vision and, in some, by loss of central vision. Clumps of pigment appear in the retina, typically resembling spicules of bone but in some cases the retina may have a salt-and-pepper appearance.[57] Other patients may have optic atrophy, and there may be nystagmus on horizontal or vertical gaze, and esotropia. Cerebellar atrophy has been observed on neuroimaging.

What Diagnostic Tests Should Follow?

- Brain MRI
- Positron emission tomography (PET)
- Electroencephalogram (EEG)
- Nerve conduction studies
- Skin/muscle biopsy

Test Results

Brain MRI showed no atrophy of the cerebellum or brainstem. The PET scan and EEG were normal. Nerve conduction studies showed mild left peroneal nerve and peripheral motor neuropathy. An amino acid analysis (complete panel) showed a normal pattern. The skin biopsy was negative for storage disease. The muscle biopsy was negative for mitochondrial disease.

Special Explanatory Note

The presence of a mild peripheral neuropathy in the legs of this patient was typical for spastic ataxia of Charlevoix-Saguenay, whereas the absence of nystagmus was not: all of the Quebec cases had horizontal nystagmus and, occasionally, vertical nystagmus. In six of the Quebec families, the parents and unaffected siblings were normal, as were the parents of this patient. Ataxia of gait was present from the beginning of walking in all of the Quebec cases, whereas in this patient it developed when he was 10 years old. Saccadic pursuit and horizontal saccadic hypermetria seen in this patient are signs commonly present in most cases of familial spastic ataxia, and similar findings are reported in heredo-familial spinocerebellar degeneration.[58]

On balance, the diagnosis of the Charlevoix-Saguenay syndrome provides the clearest explanation of this patient's clinical syndrome.

Syndrome of the Dorsal Vermis (Lobules VI and VII)

A patient with severe gait instability is presented in Case 9-2.

CASE 9-2 Syndrome of the Dorsal Vermis: Gait Ataxia

Video Display

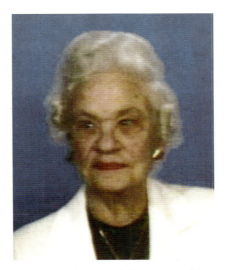

FIGURE 9-7 A seventy-two-year-old woman with gait instability.

The patient is a 72-year-old woman with a history of long-term alcohol abuse. In 1980, she presented with a 4-year history of progressive difficulty with balance, frequent falls, and unsteadiness walking (Figure 9-7). She was referred to Dr. Raymond Adams.

Analysis of the History

- What are the major presenting symptoms?
- Where are the CNS lesion(s) likely to be?

CASE 9-2 SYMPTOMS

Symptoms	Location Correlation
Progressive loss of balance	Cerebellum

The analysis guides the clinical examination.

Examination

Neurological

- Oriented ×3
- Mild impairment in recall memory
- Speech normal
- Motor strength 5/5 throughout, reflexes 1+ symmetric, absent ankle jerk, plantar responses flexor
- Mild motor/sensory peripheral neuropathy
- Titubation, truncal ataxia, and marked gait ataxia without limb ataxia
- Able to walk with a cane but showed marked ataxia on turning
- Romberg negative

Ocular Motility

- Full vertical and horizontal eye movements
- Prominent square-wave jerks disrupting fixation
- Horizontal gaze-evoked nystagmus to right and left
- Saccadic horizontal pursuit
- Smooth vertical pursuit
- Horizontal saccadic hypermetria, no vertical dysmetria
- Absent optokinetic nystagmus vertically and horizontally
- Normal convergence
- Vestibulo-ocular reflexes normal

Localization and Differential Diagnosis

Progressive cerebellar disease over a 4-year period is unlikely to be due to a paraneo-plastic syndrome so the important differential in this case is a neurodegenerative disease (e.g., Parkinson's disease or progressive sensory peripheral neuropathy).

In Parkinson's, a degree of bradykinesia is usually needed for a definite diagnosis, and watching the patient walk establishes it. The most typical patient with Parkinson's has a flexed posture and a shuffling gait, the arms do not swing naturally when walking, and there is a tendency to turn "en bloc, as if the joints are soldered" (Charcot's description).

In progressive sensory peripheral neuropathy, loss of proprioception (joint position) in the feet can lead to sensory ataxia. To test this, the patient should be asked to stand with feet together, with the eyes open and closed. If the patient can do this without falling, Romberg's sign is negative. When gait unsteadiness is due to loss of propriocep-tion, the patient loses balance with eyes closed and tends to sway from side to side and even fall; in this case Romberg's sign is positive.

What Diagnostic Tests Should Follow?

- Brain MRI (unavailable at the time)

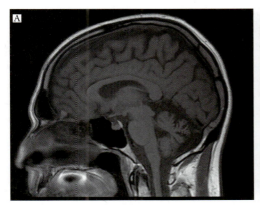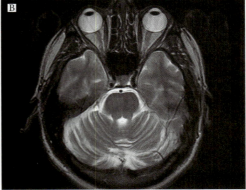

FIGURE 9-8 (A) Magnetic resonance sagittal T1 image and (B) Axial T2 image shows marked cerebellar atrophy, including involvement of the vermis, with relative preservation of cerebral volume, in a patient with significant history of alcohol abuse. Note the diminished cerebellar folia and enlarged sulci.

Courtesy of Mykol Larvie, M.D., Ph.D.

Test Results

MRI in a similar case with a history of alcohol abuse (Figure 9-8A–B), shows marked cerebellar atrophy involving the vermis, with relative preservation of cerebral volume. Atrophy of the superior vermis is reflected in the thinning of the cerebellar folia a diagnostic feature that explains gait instability.

Diagnosis: Alcoholic Degeneration of the Cerebellar Vermis with Motor-Sensory Peripheral Neuropathy

Treatment

Early intervention in alcoholism in the subclinical phase through counseling, improved nutrition, and vitamin B therapy would have been beneficial in this case.

Special Explanatory Note

Two particular forms of the alcoholic cerebellar syndrome have been recognized.[59] In the first, clinical abnormalities are limited to instability of station and gait, with individual limb movements unaffected, as in this case, and with pathological changes restricted to the anterosuperior portion of the vermis with loss of Purkinje cells.

The second type is acute and transient in nature and is due to a biochemical lesion that has not yet caused structural change.

These two forms of cerebellar disease in alcoholism are difficult to distinguish on either pathologic or clinical grounds from the cerebellar manifestations of Wernicke's disease, which is due specifically to a deficiency of thiamine. However, Victor, Adams, and Mancall's landmark paper[60] suggests that the restricted form of cortical cerebellar degeneration seen in the serious alcoholic represents a discrete clinical pathological entity, and this patient's history and clinical signs match these authors' very detailed description of the disease.

The Syndrome of the Flocculus/Paraflocculus (Tonsil)

The *Chiari malformation* is a congenital anomaly in which the cerebellar tonsils (paraflocculus) and the lower brainstem herniate into the cervical canal. The malformation was described by Arnold Chiari, first in 1891, and then in more detail in 1896. He was among the first to recognize multiple hindbrain malformations associated with congenital hydrocephalus.

There are four types of Chiari malformation, each characterized by a different degree of herniation:

- Chiari type I malformation is a downward displacement of the cerebellum and cerebellar tonsils.
- Chiari type II is a complex malformation that includes downward displacement of the cerebellar vermis and tonsils and is encountered in the vast majority of patients with myelomeningocele.
- Chiari type III is an encephalocervical meningocele.
- Chiari type IV refers to hypoplasia of the cerebellum.

The major additional morphological features include elongation of the medulla and pons, a narrowed cerebral aqueduct, and displacement of the medulla and cerebellum, which occludes the foramen magnum.

All of these factors combine to develop obstructive hydrocephalus[61,62] and downbeat nystagmus,[63–65] the syndrome's principal clinical features. The case presented here is a striking example of Chiari type I.

CASE 9-3 Syndrome of the Flocculus: Downbeat Nystagmus

Video Display

The patient is a 59-year-old woman with a congenital anomaly of the occipitocervical junction with occipitalization of the C1 ring. In 1957, at the age of 24, she presented with headache, "jumping vision" (oscillopsia), and progressive unsteadiness with a tendency to fall to the right. She was given a misdiagnosis of multiple sclerosis.

In March 1992, the patient consulted a neurologist for evaluation of headaches. (Figure 9-9). He referred her to the Neurosurgery Clinic at the Massachusetts General Hospital.

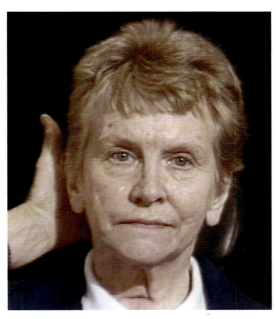

FIGURE 9-9 A fifty-nine-year-old woman with downbeat nystagmus.

Her past history was notable for basal cell carcinoma (1970) and a mastectomy for adenocarcinoma of the breast (1986).

Analysis of the History

- What are the major presenting symptoms?
- Where are the CNS lesion(s) likely to be?

CASE 9-3 SYMPTOMS

Symptoms	Location Correlation
Headache	Increased intracranial pressure
Oscillopsia	Vestibular system
Progressive unsteadiness	Cerebellum

The analysis guides the clinical examination.

Examination

Neurological

- Limited neck flexion and extension
- Spastic quadriparesis with 4/5 muscle strength throughout

- Hyperreflexia with extensor plantar responses
- Bilateral cerebellar ataxia on finger-nose and heel-knee-shin test
- Gait ataxia

Neuro-ophthalmological

- Visual acuity 20/60 OU;fields, pupils and fundi normal
- Downbeat nystagmus in primary gaze with vertical oscillopsia
  Larger amplitude downbeat nystagmus on lateral
  gaze right and left
  Small amplitude on downgaze
- Saccadic pursuit in all directions, particularly marked on downgaze
- Convergence insufficiency with exophoria
- Full vertical and horizontal eye movements
- Oculocephalic reflexes normal
- Bell's reflex normal—eyes deviated up under closed lids

Localization and Differential Diagnosis

Downbeat nystagmus is a distinctive feature of lesions of the flocculus/paraflocculus. The eyes drift up (slow phase) and are brought back to the fixation target by a corrective downward saccade (quick phase). Headache and downbeat nystagmus are the prominent diagnostic markers in lesions at the level of the foramen magnum associated with hydrocephalus.

What Diagnostic Tests Should Follow?

- Brain MRI and sagittal view of the craniocervical junction

An MRI with sagittal views of the craniocervical junction in Chiari type I produces a highly characteristic radiologic profile, particularly on T1-weighted images, which will show low-lying cerebellar tonsils below the foramen magnum and behind the upper cervical cord.[66–68]

Test Results

An MRI of the cervical and thoracic spine showed a craniocervical junction anomaly, basilar invagination, and a cervical-thoracic syrinx extending from C2 to T4.

An MRI in head flexion and extension showed occipitalization of the atlas and subluxation of the cerebellar tonsils further downward into the spinal canal, particularly in extension.
    Neuroimaging studies were not available for publication and images from a classic case of Chiari malformation are presented here with saggital views showing exquisite detail of the "peglike" cerebellar tonsils extending inferiorly through the foramen magnum (Figure 9-10A–B). There is no associated syrinx in this case.

Diagnosis: Chiari Type I Malformation with Cervical-Thoracic Syrinx

OCULAR MOTOR SYNDROMES
OF THE CEREBELLUM

Syndrome of the Nodulus and Uvula

The nodulus and uvula project to the vestibular nuclei and control the velocity-storage mechanism of the horizontal VOR. When this process is interrupted, PAN may occur.

CASE 9-4 Syndrome of the Nodulus and Uvula: Periodic Alternating Nystagmus

No Video Display

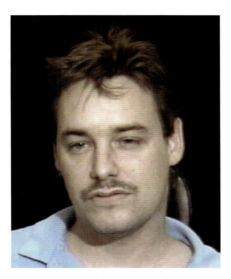

FIGURE 9-11 A thirty-year-old man with "jerking eyes."

The patient is a 30-year-old retarded man, winner of a gold medal for weight lifting in the Special Olympics, who was referred with a diagnosis of mental retardation, seizures, and ataxia.

In 1988, at the age of 24, an EEG and brainstem auditory evoked potentials were normal. In February 1989, at the age of 25, he was found to have "jerking" eyes, oscillopsia, unsteady gait, and slurred speech. A neurologist found mild terminal tremor of the upper extremities, heel-shin and gait ataxia, and hyperactive reflexes with flexor plantar responses.

In 1992, at the age of 28, he was given a diagnosis of olivopontocerebellar degeneration.

In July 1994, aged 30, the patient was admitted to a local hospital following a seizure with postictal confusion and agitation. An EEG was normal, and he was started on Tegretol 200 mg. b.i.d.

In October 1994, he was referred to the Neurovisual unit at the Massachusetts General Hospital for evaluation of "jiggly" eyes and a complaint that the visual world was moving (oscillopsia) (Figure 9-11).

Analysis of the History

· What are the major presenting symptoms?
· Where are the CNS lesion(s) likely to be?

CASE 9-4 SYMPTOMS

Symptoms	Location Correlation
Mental retardation	Cerebral cortex
Seizures	
Ataxia	Cerebellum
Oscillopsia	Vestibular pathways

The analysis guides the clinical examination.

Examination

Neurological

· Mild mental retardation
· Dysarthric speech
· Slow to obey one-step commands
· Muscle strength 5/5 throughout
· Gait wide-based and ataxic, unable to tandem walk
· Sensory examination normal
· Romberg negative

Neuro-ophthalmological

· Visual acuity (VA) 20/50 correcting to 20/25 OU
  when he placed his head in the most neutral position for his eyes
  or when he looked straight ahead and waited for the nystagmus
  to slow down before reversing direction
· Periodic alternating horizontal nystagmus with and without fixation
  the horizontal nystagmus reversed direction every
  104–110 seconds
· Saccadic pursuit in all directions of gaze
· Convergence normal
· Optokinetic nystagmus could not be elicited
· Oculocephalic reflexes normal
· Bell's reflex normal—eyes deviated up under closed lids
· Unable to suppress vestibular ocular reflex—on rotation in a chair, he was unable
  to maintain fixation on his thumb held up on his outstretched arm rotating with him

Localization and Differential Diagnosis

This ataxic and retarded patient was first seen with "jerking" eyes at the age of 24. Four years later, at age 28, he was given a diagnosis of olivopontocerebellar degeneration. The second neurological opinion, at age 30, differentially localized his trunkal ataxia to the cerebellar vermis and PAN to the cerebellar nodulus and ventral uvula.

What Diagnostic Test Should Follow?

- Brain MRI

Test Results

A Brain MR1 showed marked cerebellar atrophy affecting primarily the vermis.

Special Explanatory Note

A similar case of a 34-year-old man with slowly progressive gait instability and limb ataxia from age 15, was the third of four cases of PAN reported by Furman et al.[75] There was dysmetria during finger-to-nose and heel-knee-shin testing, and the patient's gait was ataxic. Baclofen 30 mg/day provided minimal symptomatic relief of imbalance; PAN persisted. A mid-sagittal MRI showed marked atrophy of the cerebellar hemisphere and vermis. The MRI was not retained for my own patient and I have used the MR image of Furman's third case to illustrate the syndrome (Figure 9-12).

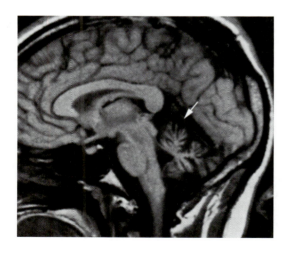

FIGURE 9-12 Midsagittal T1 magnetic resonance image shows severe atrophy of the cerebellar hemispheres and vermis (*arrow*).

Reproduced with permission.[75]

Treatment

- Baclofen (β-parachlorophenol γ-aminobutyric acid), a GABA-agonist

The patient received baclofen 10 mg. t.i.d. increasing to 20 mg. t.i.d., gabapentin 300 mg. t.i.d., and Tegretol 200 mg. t.i.d.

Four months later, his visual acuity was 20/40. He had no PAN and only primary position upbeat nystagmus visualized with the ophthalmoscope.

What were Additional Differential Diagnoses in a Complex Case Like This?

· Chiari type I malformation (ruled out by a negative brain MRI)
· Phenytoin toxicity[76] (an anticonvulsant drug not prescribed for this patient)
· Multiple sclerosis (ruled out by a negative brain MRI)

Diagnosis: Cerebellar Degeneration, Atrophy of the Cerebellar Vermis with Progressive Ataxia, and Periodic Alternating Nystagmus

An extensive list of disorders associated with PAN is shown in Table 9-1.[33]

Syndrome of the Fastigial Nucleus

Normally, a saccade is executed with remarkable precision and accuracy but with a cerebellar lesion there is a characteristic overshoot (*hypermetria*) if the deep nuclei are involved or undershoot (*hypometria*) if the vermis alone is involved. With saccadic hypermetria, pendular excursions of the eyes—referred to as *macrosaccadic oscillations*—occur when the eyes overshoot prior to final stable fixation.[77]

CASE 9-5 Syndrome of the Fastigial Nucleus: Saccadic Dysmetria

Video Display

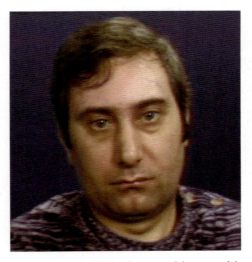

FIGURE 9-13 A thirty-six-year-old man with postoperative saccadic hypermetria.

The patient is a 36-year-old Italian man who presented in October 1967, at the age of 27, with acute dizziness and ataxia. He was evaluated in Rome. A pneumoencephalo-gram showed hydrocephalus attributed to arachnoiditis, and a ventriculo-atrial shunt was placed. Three months post shunt placement, he had a return of dizziness and ataxia accompanied by daily bioccipital headache, clumsiness, and weakness of the left arm.

In January 1968, he was readmitted, and a large tumor of the left cerebellar hemi-sphere with invasion of the vermis was biopsied. A diagnosis of glioblastoma multiforme was made, and he received radiation therapy.

In 1970, he emigrated to the United States, and, in 1971, with increasing gait ataxia and oscillopsia, he was referred to Dr. William Sweet, Chief of Neurosurgery, Massachusetts General Hospital (Figure 9-13).

Analysis of the History

· What are the major presenting symptoms?
· Where are the CNS lesion(s) likely to be?

CASE 9-5 SYMPTOMS

Symptoms	Location Correlation
Ataxia	Cerebellum
Oscillopsia	Vestibular pathways

The analysis guides the clinical examination.

Localization and Differential Diagnosis

Three years is too long a period to attribute progressive ataxia to postradiation necro-sis, and recurrent cerebellar glioblastoma multiforme is the likely diagnosis.

What Diagnostic Tests Should Follow?

· Brain MRI (not available at the time)
· Brain computed tomography (CT) scan
· Cerebral arteriography (Brian MRA and CTA not available)

Test Results

A brain CT showed an area of enhancement involving the cerebellar vermis and medial left cerebellar hemisphere with an associated cystic component consistent with recur-rent tumor. A cerebral arteriogram showed a highly vascular tumor bulging into the fourth ventricle.

Special Explanatory Note

Two types of tumors are especially common in this area of the cerebellum, the astrocytomas and the medulloblastomas. Cerebellar astrocytomas are relatively slow growing, predisposed to cyst formation, and are favorable for surgical resection. They produce nystagmus and paresis of conjugate gaze along with dysdiadochokinesis (abnormal alternating movements) and hypotonia.

The medulloblastomas are rapidly growing, usually arising in the posterior portions of the vermis, and are unfavorable for complete surgical removal. They produce primarily disturbances of equilibrium but little nystagmus (the flocculonodular syndrome). The removal of a midline cerebellar tumor that requires manipulation of the floor of the fourth ventricle may lead to a catastrophic and permanent paralysis of conjugate lateral gaze and skew deviation. This is a prime neuro-ophthalmic complication of neurosurgery in this region, and surgical splitting of the vermis to resect a cerebellar astrocytoma may carry a similar risk.

An invariably applicable and important clinical caution: the original biopsy of a brain tumor (or of any tissue) should always be brought in for review by a pathologist (Chapter 7, Case 7-5).

The slides from the original biopsy were obtained from Rome and reviewed by Dr E. P. Richardson, who confirmed the diagnosis of a high-grade astrocytoma grade 3–4.

Treatment

A posterior fossa craniotomy was performed and, the vermis was split to access the tumor. A well-demarcated tumor nodule was found extending to both sides of the cerebellum and it was possible to separate the superior borders of the tumor from the fourth ventricle. Several small branches of the posterior inferior cerebellar arteries had to be divided to devascularize the tumor, which was then carefully dissected away from the floor of the fourth ventricle. Close to a grossly total removal of the tumor as was performed and no visible tumor was left behind.

The patient was examined postoperatively.

Neurological

· Slight titubation
· Left limb ataxia on finger-nose-finger and heel-knee-shin testing
· No gait ataxia

Ocular Motility

· Full vertical and horizontal gaze
· Upbeat nystagmus in primary gaze, increased on upgaze
· Square-wave jerks

- Horizontal gaze evoked nystagmus left > right
- No nystagmus on downgaze
- Pursuit (horizontal and vertical): smooth to a very slow target; slow to initiate and markedly saccadic to a fast target
- Convergence normal
- Marked saccadic hypermetria
  - Right gaze to center, hypermetria—eyes overshoot almost fully to the left
  - Left gaze to center, hypermetria—eyes overshoot almost fully to the right
  - Upgaze to center—small amplitude hypermetria
  - Downgaze to center—small amplitude hypermetria

Localization

Saccadic dysmetria (analogous to overshoot on finger-nose-finger test with upper limb ataxia) is diagnostic of a lesion of the OMV (V, VI, VII) or the FOR.

A very similar patient, post-resection of a cerebellar cystic astrocytoma had a surgical lesion involving the fastigial nuclei and saccadic hypermetria, is shown in Figure 9-14A–B.

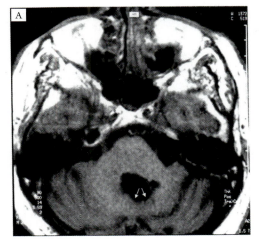
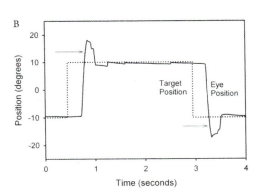

FIGURE 9-14 Cerebellar disease causing saccadic dysmetria. (A) Magnetic resonance imaging of a 50-year-old man who had undergone resection of a cystic astrocytoma, with a surgical lesion involving the fastigial nuclei (*arrows*). (B) The patient's main ocular motor deficit was saccadic hypermetria, indicated by arrows. Right eye rotations correspond to upward deflections.

Reproduced with permission.[33]

The Pancerebellar Syndrome

The pancerebellar syndrome, as its name suggests, consists of all four of the cerebellar syndromes combined. It is characterized by bilateral signs of cerebellar dysfunction affecting the trunk, limbs, and cranial musculature, as well as by disordered movements of the eyes. The syndrome is seen with certain toxic-metabolic disorders, infectious and parainfectious processes, and paraneoplastic disorders.[78-81]

CASE 9-6 Pancerebellar Syndrome: Paraneoplastic Opsoclonus

Video Display

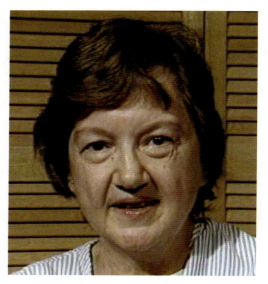

FIGURE 9-15 A fifty-six-year-old woman with carcinoma of the breast—the index case of the anti-Ri antibody.

The patient is a 56-year-old woman who presented with the acute onset of dizziness and nausea and her eyes "going out of focus" 1 month prior to admission (Figure 9-15). A vague feeling of nausea and motion sickness persisted, similar to symptoms she had experienced during an episode of dizziness 6 years previously. She consulted her doctor, who attributed them to labyrinthitis.

Five days later, she had difficulty focusing her eyes to read the newspaper, and the print appeared blurred and "moving in all directions" (oscillopsia). The next day, she had severe dizziness with eyes open and closed, and she felt that the environment was spinning around her. She saw her ophthalmologist, who commented on the presence of "marked nystagmus," and she was admitted to the Infirmary at the Massachusetts Institute of Technology with a diagnosis of acute labyrinthitis.

Four days later, she was unable to sit up in bed without falling over and unable to stand steady without support. She was transferred to the Massachusetts General Hospital.

Analysis of the History

· What are the major presenting symptoms?
· Where are the CNS lesion(s) likely to be?

CASE 9-6 SYMPTOMS

Symptoms	Location Correlation
Dizziness	Vestibular system
Oscillopsia	Vestibular pathways
Truncal ataxia	Cerebellar vermis

The analysis guides the clinical examination.

Examination

Neurological

· Titubation
· Marked truncal ataxia sitting and standing
· Gait ataxia, and unable to tandem walk
· No myoclonic jerks
· Normal coordination in the limbs
· Motor system and sensory system intact
· Reflexes 1+ throughout with flexor plantar responses

Ocular Motility

· Full horizontal eye movements disturbed by continuous bursts of rapid back-to-back saccades in all directions characteristic of opsoclonus
· Transient ocular flutter
· Clockwise rotary nystagmus on gaze left
· Right-beating horizontal nystagmus on gaze right
· Full vertical eye movements without nystagmus
· When tested between attacks of opsoclonus, smooth pursuit eye movements saccadic to a slow moving target

Localization and Differential Diagnosis

Truncal and gait ataxia localize to a midline cerebellar (vermis) lesion and/or cerebellar pathways in the brainstem. Disorders to consider in the differential diagnosis of patients with a combination of ocular flutter/opsoclonus and truncal ataxia are:

- Hyperosmolar nonketotic stupor
- Casual drugs and toxins, including amitriptyline, haloperidol, and lithium
- Myoclonic encephalopathy (dancing eyes and dancing feet syndrome)
- Paraneoplastic syndrome due to a remote malignancy

What Diagnostic Tests Should Follow?

- Tox screen
- EEG
- Blood studies including paraneoplastic markers
- Spinal tap
- Chest x-ray
- Brain MRI
- Search for Occult malignancy

Test Results

The tox screen was negative, the EEG showed no seizure activity and blood test negative for paraneoplastic antibodies.

The results of the spinal tap under fluoroscopy were as follows:

- Cerebrospinal fluid (CSF) protein 70 mg/dL
- Glucose 73 mg%
- RBC 0/ mm^3
- WBC 8/ mm^3
- 93% lymphocytes
- Cytology negative
- IgG 6.4
- Albumin 4.1 and multiple oligoclonal bands

A chest x-ray showing a tiny nodular density in the right middle lobe adjacent to the major fissure was thought to represent a granuloma. A neoplasm could not be ruled out.

Brain MRI (July and October 1986) T1 T2 images showed a small area of hyperintensity in the dorsal midbrain bilaterally, more obvious on the right (Figure 9-16A–C).

A CT scan of the abdomen and pelvis was normal, and a bone scan was also normal. Mammography (delayed for weeks because of the patient's inability to stand) revealed a small suspicious lesion in the upper outer quadrant of the right breast. A breast biopsy performed under fluoroscopy was positive for intraductal adenocarcinoma of the breast.

Diagnosis: Paraneoplastic Cerebellar Syndrome with Opsoclonus/Flutter and Intraductal Adenocarcinoma of the Breast

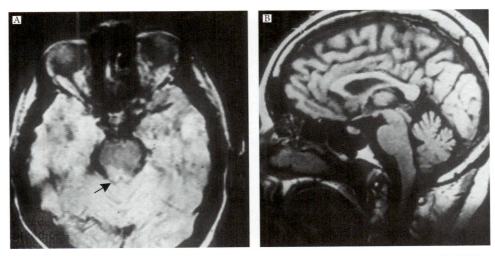

FIGURE 9-16 Brain magnetic resonance imaging (MRI). (A) Fluid attenuated (FLAIR) image shows a bilateral hyperintensity in the dorsal midbrain more extensive on the right side. (B) Sagittal T1 image shows mild-cerebellar atrophy.

Treatment

The approach to treatment in paraneoplastic syndromes includes:[82]

Appropriate therapy for the cancer

- Surgery
- Chemotherapy and/or radiation
- Immune modulation
- Plasma exchange
- Immunoadsorbent therapy
- Intravenous immunoglobulin
- Steroids

Symptomatic treatment for vertigo and other symptoms.

The patient chose to have a segmental mastectomy followed by radiation. 5/9 lymph nodes were positive and chemotherapy was also recommended.

In the absence of anti-CNS antibodies, she was turned down for treatment with plasma exchange.

Her vertigo, opsoclonus, titubation, truncal ataxia, and anxiety were variable throughout her hospital course. Multiple combinations of medications were tried to relieve vertigo, and the most effective were baclofen and meclizine. She received Xanax for anxiety. Prednisone (20 mg p.o., t.i.d.) and ranitidine (150 mg p.o., b.i.d.) were prescribed and taken for a period of 6–8 weeks.

In October 1986, she received a chemotherapeutic cocktail of Cytoxan, Adriamycin, and 5 Fluorouracil units weekly for a period of 6 months, followed by local radiation therapy.

Prognosis

Over the next 2 months, she slowly improved and, on completion of her chemotherapy, she reported that she was "back in the land of the living," able to walk with a cane, climb one flight of stairs, go riding in a car, out for lunch, and generally doing much better. Visual blurring was less marked, and she was able to read. She was considerably encouraged and cheerful at that time even though she was still experiencing occasional bursts of opsoclonus.

By January 1987, she had made a complete recovery and remained well until 1993 when she was diagnosed with cancer of the bladder. She received treatment and again made a complete recovery. I continued to follow her annually until September 2002, when she transferred her care to the University of Massachusetts to be near to her home.

Special Explanatory Note

This case is a notable example of "transitional medicine" in reverse—from bedside to bench. The American Academy of Neurology met in Boston when this patient was in the Massachusetts General Hospital, and Dr. Jerome Posner gave a talk on "Paraneoplastic Syndromes and Marker Antibodies." After the lecture, I asked Dr. Posner if he would be willing to study my patient. He agreed, and I sent him tumor tissue and samples of CSF and serum. Dr. Posner and his colleagues discovered a new and highly specific anti-CNS nuclear neuronal antibody in the serum and CSF through dilutions of 1:1,000 and 1:50 respectively[83] The patient's serum recognized two groups of antigens with molecular weights of 53–61 kDa and 79–84 kDa in immunoblots of Purkinje and cerebral cortex neurons. The antibody was named anti-Ri, Ri being the first two letters of the patient's surname.

The anti-Ri antibody identifies a subset of patients with paraneoplastic ataxia and usually opsoclonus, most of whom have an associated carcinoma of the breast or other gynecological cancer. The anti-Ri antibody has not been found in serum of patients with paraneoplastic opsoclonus associated with neuroblastoma or small-cell lung cancer.

The pathological lesion of paraneoplastic opsoclonus is unknown, and the absence of pathological findings in the brain of patients who have come to autopsy may explain why, in contrast to paraneoplastic cerebellar degeneration and loss of Purkinje cells associated with the anti-Yo antibody syndrome, many patients with paraneoplastic opsoclonus with the anti-Ri antibody undergo spontaneous remission.

Table 9-2 shows the clinical features of seven patients with paraneoplastic opsoclonus. Patient 7 is the case presented here.

TABLE 9-2: Clinical Features of Seven Patients with Paraneoplastic Opsoclonus

Patient No.	Age	Sex	Tumor	Opsoclonus	Truncal Ataxia	Myoclonus	Encephalopathy
1	10 mos	F	Neuroblastoma	+	+	+	0
2	48 yrs	F	Lung (small cell)	+	+	+	+
3	46 yrs	M	Lung (small cell)	+	+	+	+
4	53 yrs	F	Lung (small cell)	+	+	0	+
5	59 yrs	M	Lung (small cell)	+	+	+	0
6	29 yrs	M	Thyroid (medullary carcinoma)	+	+	+	+
7	58: yrs	F	Breast	+	+	0	0

Reproduced with permission.[83]

SELECTED REFERENCES

1. Blumenfeld H. *Neuroanatomy Through Clinical Cases.* 2nd ed. Sunderland, MA: Sinauer Associates; 2010.
2. Horn AKE, Leigh RJ. The anatomy and physiology of the ocular motor system. In: Kennard C, Leigh RJ, eds. *Neuro-ophthalmology.* Vol. 102. 3rd series: *Handbook of Clinical Neurology.* Amsterdam: Elsevier B.V.; 2011.
3. Fuchs AF, Robinson FR, Straube A. Role of the caudal fastigial nucleus in saccade generation: I. Neuronal discharge patterns. *J Neurophysiol.* 1993;70:1723–1740.
4. Robinson FR, Fuchs AF. The role of the cerebellum in voluntary eye movements. *Annu Rev Neurosci.* 2001;24:981–1004.
5. Brodal P. Further observations on the cerebellar projections from the pontine nuclei and the nucleus reticularis tegmenti pontis in the rhesus monkey. *J Comp Neurol.* 1982;204:44–55.
6. Thielert CD, Thier P. Patterns of projections from the pontine nuclei and the nucleus reticularis tegmenti pontis to the posterior vermis in the rhesus monkey: a study using retrograde tracers. *J Comp Neurol.* 1993;337:113–126.
7. Helmchen C, Straube A, Büttner U. Saccade-related activity in the fastigial oculomotor region of the macaque monkey during spontaneous eye movements in light and darkness. *Exp Brain Res.* 1994;98:474–482.
8. Noda H, Fujikado T. Topography of the oculomotor area of the cerebellar vermis in macaques as determined by microstimulation. *J Neurophysiol.* 1987;58:359–378.
9. Barash S, Melikyan A, Sivakov A, Zhang M, Glickstein M, Their P. Saccadic dysmetria and adaptation after lesions of the cerebellar cortex. *J Neurosci.* 1999;19:10931–10939.
10. Thier P, Dicke P, Hass R, Barash S. Encoding of movement time by population of cerebellar Purkinje cells. *Nature.* 2000;405:72–76.
11. Robinson FR, Straube A, Fuchs AF. Role of the caudal fastigial nucleus in saccade generation. 2. Effects of muscimol inactivation. *J Neurophysiol.* 1993;70:1741–1758.
12. Vahedi K, Rivaud S, Amarenco P, Pierrot-Deseilligny C. Horizontal eye movement disorders after posterior vermis infarctions. *J Neurol Neurosurg Psychiat.* 1995;58:91–94.
13. Belton T, McCrea RA. Role of the cerebellar flocculus region in the coordination of eye and head movements during gaze pursuit. *J Neurophysiol.* 2000;84:1614–1626.
14. Zee DS, Yamazaki A, Butler PH, Gücer G. Effects of ablation of flocculus and paraflocculus on eye movements in primate. *J Neurophysiol.* 1981;46:878–899.
15. Rambold H, Churchland A, Selig Y, Jasmin L, Lisberger SG. Partial ablations of the flocculus and ventral paraflocculus in monkeys cause linked deficits in smooth pursuit eye movements and adaptive modification of the VOR. *J Neurophysiol.* 2002;87:912–924.

16. Rubertone JA, Haines DE. Secondary vestibulocerebellar projections to flocculonodular lobe in a prosimian primate, *Galago senagalensis. J Comp Neurol.* 1981;200:255–272.

17. Voogd J. The human cerebellum. *J Chem Anat.* 2003;26:243–252.

18. Walberg F, Dietrichs E. The interconnection between the vestibular nuclei and the nodulus: a study of reciprocity. *Brain Res.* 1988;449:47–53.

19. Solomon D, Cohen B. Stimulation of the nodulus and uvula discharges velocity storage in the vestibulo-ocular reflex. *Exp Brain Res.* 1994;102:57–68.

20. Waespe W, Cohen B, Raphan T. Dynamic modification of the vestibulo-ocular reflex by the nodulus and uvula. *Science.* 1985;228:199–202.

21. Garbutt S, Thakore N, Rucker JC, Han Y, Kumar AN, Leigh RJ. Effects of visual fixation and convergence in periodic alternating nystagmus due to MS. *Neuro-ophthalmol.* 2004;278:221–229.

22. Leigh RJ, Robinson DA, Zee DS. A hypothetical explanation for periodic alternating nystagmus: Instability in the optokinetic-vestibular system. *Ann NY Acad Sci.* 1981;374:619–635.

23. Shallo-Hoffmann J, Faldon M, Tusa RJ. The incidence and waveform characteristics of periodic alternating nystagmus in congenital nystagmus. *Invest Ophthalmol Vis Sci.* 1999;40:2546–2553.

24. Shallo-Hoffmann J, Riordan-Eva P. Recognizing periodic alternating nystagmus. *Strabismus.* 2001;9: 203–215.

25. Halmagyi GM, Rudge P, Gresty MA, Leigh RJ, Zee DS. Treatment of periodic alternating nystagmus. *Ann Neurol.* 1980;8:609–611.

26. Solomon D, Shepard N, Mishra A. Congenital periodic alternating nystagmus: response to baclofen. *Ann NY Acad Sci.* 2002;956:611–615.

27. Gradstein L, Reinecke RD, Wizov SS, Goldstein HP. Congenital periodic alternating nystagmus. Diagnosis and management. *Ophthalmology.* 1997;104:918–928.

28. Wong AME. *Eye Movement Disorders.* New York: Oxford University Press, 2008.

29. Ohtsuka K, Noda H. Saccadic burst neurons in the oculomotor region of the fastigial neurons in macaque monkeys. *J Neurophysiol.* 1992;65:1422–1434.

30. Fuchs AF, Robinson FR, Straube A. Participation of the caudal fastigial nucleus in smooth-pursuit eye movements. I. Neuronal activity. *J Neurophysiol.* 1994;72:2714–2728.

31. Gonzalo-Ruiz A, Leichnetz GR, Smith DJ. Origin of cerebellar projections to the region of the oculomotor complex, medial pontine reticular formation, and superior colliculus in new world monkeys: A retrograde horseradish peroxidase study. *J Comp Neurol.* 1988;268:508–526.

32. Noda H, Sugita S, Ikeda Y. Afferent and efferent connections of the oculomotor region of the fastigial nucleus in the macaque monkey. *J Comp Neurol.* 1990;302:330–348.

33. Leigh RJ, Zee DS. *The Neurology of Eye Movements.* 4th ed. New York: Oxford University Press; 2006.

34. Leigh RJ, Zee DS. with permission 2013.

35. Gilman S, Bloedel J, Lechtenerg R. *Disorders of the Cerebellum.* Philadelphia: Davis 1980; 159–177.

36. Hallett M, Berardelli A, Matheson J, Rothwell J, Marsden CD. Physiological analysis of simple rapid movement in patients with cerebellar deficits. *J Neurol Neurosurg Psychiat.* 1991;53:124.

37. Urban PP, Marx J, Hunsche S, Gawehn J, Vucurevic G, Wicht S, Massinger C, Stoeter P, Hopf HC. Cerebellar speech representation: lesion topography in dysarthria as derived from cerebellar ischemia and functional magnetic resonance imaging. *Arch Neurol.* 2003;60:965–972.

38. Robitaille Y, Lopes-Cendes I, Becher M, Rouleau G, Clark AW. The neuropathology of CAG repeat diseases: review and update of genetic and molecular features. *Brain Pathol.* 1997;7:901–926.

39. Zoghbi HY, Orr HT. Glutamine repeats and neurodegeneration. *Annu Rev Neurosci.* 2000;23:217–247.

40. Wadia NH. Heredo-familial spinocerebellar degeneration with slow eye movements: another variety of olivopontocerebellar degeneration. *Neurol India.* 1977;25:147–160.

41. Zee DS, Yee RD, Cogan DG, Robinson DA, Engel WK. Ocular motor abnormalities in hereditary cerebellar ataxia. *Brain.* 1976;99:207–234.

42. Büttner N, Geschwind D, Jen JC, Perlman S, Pulst SM, Baloh RW. Oculomotor phenotypes in autosomal dominant ataxias. *Arch Neurol.* 1998;55:1353–1357.

43. Burk K, Fetter M, Abele M, Laccone F, Brice A, Dichgans J, Klockgether T. Autosomal dominant cerebellar ataxia type I: oculomotor abnormalities in families with SCA1, SCA2 and SCA3. *J Neurol.* 1999;246(9):789–797.

44. Wadia NH, Swami RK. A new form of heredo-familial spinocerebellar degeneration with slow eye movements. *Brain.* 1971;94:359–374.

45. Rub U, Brunt ER, Gierga K, Schultz C, Paulson H, de Vos RAI, Braak H. The nucleus raphe interpositus in spinocerebellar ataxia type 3 (Machado-Joseph disease). *J Chem Neuroanat.* 2003;25:115–127.

46. Rub U, Burk K, Schols L, Brunt ER, de Vos RAI, Orozco Diaz G, Gierga K, Ghebremedhin E, Schultz C, Del Turco D, Mittelbronn M, Auburger G, Deller T, Braak H. Damage to the reticulotegmental nucleus of the pons in spinocerebellar ataxia type 1, 2, and 3. *Neurology.* 2004;63:1258–1263.

47. Harding AE. Friedreich's ataxia: a clinical and genetic study of 90 families with an analysis of early diagnostic criteria and intrafamilial clustering of clinical features. *Brain.* 1981;104:589–620.

48. Gorman WF, Brock S. Periodic alternating nystagmus in Friedreich's ataxia. *Am J Ophthalmol.* 1950;33:860–864.

49. Furman JM, Perlman S, Baloh RW. Eye movements in Friedreich ataxia. *Arch Neuro.* 1983;40:343–346.

50. Stell R, Bronstein AM, Plant GR, Harding AE. Ataxia telangiectasia: a reappraisal of the ocular motor features and their value in the diagnosis of atypical cases. *Mov Disord.* 1989;4:320–329.

51. Louis-Bar D. Sur un syndrome progressif cormprenant des telangiectasies capillaires cutanees et conjonctivales symetriques, a disposition naevoide et des troubles cerebelleux. *Confinia Neurologica.* 1941;4:32–42

52. Boder E, Sedgwick RP. Ataxia-telangiectasia: a familial syndrome of progressive cerebellar ataxia, oculocutaneous telangiectasia and frequent pulmonary infection. *Pediatrics.* 1958;21(4):526–554.

53. Bouchard JP, Barbeau A, Bouchard R, Paquet M, Bouchard RW. A cluster of Friedreich's ataxia in Rimouski, Quebec. *Can J Neurol Sci.* 1979;6(2):205–208.

54. Bouchard JP, Barbeau A, Bouchard R, Bouchard RW. Autosomal recessive spastic ataxia of Charlevoix-Saguenay. *Can J Neurol Sci (Winnipeg).* 1978;5(1): 61–69.

55. Narayanan V, Rice SG, Olfers SS, Sivakumar K. Autosomal recessive spastic ataxia of Charlevoix-Saguenay: compound heterozygotes for nonsense mutations of the SACS gene. *J Child Neurol.* 2011;26(12):1585–1589.

56. Vanier MT, Millat G. Niemann-Pick disease Type C. *Clin Genet.* 2003;64:269–281.

57. Kerrison JB, Biousse V, Newman NJ. Retinopathy of NARP syndrome. *Arch Ophthalmol.* 2000;118:298–299.

58. Wadia NH. Heredo-familial spinocerebellar degeneration with slow eye movements: another variety of olivopontocerebellar degeneration. *Neurol India.* 1977;25:147–160.

59. Yokota O, Tsuchiya K, Terada S, Oshima K, Ishizu H, Matsushita M, Kuroda S, Akiyama H. Frequency and clinicopathological characteristics of alcoholic cerebellar degeneration in Japan: a cross-sectional study of 1,509 postmortems. *Acta Neuropathol (Berl).* 2006;112:43–51.

60. Victor M, Adams RD, Mancall EL. A restricted form of cerebellar degeneration occurring in alcoholic patients. *Arch Neurol.* 1959;1:579–688.

61. Vrabec TR, Sergott RC, Savino PJ, Bosley TM. Intermittent obstructive hydrocephalus in the Arnold-Chiari malformation. *Ann Neurol.* 1989;26:401–404.

62. Dyste GN, Menezes AH, VanGilder JC. Symptomatic Chiari malformations. An analysis of presentation, management, and long-term outcome. *J Neurosurg.* 1989;71:159–168.

63. Yee RD, Baloh RW, Honrubia V. Episodic vertical oscillopsia and downbeat nystagmus in a Chiari malformation. *Arch Ophthalmol.* 1984;102:723–725.

64. Cogan DG. Downbeat nystagmus. *Arch Ophthalmol.* 1968;80:757–768.

65. Halmagyi GM, Rudge P, Gresty MA, Sanders MD. Downbeating nystagmus: a review of 62 cases. *Arch Neurol.* 1983;40:777–784.

66. Bronstein AM, Miller DH, Rudge P, Kendall BE. Downbeating nystagmus: magnetic resonance imaging and neuro-otological findings. *J Neurol Sci.* 1987;81:173–184.

67. Pinel JF, Larmande P, Guegan Y, Iba-Zizen MT. Downbeat nystagmus: case report with magnetic resonance imaging and surgical treatment. *Neurosurgery.* 1987;21(5):736–739.

68. Bosley TM, Cohen DA, Schatz NJ, Zimmerman RA, Bilaniuk LT, Savino PJ, Sergott RS. Comparison of metrizamide computer tomography and magnetic resonance imaging in the evaluation of lesions at the cervicomedullary junction. *Neurology.* 1985;35:485–492.

69. Baloh RW, Spooner JW. Downbeat nystagmus: a type of central vestibular nystagmus. *Neurology.* 1981;31:304–310.

70. Mossman SS, Bronstein AM, Gresty MA, Kendall B, Rudge P. Convergence nystagmus associated with Arnold-Chiari malformation. *Arch Neurol.* 1990;47:357–359.

71. Straumann D, Muller E. Torsional rebound nystagmus in a patient with type I Chiari malformation. *Neuro-ophthalmology.* 1994;14:79–84.

72. Pujol J, Roig C, Capdevila A, Pou A, Marti-Vilalta JL, Kulisevsky J, Escartin A, Zannoli G. Motion of the cerebellar tonsils in Chiari type I malformation studies by cine phase-contrast MRI. *Neurology.* 1995;45:1746–1753.

73. Spooner JW, Baloh RW. Arnold-Chiari malformation. Improvement in eye movements after surgical treatment. *Brain.* 1981;104:51–60.

74. Pedersen RA, Troost BT, Abel LA, Zorub D. Intermittent downbeat nystagmus and oscillopsia reversed by suboccipital craniectomy. *Neurology.* 1980;30:1239–1242.

75. Furman JM, Wall C III, Pang D. Vestibular function in periodic alternating nystagmus. *Brain.* 1990;113:1425–1439.

76. Campbell WW. Periodic alternating nystagmus in phenytoin intoxication. *Arch Neurol.* 1980;37:178–180.

77. Crino PB, Galetta SL, Sater RA, Raps EC, Witte A, Roby D, Rosenquist AC. Clinicopathologic study of paraneoplastic brainstem encephalitis and ophthalmoparesis. *J Neuro-ophthalmol.* 1996;16(1):44–48.

78. Ko MW, Dalmau J, Galetta SL. Neuro-ophthalmologic manifestations of paraneoplastic syndromes. *J Neuro-Ophthalmol.* 2008;28:58–68.

79 Wray SH, Dalmau J, Chen A, King S, Leigh RJ. Paraneoplastic disorders of eye movements. *Ann N.Y. Acad Sci.* 2011;1233:279–284.

80 Dalmau JO, Posner JB. Paraneoplastic syndromes. *Arch Neurol.* 1999;56(4):405–408.

81. Bataller L, Dalmau J. Paraneoplastic Neurologic Syndromes: Approaches to Diagnosis and Treatment. *Semin Neurol.* 2003;23:215–224.

82. Budde-Steffen C, Anderson NE, Rosenblum MK, Graus F, Ford D, Synek BJL, Wray SH, Posner JB. An anti-neuronal autoantibody in paraneoplastic opsoclonus. *Ann Neurol.* 1988;23:528–531.

83. Luque AF, Furneaux HM, Ferziger R, Rosenblum MK, Wray SH, Schold SC Jr, Glantz MJ, Jaeckle KA, Biran H, Lesser MK, Paulsen WA, River ME, Posner JB. Anti-Ri: an antibody associated with paraneoplastic opsoclonus and breast cancer. *Ann Neurol.* 1991;29:241–251.

| 10 |

OSCILLOPSIA, NYSTAGMUS, SACCADIC OSCILLATIONS, AND INTRUSIONS

OSCILLOPSIA

Oscillopsia is an illusion of movement in the visual world. Because clear vision is possible only if the image is held steady in the foveal area of the retina, a slip of the image away from foveal fixation (retinal slip) will cause vision to blur. When the slip is excessive, continuous oscillopsia develops and it is "like a television that has lost its vertical hold...the visual world is rolling over vertically in front of me". This vivid description of vertical oscillopsia was the presenting symptom in a 58-year-old engineer who had downbeat nystagmus. He had no oscillopsia lying in bed, sitting still, or moving his head slowly, but an illusion of motion was provoked by rapid head turning, for instance, when reversing his car or moving his head suddenly while driving.

The disruption of fixation that causes oscillopsia is essentially the consequence of one or the other of two possibilities: either the eyes do not move adequately when they should—the—eye movements fail to compensate for the patient's head movements because the vestibulo-ocular reflex (VOR) is defective, as in the case of the engineer; or the eyes move excessively when they should be steady—because the patient has spontaneous nystagmus or saccadic oscillations.

Oscillopsia occurring only with movements of the head, suggests an abnormality of the VOR. Patients with symmetrical loss of VOR function, for example due to gentamicin ototoxicity, are unable to fixate on objects when walking because the surroundings appear to be bouncing up and down.[1] The head oscillates in the vertical plane, and the visual pursuit system cannot compensate for the loss of vestibular function to stabilize gaze. To see the faces of passers-by, patients learn to stop and hold their head still. This can present difficulty in something as ordinary and everyday as supermarket shopping: labels can be read clearly only if the patient stands still. When reading, these patients learn to stabilize the head by placing their hand on their chin to prevent even the slight movements associated with pulsatile cerebral blood flow.

Patients with cerebellar lesions cannot suppress their VOR *without* fixation. They experience a brief sensation of oscillopsia after each rapid head movement owing to a transient, unwanted vestibular nystagmus. These patients typically have gaze-evoked nystagmus on lateral or vertical gaze, and they may experience oscillopsia with both head and eye movements.[2,3]

THE OSCILLOPSIA HISTORY

Patients with oscillopsia describe their problem in many different ways, for example "blurred vision," "difficulty in focusing," "shimmering vision," and for diagnostic purposes the examiner should always ask:

- Is your vision moving, oscillating, jumping, or wobbly?
- In one eye or both eyes?

A positive answer will indicate either *monocular* or *binocular* oscillopsia.

Oscillopsia with Movements of the Head

These questions tell the examiner whether oscillopsia occurs during head movements or whether head movements trigger oscillopsia:[4]

- Does oscillopsia occur during movements of the head?
- Is it triggered by specific head movements?
- Do you get oscillopsia turning over in bed?
- Is your vision clear and steady when you sit still or lie down?

Affirmative answers suggest a loss of vestibular function, and the symptomatic results of this vary with the actual cause. Fortunately, the severity of oscillopsia in patients with bilateral and permanent VOR failure tends to diminish with time.

Oscillopsia at Rest

When patients report that oscillopsia is completely unrelated to movement or head position and is present at rest, the next important question is:

- Is the oscillopsia constant and continuous or is it paroxysmal?

Constant and continuous oscillopsia is a disabling symptom, difficult to relieve and invariably associated with acquired spontaneous nystagmus. It is usually a sign of vestibular, brainstem, or cerebellar involvement, and, in rare cases, it can be caused by paralysis of the eye muscles or a lesion in the cortical visual association areas.

Constant oscillopsia associated with unilateral *peripheral* vestibular lesions is usually transient, disappearing as the acute vertigo and spontaneous nystagmus disappear. Patients with spontaneous nystagmus due to lesions of the *central* vestibular pathways often report their eyes flicking back and forth, accompanying the fast component of the nystagmus, and they illustrate the movement with their hands, particularly if it is upbeat or downbeat nystagmus. These patients have associated symptoms and signs of brainstem dysfunction (see Chapter 9, Case 9-3).

Paroxysmal oscillopsia, characterized by frequent episodes of shaking visual images lasting for seconds only, is almost always seen with transient nystagmus or obtrusive oscillations. It can be caused by extra-axial lesions impinging on the vestibular nerve with or without vertigo. Vascular compression of the eighth cranial nerve has also been suggested as the cause of the syndrome vestibular paroxysmia (disabling positional vertigo) (Chapter 8). However, its sporadic nature, lack of a well-defined syndrome and of a reliable diagnostic test, can make parosysmal oscillopsia difficult for the non-surgical clinician to identify.[5]

When paroxysmal oscillopsia is monocular, superior oblique myokymia is the leading cause. Superior oblique myokymia is a high-frequency monocular oscillation (microtremor) produced

TABLE 10-1: Diagnosing Oscillopsia

Oscillopsia	Symptomatic Result	Cause
During movements of the head	Bilateral loss of vestibular function	Absent VOR Postmeningitic sequelae Ototoxicity Idiopathic
Triggered by movements of the head	Central positional nystagmus	Brainstem-cerebellar disease
At rest, head still		
Continuous	Spontaneous nystagmus 　Upbeat 　Downbeat	Brainstem-cerebellar disease
	Torsional 　Pendular 　Pendular pseudonystagmus	Head tremor + absent VOR
Paroxysmal	Tullio phenomenon (sound-induced)	Superior canal dehiscence
	Vestibular paroxysms	Vestibular nerve: vestibular paroxysmia Vestibular nuclear lesions
	Paroxysmal ocular oscillations	Ocular flutter Microflutter Voluntary nystagmus Monocular: superior oblique myokymia

VOR: vestibulo-ocular reflex

Reproduced with permission.[13]

by spontaneous firing of the superior oblique muscle,[6,7] and it is characterized by very brief (seconds only) episodes of monocular vertical oscillopsia occurring at irregular intervals. The diagnosis is made by asking the patient to look down and intort the eye in the field of action of the superior oblique muscle while viewing the eye with an ophthalmoscope to visualize torsional oscillations. This disorder is usually idiopathic but if symptoms persist, neuroimaging of the brain is indicated since some cases may be caused by microvascular compression of the trunk (root exit zone) of cranial nerve (CN) IV by branches of the superior cerebellar artery.[8,9] Microvascular decompression of CN IV has been used to alleviate paroxysmal oscillopsia, but this procedure carries with it the risk of a superior oblique palsy.[10] Medications such as gabapentin, baclofen, and memantine should be tried first.[11,12]

Guidelines to diagnosing oscillopsia are shown in Table 10-1.[13]

NYSTAGMUS

Nystagmus is an involuntary, repetitive, rhythmic to-and-fro movement of the eyes initiated by a slow-phase (or slow-drift) that shifts an image off the fovea. Its cause can be physiological, congenital, or acquired.

A flow chart for classifying and distinguishing between types of acquired nystagmus is shown in Figure 10-1.[14]

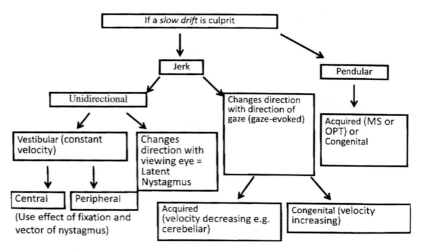

FIGURE 10-1 Flow chart for classifying acquired nystagmus.

Reproduced with permission.[14]

This chart helps to visualize nystagmus initiated by a slow drift of the eyes away from fixation. This slow phase is the fundamental "driving" component of both jerk nystagmus and pendular nystagmus, and it is worth repeating that *analysis of the slow phase is the most helpful factor in locating and identifying the lesion* of the ocular motor subsystem that has caused it. The slow eye movement may be due to defects in the vestibulo-ocular, smooth pursuit, optokinetic, or gaze-holding systems, or, more rarely, in the vergence system.

Four common slow-phase nystagmus waveforms contribute to lesion localization:

- First, a constant-velocity drift of the eyes that occurs in nystagmus caused by *peripheral or central vestibular disease* and that is also associated with lesions of the cerebellar flocculus (Figure 10-2A).
- Second, a decreasing velocity drift of the eyes back from an eccentric orbital position toward the midline that is characteristic of gaze-evoked nystagmus (Figure 10-2B). This waveform reflects an unsustained eye position signal caused by an *impaired neural integrator*.
- Third, an increasing velocity drift of the eyes from the central position that may be due to an unstable neural integrator—this is seen in the horizontal plane in congenital nystagmus and in the vertical plane in *cerebellar disease* (Figure 10-2C).
- Fourth, slow-phase oscillations, or pendular nystagmus, which may be congenital or acquired (Figure 10-2D).

The waveforms of nystagmus are shown in Figure 10-2A–D.[15]

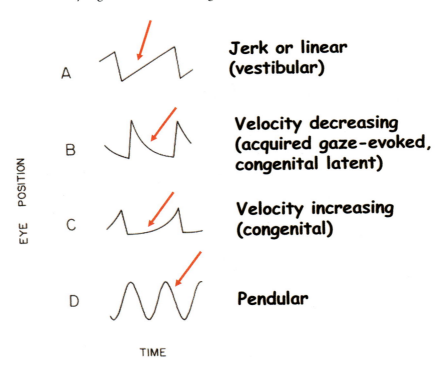

FIGURE 10-2 Steps to take in Evaluating Nystagmus: Four common slow-phase waveforms of nystagmus. (A) Constant-velocity drift of the eyes. The added quick phases give a "sawtooth" appearance. (B) Drift of the eyes back from an eccentric orbital position toward the midline (gaze-evoked nystagmus). The drift shows a negative exponential time course, with decreasing velocity. (C) Drift of the eyes away from the central position with a positive exponential time course (increasing velocity). This waveform suggests an unstable neural integrator and is encountered in the horizontal plane in congenital nystagmus and in the vertical plane in cerebellar disease. (D) Pendular nystagmus, which may be congenital or acquired.

Reproduced with permission.[15]

On the basis of etiology, nystagmus is classified as neurologic, otologic, ocular, or labyrinthine and on the basis of direction of movement, horizontal or vertical nystagmus describe themselves. The direction of torsional jerk nystagmus, however, is most clearly described by saying that the nystagmus beats torsionally toward the left or the right shoulder (not clockwise or counterclockwise).

Most often, nystagmus is described by the direction of the fast phase: for example, right-beating, left-beating, upbeat, or downbeat nystagmus. However, *the initial slow phase of nystagmus reflects the underlying disorder,* and the clinician must be extremely careful to note the characteristics of every phase. An important first step is to recognize the difference between nystagmus and saccadic intrusions, which superficially mimic nystagmus but actually differ from it because the initial movement taking the eye away from fixation is a fast saccade instead of a slow drift.

The Nystagmus Examination

A systematic examination of the ocular motor system is extremely important for evaluating nystagmus and interpreting the meaning of the sign.

Steps to Take in Evaluating Nystagmus

- Note any abnormality of head posture.
- Determine whether there is a full range of movement of each eye.
- Observe the stability of gaze by asking the patient to fix on a stationary target (such as letter X) at a viewing distance greater than 2 m.
- Determine if there is any nystagmus when the eyes are in central gaze.
- For each eye, note the direction in which the fast-phase of nystagmus occurs: right-beating, left-beating, upbeat, downbeat, torsional, or mixed.
- Compare the nystagmus in each eye—does the direction or size of movement in each eye differ? Is there any asynchrony?
- If the *size* of oscillations differs in each eye, it is referred to as *dissociated nystagmus.*
- If the *direction* of the oscillations in each eye differs, it is called *disconjugate* or *disjunctive* nystagmus.
- Cover each eye in turn to check for latent nystagmus.
- Repeat each of these observations as the eyes are brought into the right, left, up-, and down-gaze positions (as viewed by the examiner) and during sustained convergence.
- Observing nystagmus with the patient supine, prone, and lying on either side will show whether the nystagmus is either beating toward the earth (*geotropic*) or beating away from the earth (*apogeotropic*) (see Chapter 8, Case 8-3).[16]
- If there is no visible nystagmus, examine the effect of removing fixation and do additional positional testing and provocative maneuvers—head-shaking in the horizontal or vertical plane,[17] hyperventilation, the Valsalva maneuver, the Dix-Hallpike maneuver, and/or caloric stimulation with ice water (Chapter 6).

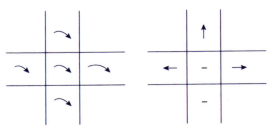

Peripheral Spontaneous   Symmetric Gaze-evoked

FIGURE 10-3 Method for describing the effect of eye position on nystagmus amplitude and direction. Arrows indicate direction of the fast phase in each eye position for peripheral spontaneous nystagmus and symmetric gaze-evoked nystagmus.

Reproduced with permission.[18]

All of this information should be noted for use in fully evaluating the clinical implications of the nystagmus. The examination completed, make a box diagram of the nystagmus in which arrows denote the trajectory and quick-phase direction of the eye movement and line length depicts intensity (amplitude × frequency) in each gaze position as viewed by the examiner (Figure 10-3).[18]

■ **Clinical Points to Remember About Nystagmus**

- Peripheral vestibular nystagmus is usually suppressed by fixation.
- During ophthalmoscopy, the direction of horizontal or vertical (upbeat or downbeat) nystagmus is inverted when viewed through the ophthalmoscope.
- Patients with a head tremor do not show motion of the retina during ophthalmoscopy unless they have lost their VOR—in which case they have pseudonystagmus.
- Nystagmus that appears horizontal in the straight-ahead position but torsional on looking up indicates that the eyes are rotating around the rostral-caudal axis relative to the head. This is characteristic of vestibular nystagmus.
- Nystagmus that appears horizontal in the straight-ahead position and still appears "horizontal" on looking up indicates the eyes are rotating around an eye fixed axis, a characteristic of congenital nystagmus. ■

PHYSIOLOGICAL NYSTAGMUS

Nystagmus may be physiological. Optokinetic nystagmus (OKN) is an example of physiological nystagmus. It occurs naturally during rapid full-field stimulation; for example, the countryside flashing past while sitting in a fast-moving car can produce physiological jerk nystagmus. Both the smooth pursuit and optokinetic systems contribute to this response.

Optokinetic nystagmus can be easily evaluated clinically by asking patients to count the black lines on a black-and-white striped optokinetic drum rotated in front of them. If the speed of the drum rotating horizontally is too fast, or the interval between the stripes is too small, nystagmus does not occur. If the response is normal, the eyes will involuntarily follow one or more of the stripes to the edge of the drum and then make a quick corrective movement in the opposite direction to fixate on another set of stripes. Although this response is normal, it is nonetheless classified as OKN, a jerk nystagmus. Its slow component corresponds in speed and direction to the rotating drum, whereas the fast component, a corrective movement (saccade) to bring the eyes back to their original position, is independent of the drum. The slow and fast phases of OKN are thus distinct and separate, and the slow phase is involuntary in the sense that the eyes cannot voluntarily be kept stationary while the gaze is fixed on the stripes.

The relationship of disturbances in OKN to cerebral lesions is most important. As a general rule, abnormalities of optokinetic slow components parallel abnormalities in smooth pursuit, and abnormalities of optokinetic fast components correlate with abnormalities of voluntary saccades. Focal lateralized disease of the parietal occipital region, brainstem, and cerebellum results in absent (or asymmetric) OKN when the stimulus moves toward the side of the lesion.[19,20] This asymmetric response is most frequently seen with a unilateral parieto-occipital lesion, with and without hemianopia. Not all occipito-parietal lesions are accompanied by a defective OKN response, however. Although rare, an inverse or paradoxic response may be seen in which the fast phase of the response moves in the same direction as the moving stimulus, and it may be vertical when the field is rotated horizontally. The inverse OKN response is seen in children with congenital nystagmus and the vertical response in patients with brainstem disease.[21]

CONGENITAL NYSTAGMUS

The classification of infantile nystagmus (IN) into one single syndrome caused by one underlying mechanism is now outdated. Genetic methods and other new diagnostic tools such as optical coherence tomography (OCT) allow sensory abnormalities associated with IN to be characterized with far greater clarity. Analysis of specific diseases, such as albinism and achromatopsia, as well as known genetic abnormalities, such as *FRMD7* and *PAX 6* mutations, permit clearer segregation of IN groupings, with eye movement recordings to accurately characterize oculomotor abnormalities. Albinism, for example, as well as causing nystagmus, is associated with a number of other visual system deficits including an abnormal axonal crossing pattern at the optic chiasm that is considered to be the underlying motor cause of IN in this disorder. In contrast, achromatopsia has a primary cause that is purely sensory since it is directly caused by defects in the retinal photo-transduction pathway.[22] As OCT improves in quality and image acquisition, and as genetic profiling becomes more affordable, a fuller understanding of IN will undoubtedly lead to a classification based on the pathogenesis of IN subgroupings.

Infantile Nystagmus

Infantile nystagmus may be present at birth, but typically it develops during the second through fourth months of life when visual fixation normally develops.[23] The nystagmus is usually horizontal, almost never vertical, with a jerk waveform in albinism and in idiopathic nystagmus associated with mutations in *FRMD7*. It persists throughout life, affecting the two eyes conjugately. In infants with *PAX6* mutations, the nystagmus characteristics are variable—horizontal, vertical, or gaze-evoked. In achromatopsia, which has a distinct foveal morphology and is primarily a retinal disease, the nystagmus is variable as well. Albinism or *PAX6* mutations have similar OCT features but different nystagmus waveforms.

Infantile pendular nystagmus (so-called because the eyes move from side to side like pendulums) can be caused by congenital disorders including spasmus nutans. Elliptical pendular nystagmus together with upbeat nystagmus may occur in Pelizaeus-Merzbacher disease, a rare X-linked recessive neurodegenerative condition in young children; the disease primarily affects the white matter of the central nervous system (CNS), and pendular nystagmus accompanied by visual loss and optic atrophy may be the initial manifestation. Other childhood white matter disorders with a similar presentation include adrenoleukodystrophy and Cockayne's syndrome.

Infantile pendular nystagmus frequently converts into a jerk nystagmus on lateral gaze. The null point, or zone where nystagmus is minimal and vision best, may be in primary gaze or in an eccentric position (the foveation period allows normal visual development). To either side of the null point, a relatively coarse jerk nystagmus develops with the fast phase toward the direction of gaze. Convergence dampens IN, and head turns are common to bring the eye and the orbit close to the null point to clarify vision. Some children with IN also have head oscillations[24]—these head movements are not compensatory and tend to increase when the child pays attention to an object, which also increases the nystagmus. In most affected children, these head and ocular oscillations may be caused by a common neural mechanism.

Autosomal dominant and sex-linked recessive forms of inheritance are reported in familial IN.[25] In X-linked forms, the mother may show subtle ocular motor abnormalities. In a personal case of familial IN, the infant son had pendular nystagmus in primary gaze, jerk nystagmus on lateral gaze, and no head tilt or latent nystagmus. The mother had pendular nystagmus.

Latent Nystagmus

Infantile nystagmus and latent nystagmus occasionally coexist. *Latent nystagmus* is characterised by a jerk nystagmus that is absent when both eyes are viewing but appears when one eye is covered. Latent nystagmus may be produced by an imbalance of visual inputs to the vestibular system and occurs in some children who have congenital monocular visual loss. This suggests that other factors beyond visual deprivation are responsible for the latent nystagmus.

When both eyes are open, a clear image is seen and no nystagmus is present. Covering one eye (or blurring the image of one eye or shining a bright light into one eye) results in a conjugate slow drift of the eyes toward the side of the covered (or illuminated) eye, with a fast corrective phase toward the side of the uncovered (or nonilluminated) eye. The nystagmus is least when the gaze is directed toward the side of the covered eye and greatest when the gaze is directed toward the side of the uncovered eye. In some children with latent nystagmus, there is upward deviation of whichever eye is under cover—*dissociated vertical deviation*. The monocular upward drift may also occur spontaneously during periods of inattention. The disorder is unexplained, but usually it is associated with esotropia and latent nystagmus.

Latent nystagmus is usually present bilaterally, and these patients may fail routine eye tests because oscillopsia, induced during monocular patching, reduces visual acuity in the seeing eye. With both eyes open, visual acuity is improved. However, cases have been reported in which the nystagmus is present in one eye only, and latent nystagmus may become manifest when neither eye is occluded because the patient chooses to fixate with one eye.

Latent nystagmus is a relatively benign condition. It is due to disruption of binocular vision during the critical period of development in early infancy and is associated with infantile esotropia. It is usually not associated with neurological abnormalities, and, when the clinical findings are typical, neuroimaging of the brain is not indicated.

Spasmus Nutans Syndrome

Spasmus nutans is a transient ocular motility disorder that develops in the first year of life and is characterized by the triad—nystagmus, head nodding, and unusual head position such as torticollis.[26] Nystagmus is its most consistent feature, and it is detected more readily in the abducting eye on lateral gaze than in primary gaze, where it can be easily missed. The nystagmus of spasmus nutans is predominantly horizontal, intermittent, small amplitude, and shimmering, but it can have vertical, torsional, or pendular components. It may be brought out by convergence; this is the "near-evoked" nystagmus of Chrousos, Ballen, Matsuo, and Cogan who observed it in two children with spasmus nutans.[27] Monocular or dissociated nystagmus can also occur in spasmus nutans but irregular head nodding with horizontal and vertical components may be the first sign. Some children have an additional head tilt or turn, which may be an adaptive strategy to reduce or turn off the nystagmus as it develops.

One important distinguishing feature of spasmus nutans is the variability in amplitude of the oscillations in the two eyes. Over the course of a few minutes, the oscillations may be conjugate, disconjugate, disjunctive, and purely monocular.

Spasmus nutans is no longer regarded as a benign entity. A spasmus nutans-like nystagmus, which occurs in children with optic glioma, parasellar and hypothalamic tumors, and certain retinal disorders, must always be accounted for. It is important to obtain a brain magnetic resonance imaging (MRI) or a computed tomography (CT) scan of the visual pathways to rule out serious structural lesions.[28–30]

ACQUIRED NYSTAGMUS

Gaze-Evoked Nystagmus

Gaze-evoked nystagmus is the commonest form of nystagmus and the most important form to understand. Such nystagmus can occur in the horizontal or vertical plane. It can be symmetric, asymmetric, rebound, or dissociated. or Gaze-evoked nystagmus *changes direction* with direction of gaze and occurs only when the eyes are moved into eccentric gaze, especially into lateral and upgaze.

Gaze-evoked nystagmus is caused by impairment of the gaze-holding mechanism To visualize it, think of a patient whose head is still but who has, on gaze to the right, a right-jerk waveform nystagmus that is present only during attempted eccentric fixation; on gaze to the left, he has a left-jerk waveform nystagmus but, again, only on eccentric fixation. Normally, a properly functioning neural integrator generates the position signal to hold the eyes in eccentric orbital position but when the function of the neural integrator(s) is impaired, the position signal is too weak to oppose the elastic restoring forces of the orbit and the eyes drift toward the orbit's center (pulse-step mismatch: normal pulse, poorly sustaind step (Chapter 1, Figure 1-16)). Corrective saccades (quick phases) are then needed to bring them back to eccentric position. Crucial structures for horizontal gaze holding are the nucleus prepositus hypoglossi and the medial vestibular nucleus, and, for vertical gaze holding, the interstitial nucleus of Cajal (INC).

Symmetric gaze-evoked nystagmus (equal amplitude to the left and to the right) on lateral gaze is clinically important although it has limited localizing value. It occurs most commonly as a side effect of sedatives (barbituates), anticonvulsants (phenytoin, carbamazepine), antidepressants (lithium), diazepam, and alcohol. The nystagmus initially appears at extreme horizontal gaze positions and moves toward the midposition with higher drug levels—a rough correlation exists between nystagmus amplitude and the blood drug level.[31,32]

Symmetric gaze-evoked nystagmus also commonly occurs in spinocerebellar atrophy, multiple sclerosis (MS), and posterior fossa tumors[33] when lesions in the cerebellum (especially the flocculus) and its projection to the brainstem are involved.

In the ER, symmetric gaze-evoked nystagmus with inability to tandem walk should prompt toxicity screening. If a complete neurological examination reveals other signs of cerebellar disease, MRI is necessary to look for a structural lesion—for example cerebellar atrophy or the focal white matter lesions of MS.

■ **Clinical Points to Remember About Symmetric Gaze-Evoked Nystagmus**

- *Pathological symmetric gaze-evoked nystagmus* must always be distinguished from its pathological variants—end-point nystagmus and fatigue nystagmus.
- *End-point nystagmus* is frequently described in normal subjects.[34] It looks very similar to gaze-evoked nystagmus, but it is low amplitude, low frequency, poorly sustained, and not associated with abnormal ocular motor or cerebellar signs.
- *Fatigue nystagmus* is seen in patients who cannot maintain conjugate gaze to one side or the other due to muscle weakness (typically paresis of cranial nerves III, IV, and VI) or disease of the neuromuscular junction.[35] The direction of the nystagmus is always toward the side of the weakness. Fatigue nystagmus is frequently present in patients with myasthenia gravis after prolonged gaze to the same side.[36]

  Fatigue nystagmus also appears in other fatigue states, in effort syndromes, in alcohol intoxication, and often in patients recovering from anesthesia. In these cases, it is usually symmetrical when present on gaze to either side. More than any other, this type of nystagmus depends on the attention of the patient: because it is gaze-evoked, as soon as attention is relaxed, the eyes drift away from their eccentric position and nystagmus ceases. ■

Asymmetric horizontal gaze-evoked nystagmus *always* indicates a structural brain lesion. When it is caused by a focal lesion of the brainstem or cerebellum, the larger amplitude nystagmus is usually directed toward the side of the lesion. *Brun's nystagmus, for example,* is caused by large posterior fossa tumors in the cerebellopontine angle that compress the brainstem and cerebellum and cause asymmetric gaze-evoked nystagmus. In Brun's, a low-frequency, large-amplitude, horizontal gaze nystagmus due to defective gaze holding, occurs when the patient looks toward the side of the lesion. A high-frequency, small-amplitude nystagmus due to vestibular imbalance is present when the patient looks away from the side of the lesion.

Rebound nystagmus is seen in some patients with gaze-evoked nystagmus and can occur in normal subjects after prolonged eccentric gaze. On sustained eccentric gaze (>30 seconds), the nystagmus decreases in amplitude, or it may even reverse direction so that the eyes begin to drift centrifugally (away from primary position), resulting in a *centripetal nystagmus* (beating toward primary position). When the eyes return to primary gaze, rebound nystagmus occurs, with quick phases beating in the opposite direction to the eyes in eccentric gaze. Rebound nystagmus lasts for a few seconds only and typically occurs in patients with disease affecting the vestibulo-cerebellum, particularly patients with cerebellar atrophy and focal cerebellar lesions. It is the only variety of nystagmus thought to be specific for cerebellar involvement[37] (Chapter 9).

Dissociated or *disconjugate* gaze-evoked nystagmus commonly results from lesions of the medial longitudinal fasciculus (MLF), which cause paresis of adduction ipsilateral to the lesion and dissociated gaze-evoked nystagmus of the contralateral abducting eye—an internuclear ophthalmoplegia (Chapter 6, Case 6-6).

See-saw nystagmus, a form of pendular nystagmus, is an unusual type of dissociated nystagmus. See-saw nystagmus is a torsional-vertical nystagmus in which, in one half cycle, one eye elevates and intorts as the other depresses and extorts, followed by the next half cycle, when the vertical and torsional movements reverse, thus giving the appearance of a "see-saw."[38,39] The see-saw movement is best visualized by having the patient look at the bridge of the nose: the nystagmus becomes smaller and faster on upgaze and larger and slower on downgaze. It disappears in the dark and on eye closure.

See-saw nystagmus may be congenital but most often it is associated with visual loss due to head trauma causing bitemporal field defects or to parasellar lesions, such as a pituitary tumor with a bitemporal hemianopia implicating crossing fibers of the optic nerves in its pathogenesis. In patients with progressive retinitis pigmentosa, loss of vision may result in see-saw nystagmus (Figure 10-4).[40]

Hemi-see-saw nystagmus, a jerk nystagmus, usually occurs because of a unilateral midbrain lesion in the region of the INC. It may be associated with a contralateral tonic ocular tilt reaction (OTR) or

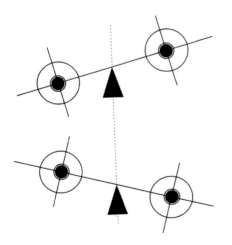

FIGURE 10-4 Schematic illustration of see-saw nystagmus, showing that during one half cycle, the left eye rises and intorts, while the right eye falls and extorts. During the next half cycle, the opposite occurs. In pendular see-saw nystagmus, both half cycles are smooth (slow-phase) movements, whereas in hemi- (or jerk) see-saw nystagmus, one half cycle is a slow phase and the other is a quick phase.

Reproduced with permission.[40]

> ■ **Clinical Points to Remember About See-Saw and Hemi-See-Saw Nystagmus**
> - See-saw and hemi-see-saw nystagmus are *associated with visual loss* and may occur with parasellar tumor, head trauma causing bitemporal visual field defects, lack or loss of crossing fibers in the optic chiasm (e.g., achiasma, septo-optic dysplasia, chiasmal compression), MS, and progressive visual loss (e.g., due to optic neuropathy or retinitis pigmentosa).
> - Hemi-see-saw nystagmus may occur with medullary lesions—syringobulbia and the Chiari malformation.
> - Bow-tie and upbeat nystagmus evolving into hemi-see-saw nystagmus is reported in cases of medial medullary infarction. ■

an ipsilateral paroxysmal OTR. In the paroxysmal form, the head tilt is ipsilateral to the INC lesion, and some of these patients also show corresponding paroxysms of jerk see-saw nystagmus.

The types, characteristics, localization and common causes of gaze-evoked nystagmus are shown in Table 10-2.[18]

TABLE 10-2: Type, Characteristics, Localization, and Common Causes of Gaze-Evoked Nystagmus

Type	Characteristics	Localization	Common Causes
Physiologic endpoint	Jerk, small amplitude, intermittent, extremes of horizontal and upgaze	Physiologic	
Gaze-paretic (symmetric)	Jerk (decreasing velocity slow components) at 30 degrees eccentric gaze	Nonlocalizing	Drugs, alcohol Metabolic disorders Fatigue
Gaze-paretic (asymmetric)	Jerk (decreasing velocity slow components), horizontal, at 30 degrees eccentric gaze, larger amplitude toward side of lesion	Lesions of brainstem, cerebellum, cerebral hemisphere	Multiple sclerosis
Rebound	Jerk, horizontal, decreases and direction can reverse in eccentric gaze, transient jerk nystagmus on return to primary gaze, fast components beating toward eccentric gaze	Cerebellum	Cerebellum—tumor, infarction, atrophy
Dissociated	Jerk, horizontal beating in abducting eye	Medial longitudinal fasciculus	Lesions of the brainstem—infarction, multiple sclerosis
Myasthenia gravis	Jerk, horizontal or vertical, gradual onset in prolonged eccentric gaze	Myoneural junction (fatigue-increasing transmission block)	

Modified and reproduced with permission.[18]

CENTRAL VESTIBULAR NYSTAGMUS

Central vestibular nystagmus is due to disease of the CNS. The lesion creates an imbalance in the vestibular system resulting in nystagmus that is purely *vertical*—downbeat, upbeat, and torsional nystagmus.

In the horizontal vestibular system, the activities of the left and right horizontal semicircular canals balance each other. In the vertical vestibular system, by contrast, the activity of the anterior canal on one side is balanced by the activity of the posterior canal on the other side. Because the central pathways for the anterior and posterior canals differ, the vertical nystagmus produced will differ—inhibition of the anterior canal pathways causes downbeat nystagmus, and inhibition of the posterior canal pathways causes upbeat nystagmus—these are two of the vestibulo-ocular system's three unmistakable nystagmus signs (Chapter 8).

Downbeat and Upbeat Nystagmus

Both downbeat nystagmus and upbeat nystagmus are due to central vestibular dysfunction affecting the superior vestibular nucleus and the ventral tegmental tract. The ventral tegmental tract is an ascending vestibular tract that connects the superior vestibular nucleus, a major relay center for ocular reflexes mediated by the semicircular canals, to the superior rectus and to the inferior oblique motor neurons in the CN III nucleus.[41]

Downbeat nystagmus is usually associated with lesions of the vestibulo-cerebellum and underlying medulla, which result in hyperactivity of the superior vestibular nucleus and the ventral tegmental tract pathway. Focal lesions causing downbeat nystagmus affect the cerebellar flocculus and/or paraflocculus and appear to tonically inhibit the superior vestibular nucleus and the ventral tegmental tract pathway (Chapter 9).

Upbeat nystagmus, is commonly due to lesions of the dorsal central medulla that affect the perihypoglossal nuclei, the adjacent medial vestibular nucleus and nucleus intercalates, and directly or indirectly cause hypoactivity of the superior vestibular nucleus-ventral tegmental tract pathway. Less frequently, upbeat nystagmus is due to a lesion in the central part of the mid pons or the rostral pons, and, rarely, to a small unilateral lesion in the dorsal tegmentum in the caudal pons.[42] Pontine upbeat nystagmus may disappear after 2–3 months, suggesting that a central adaptive mechanism can ultimately nullify this type of vertical nystagmus. In patients with medullary lesions, improvement or disappearance of upbeat nystagmus has a variable range of between a few weeks and a few months, but it has also been reported to persist for as long as 2 years in one patient.

The hypothetical pathophysiology of vertical nystagmus is depicted in Figure 10-5A–D. Only one side of the cerebello-brainstem pathway, which is assumed to be principally involved in primary position upbeat or downbeat nystagmus, is shown: (A) shows upbeat nystagmus due to a pontine lesion, (B) downbeat nystagmus due to floccular lesions, (C) upbeat nystagmus due to caudal medullary lesions, and (D) the normal circuit.[43]

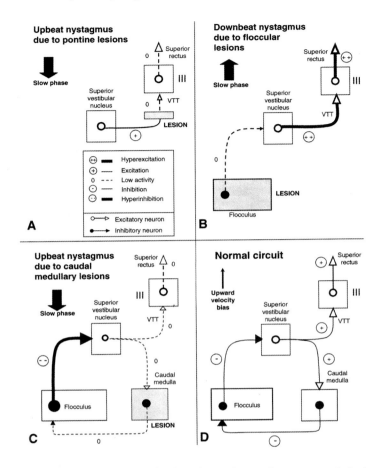

FIGURE 10-5 The hypothetical pathophysiology of vertical nystagmus. Only the cerebellar-pathway (on one side), assumed to be mainly involved in primary position upbeat nystagmus (UBN) or downbeat nystagmus (DBN) is shown. (A) UBN due to pontine lesions: the ventral tegmental tract (VTT), originating in the superior vestibular nucleus (SVN), is probably impaired (bilaterally), with consequently relative hypoactivity of the elevator muscle motoneurons with respect to the unchanged downward system, eliciting a downward slow eye deviation. (B) DBN due to floccular lesions. Since the flocculus normally inhibits the SVN, the lesion results in disinhibition of the downstream pathway, with consequently relative hyperexcitation of the elevator muscle motoneurons, compared with the unchanged downward system, eliciting an upward slow eye deviation. (C) UBN due to caudal medullary lesions. The caudal medulla (nucleus of Roller and/or a cell group of the paramedian tracts), which could receive a collateral branch from the SVN and project to the flocculus via a probably inhibitory pathway, is impaired. The result is disinhibition of the inhibitory flocculovestibular neurons, which are then overactivated, eliciting overinhibition of the downstream pathway (VTT); that is, low activity with respect to the downward system, with consequently (as in A) a slow downward deviation of the eye. (D) Normal circuit, derived from the clinical results observed in A, B, and C and anatomical experimental data known for the cat and the monkey. This circuit could specifically be involved in the upward vestibular system and does not appear to have a role in the downward system; the result could be a slight upward velocity bias in the normal state.

Reproduced with permission.[43]

■ **Clinical Points to Remember About Downbeat Nystagmus**

- Downbeat nystagmus is due to lesions of the vestibulo-cerebellum—the flocculus and paraflocculus.
- Downbeat nystagmus is poorly suppressed by fixation.
- Downbeat nystagmus is precipitated, exacerbated, or changed in direction by altering head position or vigorous head shaking.
- Convergence may increase or suppress nystagmus or convert downbeat nystagmus to upbeat nystagmus.
- Downbeat nystagmus is usually associated with other signs of vestibulo-cerebellar involvement and, rarely, with a caudal brainstem lesion.
- The most common causes of downbeat nystagmus include the Chiari malformation, cerebellar atrophy, infarction of the brainstem and cerebellum, MS, paraneoplastic encephalitis, and the GAD antibody syndrome.
- Toxic-metabolic disorders known to cause downbeat nystagmus are:
  - Anticonvulsant medication
  - Lithium intoxication
  - Alcohol intoxication and induced cerebellar degeneration
  - Wernicke's encephalopathy
  - Toluene abuse
- Recommended treatment:
  - 4-aminopyridine (5–10 mg t.i.d.)
  - 3,4-diaminopyridine (10–20 mg t.i.d.)
  - Baclofen (5 mg t.i.d.)
  - Clonazepam (0.5 mg t.i.d.)   ■

■ **Clinical Points to Remember About Upbeat Nystagmus**

- Central vestibular lesions generate pure spontaneous upbeat nystagmus.
- Upbeat nystagmus is frequently due to medullary lesions that affect the perihypoglossal nuclei.
- Upbeat nystagmus is rarely due to a unilateral lesion of the brachium conjunctivum (superior cerebellar peduncle).
- Upbeat nystagmus may resolve after 2–3 months due to central adaptation.
- Upbeat nystagmus is poorly suppressed by fixation.
- Convergence may increase or suppress nystagmus or convert upbeat nystagmus to downbeat nystagmus.
- Upbeat nystagmus is associated with abnormal smooth pursuit and square-wave jerks that produce *bow-tie nystagmus*.
- The most common causes of upbeat nystagmus include infarction of the medulla or cerebellum, infiltrating tumors, MS, brainstem encephalitis, and Creutzfeldt-Jakob disease.
- Recommended treatment:
  - Baclofen (5–10 mg t.i.d.)
  - 4-aminopyridine (5–10 mg t.i.d.)   ■

Other causes of upbeat nystagmus will undoubtedly be identified over time. A possible addition to the known list is the case presented here.

CASE 10-1 Upbeat Nystagmus: Wernicke's Encephalopathy

Video Display

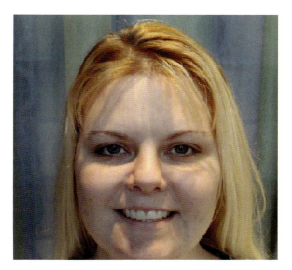

FIGURE 10-6 A thirty-three-year-old woman post gastric bypass surgery for morbid obesity.

The patient is a 33-year-old single mother with a past history of morbid obesity treated in 2005 by gastric bypass with a weight change from 270 to 170 pounds (Figure 10-6). She drinks 2–3 glasses of wine per night.

In January 2008, she was admitted to hospital as an emergency complaining of pressure headache, photophobia and phonophobia, night sweats, transient double vision lasting seconds only, intermittent numbness and paresthesia in the legs, and unsteady gait. She was afebrile, and dehydrated, with persistent nausea and vomiting. Hematological studies showed elevated lipase/normal amylase without clinical evidence of pancreatitis. Abnormal liver function studies were attributed to fatty infiltration of the liver due to a high body mass index and alcohol excess. An upper endoscopy revealed patent gastric jejunal anastomosis.

A laparoscopic cholecystectomy and cholangiogram was performed.

On the day following surgery, immediately on waking, she noted "jumping eyes," blurred vision, and transient episodes of diplopia lasting seconds only.

Her past medical history was notable for migraine with photophobia and phonophobia (onset at age 25) and a GI bleed in 2006 (stomach artery cauterized; attributed to ibuprofen use).

The patient was discharged home only to return the next day complaining of jumping vision, unsteadiness walking, and severe generalized fatigue. Examination of the spinal fluid showed cerebrospinal fluid (CSF) glucose 63 mg/dL, protein 81.5 mg/dL, and one white blood cell.

The patient was readmitted to the hospital and transferred the same day to the Massachusettes General Hospital.

Analysis of the History

· What are the major presenting symptoms?
· Where are the CNS lesion(s) likely to be?

CASE 10-1 SYMPTOMS

Symptoms	Location Correlation
Paresthesia in her legs	Sensory neuropathy
Unsteady gait	Cerebellum
Oscillopsia	Vestibular pathways
Transient diplopia for seconds only	Decompensated phoria

The analysis guides the clinical examination.

Examination

Neurological

· Alert, fully oriented, attentive and cooperative
· Short-term memory 0 out of 3 recall at 2 minutes
· Long-term memory intact for world events
· Sensory peripheral neuropathy in the legs
  · Proprioception impaired in the feet
  · Vibration sense impaired at the ankles
· Reflexes 1+ with reinforcement
· Plantar responses flexor
· No titubation or limb ataxia
· Mild gait ataxia
· Romberg negative

Neuro-ophthalmological

· Visual acuity, visual fields, pupils, and fundus examination normal
· No ptosis
· Spontaneous upbeat nystagmus
· Lid nystagmus
· Upbeat nystagmus visible under closed eyelids
· Full eye movements
· Normal convergence
· Saccadic smooth pursuit in all directions
· Normal oculocephalic reflexes

Localization and Differential Diagnosis

Sensory peripheral neuropathy with mild gait ataxia are signs consistent with nutritonal deficiency. The presence of upbeat nystagmus leave little doubt that this patient has Wernicke's encephalopathy, a potentially reversible metabolic brain dysfunction resulting from thiamine deficiency. Nystagmus is a characteristic early feature of Wernicke's encephalopathy. It can be horizontal or vertical, with horizontal more common. Wernicke's encephalopathy typically causes ataxia, ophthalmoplegia, and global confusion.

What Diagnostic Tests Should Follow?

· Hematological tests
· Brain MRI

Special Explanatory Note

Although the diagnosis of Wernicke's encephalopathy is generally considered to be a clinical one, supporting laboratory tests such as liver profile, serum electrolytes, renal function, urinalysis, and neuroimaging are all important. Serum thiamine levels may be misleading and should not be used for diagnosis.

Brain MRI is mandatory because both the medial thalamic and periaqueductal lesions can be readily demonstrated on the fluid attenuated FLAIR and T2 images.[44-46] The distinct pattern of the lesions, when also demonstrable *on diffusion-weighted sequences, is diagnostic of* Wernicke's encephalopathy.

Test Results

Hematological tests were normal. Brain MR FLAIR images showed symmetrical bilateral hyperintense signals in the hypothalamus and periaqueductal gray (Figure 10-7).

Diagnosis: For a diagnosis of Wernicke's encephalopathy to be made two of the following criteria must be met:[47]

· Dietary deficiency
· Oculomotor abnormality
· Cerebellar dysfunction
· Altered mental state or mild memory impairment
· Brain MRI sequences pre- and post-contrast (gadolinium) showing hyperintense signals bilaterally in the medial thalamus and mammillary bodies.

The oculomotor signs are:

· Gaze-evoked nystagmus (both horizontal and vertical)
· Unilateral or bilateral CN VI palsy with weaknes or absent abduction (lateral rectus)
· Horizontal or vertical conjugate gaze palsy (only rarely involving down gaze)

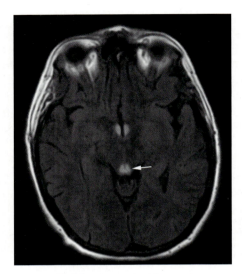

FIGURE 10-7 Fluid attenuated inversion recovery (FLAIR) magnetic resonance image shows bilateral hyperintensities in the hypothalamus and periaqueductal gray matter (*arrow*).

Confirmed Diagnosis: Wernicke's Encephalopathy

Treatment

Although 2–3 mg of thiamine may be sufficient to modify the ocular signs, much larger doses are needed to sustain improvement and replenish the depleted thiamine stores.

Thiamine replacement with 100 mg/d intravenously (IV) *or* intramuscularly (IM) may reverse signs and symptoms of Wernicke's encephalopathy and prevent further deterioration. Typically the dosage is 50 mg IV and 50 mg IM the latter dose being repeated each day until the patient resumes a normal diet. This patient received replacement thiamine *and* magnesium and steadily improved. The upbeat nystagmus resolved over the course of a day. The disappearance of nystagmus within hours of the administration of thiamine confirms the diagnosis. The peripheral sensory neuropathy persisted. The patient was discharged to a rehabilitation hospital.

Special Explanatory Note

Wernicke's encephalopathy can occur between 4 and 12 weeks after bariatric surgery, especially in young women with concomitant vomiting.[48-50] The half-life of thiamine is 10–20 days, and the occurrence of symptoms 4–12 weeks after surgery would reflect severe depletion of thiamine stores. The highest index of suspicion should be for patients who present with concomitant vomiting since vomiting limits thiamine uptake and/ in those patients receiving IV dextrose/ saline with or without a history of alcohol abuse.

Torsional Nystagmus

Spontaneous torsional nystagmus—the vestibulo-ocular system's third significant nystagmus sign—is yet another form of central vestibular nystagmus.[51,52] It is relatively rare and when present infarction of the brainstem, primarily in the dorsolateral medulla (Wallenberg's syndrome) should be suspected. Wallenberg's syndrome presents with acute vertigo and nystagmus, which is usually horizontal or mixed-horizontal torsional, with a small vertical component indicating disruption of central pathways from the horizontal, anterior, and posterior semicircular canals on the same side. In primary gaze, the slow phase is directed toward the side of the lesion[53] (Chapter 8, Case 8-4).

■ **Clinical Points to Remember About Torsional Nystagmus**

- Torsional nystagmus is a form of central vestibular nystagmus.
- Infarction of the medulla—Wallenberg's syndrome—is a common cause.
- Midbrain lesions affecting the rostral interstitial nucleus of the MLF and the INC are less common and cause vertical and torsional gaze-evoked nystagmus.
- Other causes of torsional nystagmus include the Chiari malformation (Chapter 9, Case 9-3), brainstem arteriovenous malformation (Chapter 8, Case 8-5), MS, oculopalatal tremor (Chapter 8, Case 8-1), and head trauma.   ■

Acquired Pendular Nystagmus

Acquired pendular nystagmus (APN) is frequently associated with visual loss[55] and disorders of central myelin, including MS,[54,55] Pelizaeus-Merzbacher disease which has its onset in the first few months, beginning with nystagmus, Cockayne's syndrome involving the CNS and multiple organs, and peroxisomal assembly disorders for example, neonatal adrenoleukodystrophy and Refsum disease), and toluene abuse.

CASE 10-2 Acquired Pendular Nystagmus Multiple Sclerosis

Video Display

The patient is a 56-year-old woman with a history of retrobulbar neuritis in the left eye (Figure 10-8). Eight years, after her first attack she developed difficulty focusing, unsteadiness walking, and numbness of the left side of her face. Taste was impaired.

Analysis of the History

- What are the major presenting symptoms?
- Where are the CNS lesion(s) likely to be?

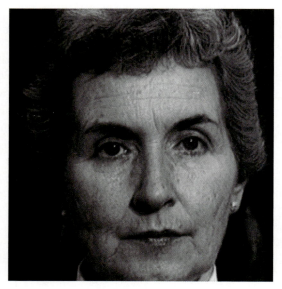

FIGURE 10-8 A fifty-six-year-old woman with multiple sclerosis.

CASE 10-2 SYMPTOMS

Symptoms	Location Correlation
Oscillopsia	Vestibular pathways
Unsteady gait	Cerebellum or cerebellar pathways
Left facial sensory loss	Trigeminal nucleus/nerve CN V, in the medulla

---

The analysis guides the clinical examination.

Examination

Neurological

- Left facial sensory loss to pain and temperature CN V (V2, V3 divisions)
- Motor system 5/5 throughout, symmetric hyperreflexia, flexor plantar responses
- Bilateral ataxia heel-knee-shin and gait ataxia
- Romberg test negative

Neuro-ophthalmic

- Visual acuity 20/20 OD, 20/40 OS
- Visual fields full OD, central scotoma OS
- Pupils equal, OD normal reflexes, OS afferent pupil defect
- Fundus examination OD normal, OS mild optic atrophy

Ocular Motility

- Pendular nystagmus in primary gaze (asymmetrical, most prominent in the left eye)
- Gaze-evoked horizontal nystagmus
- Upbeat nystagmus on full upgaze
- Full eye movements in all directions of gaze
- Saccadic pursuit in all directions of gaze
- Normal convergence
- Absent OKN

Special Explanatory Note

Acquired pendular nystagmus is characterized by smooth, pendulum-like oscillations of the eyes, without corrective quick phases. It usually has a combination of horizontal, vertical, and torsional components and when:

- If the horizontal and vertical components are in phase, the trajectory is oblique.
- If the horizontal and vertical components are 180 degrees out of phase, the trajectory is elliptical.
- If the horizontal and vertical components are 90 degrees out of phase and have the same amplitude, the trajectory is circular.

The amplitude of the nystagmus is greater in the eye with poorer visionin this case caused by unilateral demyelinating optic neuropathy.

What Diagnostic Tests Should Follow?

- Spinal tap
- Neuroimaging of the brain with attention to the brainstem and cerebellum (unavailable at the time)

Test Results

The CSF showed a slightly elevated protein 50 mg/dL, normal sugar 55 mg/dL, an increased white cell count (15 leukocytes/mm^3, and positive oligoclonal bands.

Special Explanatory Note

Gamma globulin proteins in the CSF of patients with MS are synthesized intrathecally by the CNS. They migrate in agarose electrophoresis as abnormal discrete populations, so-called *oligoclonal bands*. The demonstration of oligoclonal bands in the CSF and not in the blood is particularly helpful in confirming the diagnosis of MS, but they are not always found following the first attack or even in the later stages of the disease. Currently, gamma globulin measured as a fraction of total protein, and oligoclonal bands in the CSF, are the most reliable chemical tests for MS.

Notably, oligoclonal bands also appear in the CSF of patients with syphilis, Lyme disease, and subacute sclerosing panencephalitis—disorders that should not be difficult to distinguish from MS.

Diagnosis: Multiple Sclerosis with Acquired Pendular Nystagmus

Treatment

- Treat the acute attack of MS with IV steroids.
- Medication options for treatment of APN are gabapentin, baclofen, memantine, valproate, or clonazepam.

The patient received a 5-day course of IV methylprednisolone to treat the underlying demyelinating disease. Medications to suppress nystagmus were not available.

Special Explanatory Note

The pathogenesis of APN is unclear.[56,57] Acquired pendular nystagmus in MS may be due to disruption of the visual-motor calibration pathway to the cerebellum. As a result, visual signals cannot be adapted and modified in response to changing visual demands, causing drifts of the eyes away from the target and thus nystagmus.

Altered gamma aminobutyric acid (GABA) transmission is suggested as the mechanism for APN, and a number of drugs have been reported to improve APN in MS including the GABA$_A$ agonist clonazepam and the GABA$_B$ agonist baclofen. One of the few double-blind, placebo-controlled studies of nystagmus treatment compared gabapentin and baclofen in 15 patients with APN and found gabapentin to be highly effective in minimizing oscillopsia and oscillations.[58] The treatment of APN with gabapentin (which increases CNS GABA levels) is based on the known role of GABA-ergic neural transmission in controlling the neural integrator, which maintains stability of the eyes in eccentric gaze positions.

Memantine, a noncompetitive N-methyl-o-aspartate receptor antagonist, has also been reported to have a beneficial effect in suppressing APN in MS,[59,60] and further trials are needed to determine if combinations of gabapentin and memantine have additive effects.

SACCADIC OSCILLATIONS

When a saccade takes the eye away from the fixation target, it causes oscillopsia and saccadic oscillations, with and without an intersaccadic interval.

Normally, steady fixation is targeted by clinically imperceptible, extremely fine movements known as *microsaccades*, which are typically less than a third of a degree in amplitude. Microsaccades are suppressed during visual tasks needing particularly steady fixation, such as threading a needle. The clinician should use an ophthalmoscope with the patient's head completely still when looking for instability of fixation and check for micromovements of the optic nerve head (optic disc). Horizontal movements of the optic disc will be in the opposite direction to the movement of the eye.

A flow chart classifying and distinguishing between types of saccadic oscillations and intrusions is shown in Figure 10-9.[14]

Ocular Flutter and Opsoclonus

Ocular flutter and opsoclonus consist of continuous, uncalled-for, back-to-back saccades *without* an intersaccadic interval. Ocular flutter is purely horizontal and opsoclonus is multidirectional.[61] These oscillations occur most often in paraneoplastic syndromes[62–64] and postinfectious encephalitis, in which the underlying etiology is thought to be an autoimmune or cross-immune mechanism. Normal subjects and patients with ocular flutter or opsoclonus may show oscillations during blinks, during eye closure, and immediately (in the case of ocular flutter) on eye opening to fixate a target.

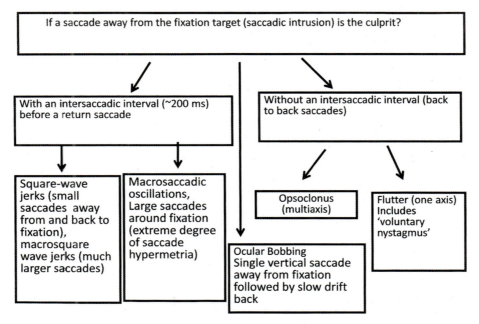

FIGURE 10-9 A flow chart of the classification of saccadic oscillations.

Reproduced with permission.[14]

CASE 10-3 Ocular Flutter: Paraneoplastic Encephalitis

Video Display

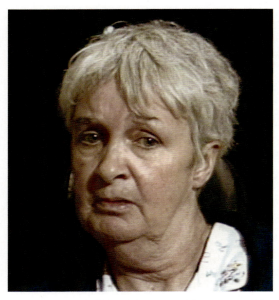

FIGURE 10-10 A fifty-eight-year-old woman with carcinoma of the lung.

The patient is a 58-year-old woman, who smoked a pack of cigarettes a day for over 30 years. She had a past history of depression and alcohol abuse (Figure 10-10). Three weeks prior to admission (PTA) she developed "dizziness" and an unsteady gait without deafness or tinnitus. Her primary care physician irrigated her ears without improvement, and her symptoms progressed. Two weeks PTA, she had a dramatic subacute change in behavior with insomnia, agitation, and depression, and spent her time wringing her hands for no apparent reason. She was seen by psychiatry in the ER with a chief complaint: "I cannot stand up, I cannot walk." A psychiatric consultant considered her unsteady gait was histrionic, related to depression and to her own perception that she was unable to walk. She was only able to walk with a walker and two assistants. She was admitted by psychiatry; the next day, she complained of intermittent difficulty focusing. A neuro-ophthalmology consult led to her transfer to neurology.

Analysis of the History

- What are the major presenting symptoms?
- Where are the CNS lesion(s) likely to be?

CASE 10-3 SYMPTOMS

Symptoms	Lesion Correlation
Acute change in behavior and agitation	Limbic system
Unsteady walking	Cerebellum or cerebellar pathways
Intermittent difficulty focusing	Oscillopsia

The analysis guides the clinical examination.

Examination

Neurological

- Disoriented in time and place
- Fluctuating level of alertness, attentiveness, and agitation
- Motor impersistence and perseveration
- Impaired short-term memory
- Failed to obey three-step commands

Cerebellum

- Dysarthria
- Titubation
- Fine tremor of the face and chin
- Marked truncal ataxia sitting and standing
- Severe ataxic gait with inability to walk without support

Ocular Motility

- Intermittent bursts of ocular flutter—conjugate horizontal saccades without a saccadic interval, particularly prominent on opening her eyes to fix a target
- Eyelid flutter
- Full vertical and horizontal gaze
- Horizontal gaze-evoked nystagmus to the right and to the left
- Saccadic pursuit, vertical and horizontal
- Normal convergence
- Normal oculocephalic reflexes

Localization and Differential Diagnosis

Dramatic subacute changes in behavior with insomnia, anxiety, depression, confusion, agitation, and a retentive memory deficiut are principal manifestations of so-called *limbic encephalitis* affecting the medial temporal lobes and adjacent nuclei.

Ocular flutter, gaze-evoked nystagmus, saccadic pursuit, titubation, and gait ataxia localize to the brainstem and cerebellum.

This formidable combination is diagnostic of an encephalitic process, primarily a paraneoplastic syndrome that, in a heavy smoker, makes cancer of the lung the first choice of an occult malignancy.

What Diagnostic Tests Should Follow?

- Tox screen
- Metabolic studies and serum electrolytes
- Search for occult malignancy
- Paraneoplastic antibodies[65]

Test Results

A tox screen was negative. Serum electrolytes were abnormal:

- Sodium 125 mmol/L (135–145)
- Potassium 2.8 mmol/L (3.4–4.8)
- Osmolality 262 mosmol/kg (280–296)

The results showed hyponatremia and low plasma osmolality indicative of the syndrome of inappropriate antidiuretic hormone (SIADH), a syndrome frequently associated with occult malignancy, most often breast or lung.

Chest x-ray and CT scan showed a well-circumscribed 6 cm mass in the left lower lobe of the lung (Figure 10-11).

Three samples of serum were tested for paraneoplastic antibodies (anti-Ri, anti-Yo, and anti-Hu). No antibodies were detected.

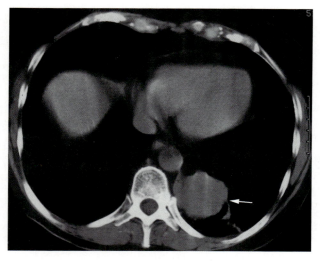

FIGURE 10-11 A thoracic computed tomogram (CT) shows a well circumscribed 6 cm mass in the left lower lobe of the lung (*arrow*).

Treatment

Treatment in paraneoplastic syndromes consists of appropriate therapy for the cancer:[66]

- Surgery
- Chemotherapy and/or radiation
- Immune modulation
- Plasma exchange
- Immunoadsorption therapy
- Intravenous immunoglobulin
- Steroids

A left lower lobe lobectomy and excision of a small-cell undifferentiated carcinoma of the lung with metastatic carcinoma in 2/5 hilar lymph nodes was performed. The patient was treated twice weekly for 3 weeks with protein-A immunoadsorption,[67] six cycles of chemotherapy, and radiation to the chest (50.4 Gy in 28 fractions).

She made a complete recovery and was followed for more than 10 years. When last seen in 2006, she was under treatment for chronic obstructive pulmonary disease and anxiety. She was still smoking one pack of cigarettes a day.

Special Explanatory Note

The diagnostic features of ocular flutter are back to back horizontal (one axis) saccades without a saccadic interval, and the diagnostic features of opsoclonus are constant, chaotic, random, multidirectional conjugate saccades without an intersaccadic interval of unequal and usually large amplitude disrupting steady fixation. Opsoclonus occurs during smooth pursuit, convergence, or blinks and typically persists under closed eyelids and during sleep. The antineuronal antibodies primarily associated with paraneoplastic opsoclonus are anti-Ri antibody (Chapter 9 Case 9-6)[68,69] (and anti-Yo markers for carcinoma of the breast, and anti-Hu for small-cell carcinoma of the lung.[70,71]

Infantile Opsoclonus

Opsoclonus in healthy preterm infants is a rare, benign, self-limiting disorder marked by back-to-back saccades almost always in the vertical plane.[72] Nevertheless, it is essential to screen infants with opsoclonus for the presence of an occult neuroblastoma. This approach was followed in the case presented here.

CASE 10-4 Opsoclonus: Neuroblastoma

Video Display

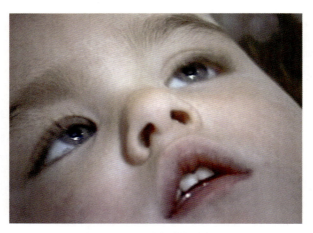

FIGURE 10-12 A two-year-old girl with progressive ataxia.

This baby girl was born after a 30-week gestation, with a birth weight of 1.25 kg. Her early developmental milestones were delayed. Bilateral esotropia was operated on at 21 months.

At 26 months, she had an upper respiratory tract infection, and, 2 weeks later, she began to fall up to five times daily. When taking 1 or 2 steps, she appeared unsteady. Eight days later, she walked "like a drunk," and 11 days later, she could not walk without assistance, and her head and upper extremities trembled when reaching for things and when she was sitting. Her pediatrician initially suspected a diagnosis of acute cerebellar ataxia, but her symptoms progressed and she was brought to the ER (Figure 10-12).

On admission she was afebrile.

Blood pressure 100/60 mm Hg
Weight 12.2 kg (50th percentile)
Height 89 cm (75th percentile)
Head circumference 49 cm (75th percentile).

She was alert, pointed to body parts, and sang a children's song intelligibly. Muscle tone was diminished throughout with dysmetria, axial and appendicular ataxia, and ataxic gait.

An MRI of the brain showed a topographic pattern of white matter changes characteristic of periventricular leukomalacia, common in premature children and probably accounting for the infant's developmental delay.

Chest x-ray, spinal fluid, and urine tests were negative for infection and toxic drugs.

She returned home only to be readmitted 4 weeks later when she began to vomit daily, and her father noted intermittent, rapid, "jiggling" movements of her eyes.

Analysis of the History

· What are the major presenting symptoms?
· Where are the CNS lesion(s) likely to be?

CASE 10-4 SYMPTOMS

Symptoms	Location Correlation
Delayed milestones	Preterm baby—immature
Upper respiratory infection Gait ataxia	Parainfectious cerebellar ataxia
"Jiggling" movements of the eyes	Cerebellum and/or brainstem vestibular pathways

---

The analysis guides the clinical examination.

Examination (Age 29 Months)

Neurological

· Gross axial hypotonia
· Truncal ataxia
  · She could only sit unsupported in the tripod position for 2–3 seconds.
  · With both hands held, she could pull herself up, stand, and take a few steps but was very unsteady.
· Brief twitching movements of the fingers interpreted as myoclonus were noted

Ocular Motility

· Sustained multidirectional saccades persisting during sleep (first 2 days)
· Spontaneous downbeat nystagmus
· Lid nystagmus
· Full random eye movements

Localization and Differential Diagnosis

The history and signs are most consistent with a subacute, relatively isolated cerebellar ataxia, a common parainfectious syndrome in children with a peak frequency in the third year of life. The disorder has an explosive onset over a period of hours, with maximal ataxia at the onset or within a day or two afterward, and recovery beginning within days. Three-quarters of affected children fully recover within 8 months.

The child's subacute progressive course called for a broader differential diagnosis. Significantly, at the time of readmission, she had opsoclonus-myoclonus-ataxia syndrome, narrowing the differential diagnosis to:

- parainfectious infantile polymyotonia (Kinsbourne'sdancing eyes, dancing feet, myoclonic encephalopathy of infants)[73]
- paraneoplastic opsoclonus-myoclonus syndrome with neuroblastoma.[74]

Only 2–3% of children with neuroblastoma present with opsoclonus-myoclonus-ataxia syndrome, and the tumor is most likely to be located in the mediastinum.

What Diagnostic Tests Should Follow?

- Urine tests for vanilmandelic and homovanillic acid
- Imaging studies to search for a neuroblastoma.

Test Results

Urine tests for vanilmandelic and homovanillic acid were negative. A thoracic scan showed no abnormality. An abdominal ultrasound showed a heterogeneous mass above the left kidney, An abdominal CT scan showed a left adrenal mass, 3.5 cm in diameter (Figure 10-13).

Treatment

The appropriate therapy for a suspected neuroblastoma is surgical excision of the tumor. Surgery to remove the tumor disclosed an encapsulated left adrenal mass. A left adrenalectomy was performed and para-aortic tissue excised, although no lymphadenopathy was evident in it. A frozen section revealed a ganglion neuroblastoma.

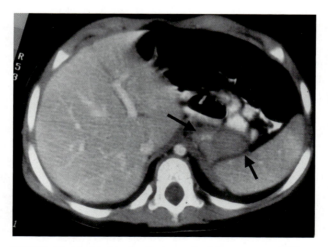

FIGURE 10–13 Abdominal computed tomogram (CT) shows a left adrenal mass (*arrows*).

Other Tests

A bone marrow biopsy under the same anesthesia was negative. No anti-Ri antibodies were detected in the serum.

Diagnosis: Ganglioneuroblastoma Paraneoplastic Opsoclonus, Downbeat Nystagmus with Cerebellar Ataxia

Treatment

High-dose steroids

The patient was started on corticotrophin IM, with improvement within 6 weeks. Within 10 weeks, she was walking independently with no ataxia, and she had no downbeat nystagmus.

There is a favorable prognosis for survival in children with coincident opsomyoclonus and neuroblastoma.[75]

Special Explanatory Note

The pathogenesis of opsoclonus remains unclear. Intrinsic ion channel dysfunction of the membrane of burst neurons may be the underlying abnormality affecting rebound firing of saccadic burst neurons after sustained inhibition (*postinhibitory rebound* (PIR)). Reciprocal inhibition between premotor excitatory and inhibitory saccadic burst neurons may be a key feature. Research studies lend support to the hypothetical role of PIR in the generation of saccadic oscillations.[76-80] For example, a selective channel blocker, ethosuximide, has been shown to affect the amplitude and frequency of saccadic oscillations evoked by eye closure in healthy subjects. A nonselective blocker, propranolol, has been reported to effectively abolish microsaccadic oscillations in a patient with the limb tremor syndrome (mSOLT). Treatment of opsoclonus with a channel blocker may ultimately be the drug of choice.

The presently known causes of ocular flutter/opsoclonus are shown in Table 10-3.[81]

Voluntary Saccadic Oscillations

Voluntary saccadic oscillations or "voluntary nystagmus" can be produced by normal subjects who can initiate saccadic oscillations with a convergence effort.[82] It is a saccadic disorder. The oscillations are high-frequency back-to-back horizontal saccades without an intersaccadic interval and are frequently accompanied by facial grimacing or eyelid flutter; which is often called *psychogenic flutter* to distinguish it from paraneoplastic ocular flutter. The oscillations are poorly sustained.

TABLE 10-3: Causes of Ocular Flutter/Opsoclonus

Parainfectious encephalitis—dancing-eyes, dancing-feet
Paraneoplastic syndromes
Cerebellar ataxia
Meningitis
Thalamic hemorrhage
Multiple sclerosis
Hydrocephalus
Hyperosmolar coma
Toxins: chlordecone, thallium, toluene
Drug side effects: lithium, amitriptyline, cocaine, phenytoin with
    Diazepam

Reproduced with permission.[81]

SACCADIC INTRUSIONS

Saccadic intrusions are uncalled-for saccades that take the eye away from fixation with an intersaccadic interval (approximately 200 ms) before a return saccade. Saccadic intrusions include saccadic dysmetria, microsaccadic flutter, macrosaccadic oscillations, square-wave jerks, macrosquare-wave jerks, and saccadic pulses. A schematic of the waveforms of saccadic oscillations and intusions is shown in Figure 10-14A–E.[15]

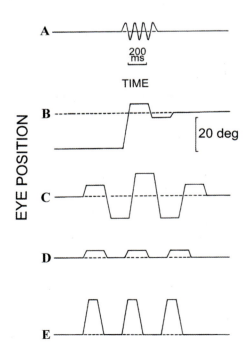

FIGURE 10-14A–E Schematic of saccadic intrusions and oscillations. (A) Ocular flutter: to-and-fro, back-to-back saccades without an intersaccadic interval. (B) Dysmetria: inaccurate saccades. (C) Macrosaccadic oscillations: Hypermetric saccades about the position of the target. (D) Square-wave jerks: small, uncalled-for saccades away from and back to the position of the target. (E) Macrosquare-wave jerks or macrosaccadic pulses: large, uncalled-for saccades away from and back to the position of the target.

Modified and reproduced with permission.[15]

Saccadic Dysmetria

Saccadic dysmetria is diagnostic of a lesion of the cerebellum: a unilateral lesion of the oculomotor vermis causes ipsilateral hypometria and contralateral hypermetria a unilateral lesion of the fastigial oculomotor region (FOR) causes ipsilateral hypermetria and contralateral hypometria; and a bilateral lesion of the FOR causes bilateral hypermetria (Chapter 9, Case 9-5).

Microsaccadic Flutter

Microsaccadic flutter (microflutter) describes rare symptomatic obtrusive horizontal saccadic oscillations with a frequency of 15–30 Hz and a very small amplitude of 0.1–0.5 degree that disrupt fixation and cause transient oscillopsia: "shimmering" vision or "jiggling," "wavy" vision. These oscillations can last from seconds to hours and are sometimes associated with dizziness or disequilibrium. They are invisible to the unaided eye and are diagnosed by ophthalmoscopy.[83,84]

Macrosaccadic Oscillations

Macrosaccadic oscillations are another form of unwanted intrusions that oscillate around the fixation point and disrupt steady fixation. They are crescendo-decrescendo runs of horizontal saccades with an intersaccadic interval of about 200 ms, typically induced by a gaze shift. They may have vertical or torsional components, and the vertical component may occasionally be clinically prominent.

These oscillations are simply due to an increase in gain of the saccadic oculomotor system. They are considered an extreme form of saccadic hypermetria since both the primary saccade that takes the eye away from fixation and the corrective saccade that returns it to the target are so hypermetric (increased gain) that they overshoot the target continuously in both directions oscillating as a result around the fixation point (Figure 10-14C). Macrosaccadic oscillations, first described in patients with cerebellar disorders, are most commonly seen with lesions that affect the fastigial nucleus and its projections.[85]

Square-Wave Jerks

Square-wave jerks, the commonest form of saccadic intrusions, are pairs of very small horizontal saccades, typically 0.5 degrees, which form a miniature square-wave pattern. A small saccade takes the eyes away from the target, and, after an intersaccadic interval of approximately 200 msec, a corrective saccade brings the eyes back to refix the target[86] (Figure 10-14D).

Square-wave jerks often occur in series and are:

- Asymptomatic
- Visible on inspection of the eyes fixing
- Easily detected during ophthalmoscopy
- Visible in normal subjects, especially the young and elderly

It is very important to bear in mind that square-wave jerks can occur in normal healthy elderly people with a frequency in the range of up to 20 per minute or greater, increasing in frequency with cigarette smoking. Persistent large-amplitude square-wave jerks (1–5 degrees) are abnormal but nonlocalizing.[87-90]

Square-wave jerks are prominent in neurodegenerative diseases affecting the basal ganglia, notably Parkinson's disease (PD), progressive supranuclear palsy (PSP), and multisystem atrophy[91,92] and they are reported following unilateral pallidotomy.[93] In a number of CNS diseases, almost continuous square-wave jerks can present as square-wave oscillations, which on occasion can be mistaken for nystagmus.

Cerebral square-wave jerks occur in patients with acute or chronic focal cerebellar lesions. (Chapter 9, Case 9-2). Low-amplitude cerebral square-wave jerks can be detected at the bedside by funduscopy.[94]

A cautionary note: Patients with dementia (in PSP or Alzheimer's disease) may show excessive distractibility in which novel visual targets evoke inappropriate saccades. This excessive distractibility disrupts steady fixation in these patients and should be distinguished from fixation instability due to square-wave jerks.

Macrosquare-Wave Jerks

Macrosquare-wave jerks are not simply enlarged square-wave jerks. They are pairs of large saccades, typically greater than 5 degrees, the first moving away from and the second back to the target, separated by a short (75–150 ms) interval and a frequency of about 2–3 Hz (Figure 10-14E). These oscillations are uncommon. They are reported in MS and multisystem atrophy and have been reported in a 21-year-old man recovering from acute encephalopathy. In his case, the oscillations were present with binocular viewing at distance and stopped when either eye was covered. Since latent nystagmus is the accepted term for a nystagmus that is absent with binocular fixation

TABLE 10-4: Type, Characteristics and Localization of Saccadic Oscillation and Intrusions

Type	Characteristics	Localization
Square-wave jerks	Horizontal, 1–5°, 200 msec intersaccadic intervals	Not localizing
Macrosquare-wave jerks	Horizontal, 10–40°, 100 msec intersaccadic intervals	Cerebellum
Macrosaccadic oscillations	Horizontal saccadic dymetria, series of hypermetric saccades, 200 msec intersaccadic intervals	Cerebellum
Voluntary 'nystagmus'	Horizontal, high frequency, low amplitude, intermittent, no intersaccadic intervals	Volitional
Saccadic pulses	Horizontal, single or double saccades with no steps	Cerebellum, lower brainstem
Ocular flutter	Horizontal, large amplitude, no intersaccadic intervals	Cerebellum, lower brainstem
Opsoclonus	Multidirectional, large amplitude, linear and curvilinear trajectories, no intersaccadic intervals	Cerebellum, lower brainstem

Modified and reproduced with permission.[81]

and present only with one eye covered, the term "inverse latent" macrosquare-wave jerks was introduced to emphasize the feature of suppression by monocular fixation.[95]

Saccadic Pulses

Saccadic pulses are brief, small eye movements away from the target followed by a rapid drift back to an object of interest. Unlike square-wave jerks, saccadic pulses allow a step change in innervation to hold the eyes in a new position, and the eyes come back to the object of interest by relatively fast drift.

The type, characteristics, and localizations of saccadic intrusions and oscillations are summarized in Table 10-4.

A FINAL CLINICAL POINT

In coming to the end of this book the most important clinical point to remember is probably this: the enormous complexity of the story that eye movements have to tell can begin only with the watchfulness of a thoughtful examiner.

The importance of the examiner's own observing eye is paramount:

- What do you see?
- What does it tell you?
- What, as a result, do you need to ask?
- How do you further refine what you see and hear?

These questions are relevant across medicine's spectrum of ailments and illness but, in the case of the eye, there is a special relevance: an eye must meet an eye and understand it more clearly than itself. There is a wonderful paradox in the challenge.

SELECTED REFERENCES

1. Crawford J. Living without a balancing mechanism. *N Engl J Med.* 1952;246:458–460.
2. Bender MB. Oscillopsia. *Arch Neurol.* 1965;13:204–213.
3. Bender MB, Feldman M. Visual illusions during head movement in lesions of the brain stem. *Arch Neurol.* 1967;17:354–364.
4. Straube A, Bronstein A, Straumann D. Nystagmus and oscillopsia. *Eur J Neurol.* 2012;19:6–14.
5. Brandt TH, Dieterich M, Danek A. Vestibular paroxysmia. *Bailliere's Clin Neurol.* 1994;3(3):565–575.
6. Hoyt WF, Keane JR. Superior oblique myokymia: report and discussion of five cases of benign intermittent uniocular microtremor. *Arch Ophthalmol.* 1970;84:461–467.
7. Suzuki Y, Washio N, Hashimoto M, Ohtsuka K. Three-dimensional eye movement analysis of superior oblique myokymia. *Am J Ophthalmol.* 2003;135(4):563–565.
8. Hashimoto M, Ohtsuka K, Hoyt WF. Vascular compression as a cause of superior oblique myokymia disclosed by thin-slice magnetic resonance imaging. *Am J Ophthalmol.* 2001;131:676–677.
9. Hashimoto J, Ohtsuka K, Suzuki Y, Minamida Y, Houkin K. Superior oblique myokymia caused by vascular compression. *J Neuro-ophthalmol.* 2004;24:237–239.

10. Scharwey K, Kizizok T, Samii M, Rosahl SK, Kaufmann H. Remission of superior oblique myokymia after microvascular decompression. *Ophthalmologica*. 2000;214(6):426–428.

11. Tomsak RL, Kosmorsky GS, Leigh RJ. Gabapentin attenuates superior oblique myokymia. *Am J Ophthalmol*. 2002;133:721–723.

12. Jain S, Farooq SJ, Gottlob I. Resolution of superior oblique myokymia with memantine. *JAAPOS*. 2008;12:87–88.

13. Bronstein AM. Oscillopsia. *Curr Opin Neurol*. 2005;18(1):1–3.

14. Leigh RJ, Zee DS. With permission 2013.

15. Leigh RJ, Zee DS. *The Neurology of Eye Movements*. 4th ed. New York: Oxford University Press; 2006.

16. Marti S, Palla A, Straumann D. Gravity dependence of ocular drift in patients with cerebellar downbeat nystagmus. *Ann Neurol*. 2005;52:712–721.

17. Perez P, Llorente JL, Gomez JR, Del Campo A, Lopez A, Suarez C. Functional significance of peripheral head-shaking nystagmus. *Laryngoscope*. 2004;114:1078–1084.

18. Baloh RW, Kerber KA. *Clinical Neurophysiology of the Vestibular System*. 4th ed. New York: Oxford University Press; 2011.

19. Baloh RW, Yee RD, Honrubia V. Optokinetic nystagmus in parietal lobe lesions. *Ann Neurol*. 1980;7:269–276.

20. Leigh RJ, Fusa EW. Disturbance of smooth pursuit caused by infarction of parieto-occipital cortex. *Ann Neurol*. 1985;17:185–187.

21. Halmagyi GM, Gresty MA, Leech J. Reversed optokinetic nystagmus (OKN): mechanism and clinical significance. *Ann Neurol*. 1980;7:429–435.

22. Proudlock F, Gottlob I. Foveal development and nystagmus. *Ann NY Acad Sci*. 2011;1233:292–297.

23. Gottlob I. Infantile nystagmus. Development documented by eye movement recordings. *Invest Ophthalmol Vis Sci*. 1997;38:767–773.

24. Brodsky MC, Wright KW. Infantile esotropia with nystagmus: a treatable cause of oscillatory head movements in children. *Arch Ophthalmol*. 2007;125:1079–1081.

25. Dell'Osso LF, Weisman BM, Leigh RJ, Abel RJ, Sheth NV. Hereditary congenital nystagmus and gaze-holding failure: the role of the neural integrator. *Neurology*. 1993;43:1741–1749.

26. Gottlob I, Wizov SS, Reinecke RD. Spasmus nutans. A long-term follow-up. *Invest Ophthalmol Vis Sci*. 1995;36:2768–2771.

27. Chrousos GA, Ballen AE, Matsuo V, Cogan DG. Near-evoked nystagmus in spasmus nutans. *J Pediatr Ophthalmol Strabismus*. 1986;23:141–143.

28. Anthony JH, Ouvrier RA, Wise G. Spasmus nutans: a mistaken identity. *Arch Neurol*. 1980;37:373–375.

29. Farmer J, Hoyt CS. Monocular nystagmus in infancy and early childhood. *Am J Ophthalmol*. 1984;98:504–509.

30. Kiblinger GD, Wallace BS, Hines M, Siatkowski RM. Spasmus nutans-like nystagmus is often associated with underlying ocular, intracranial or systemic abnormalities. *J Neuro-ophthalmol*. 2007;27:118–122.

31. Gallagher BB, Baumel IP, Mattson RH, Woodbury SG. Primidone, diphenylhydantoin and phenobarbital. Aspects of acute and chronic toxicity. *Neurology*. 1973;23:145–149.

32. Hogan RE, Collins SD, Reed RC, Remler BF. Neuro-ophthalmological signs during rapid intravenous administration of phenytoin. *J Clin Neurosci*. 1999;6(6):494–497.

33. Baier B, Dieterich M. Incidence and anatomy of gaze-evoked nystagmus in patients with cerebellar lesions. *Neurology*. 2011;76:361–365.

34. Shallo-Hoffman J, Schwarze H, Simonsz H, Muhlendyck H. A re-examination of endpoint and rebound nystagmus in normals. *Invest Ophthalmol Vis Sci*. 1990;31:388–392.

35. Abel LA, Parker L, Daroff RB, Dell'Osso LF. Endpoint nystagmus. *Invest Ophthalmol Vis Sci*. 1978;17:539–544.

36. Schmidt D, Dell'Osso LF, Abel LA, Daroff RB. Myasthenia gravis: saccadic eye movement waveforms. *Exp Neurol*. 1980;68:346–364.

37. Hood JD. Further observations on the phenomenon of rebound nystagmus. *Ann NY Acad Sci*. 1981;374:532–539.

38. Halmagyi GM, Hoyt WF. See-saw nystagmus due to unilateral mesodiencephalic lesion. *J Clin Neuro-ophthalmol*. 1991;11:79–84.

39. Halmagyi GM, Aw ST, Dehaene I, Curthoys IS, Todd MJ. Jerk-waveform see-saw nystagmus due to unilateral meso-diencephalic lesion. *Brain*. 1994;117:789–803.

40. Thurtell MJ, Leigh RJ. Nystagmus and saccadic intrusions. In: Kennard C, Leigh RJ, eds. *Neuro-ophthalmology* Vol *102, 3rd series. Handbook of Clinical Neurology,* Amsterdam: Elsevier B.V.; 2011;13:134–378.

41. Ranalli PJ, Sharpe JA. Upbeat nystagmus and the ventral tegmental pathway of the upward vestibule-ocular reflex. *Neurology.* 1988;38:1329–1330.

42. Tilikete C, Milea D, Pierrot-Deseilligny C. Upbeat nystagmus from a demyelinating lesion in the caudal pons. *J Neuro-ophthalmol.* 2008;28:202–206.

43. Pierrot-Deseilligny C, Milea D. Vertical nystagmus: clinical facts and hypotheses. *Brain.* 2005;128:1237–1246.

44. White ML, Zhang Y, Andrew LG, Hadley WL. MR imaging with diffusion-weighted imaging in acute and chronic Wernicke encephalopathy. *Am J Neuroradiol.* 2005;26:2306–2310.

45. Zuccoli G, Pipitone N. Neuroimaging findings in acute Wernicke's encephalopathy: Review of the literature. *Am J Radiol.* 2009;192:501–508.

46. Kashi MR, Henderson GI, Schenker S. Wernicke's Encephalopathy. In: McCandless DW, ed. *Metabolic Encephalopathy.* New York: Springer Science + Business Media, LLC; 2009:281–300.

47. Caine D, Halliday GM, Kril JJ, Harper CG. Operational criteria for the classification of chronic alcoholics identification of Wernicke's encephalopathy. *J Neurol Neurosurg Psychiat.* 1997;62:51–60.

48. Singh S, Kumar A. Wernicke encephalopathy after obesity surgery. A systematic review. *Neurology.* 2007;68:807–811.

49. Zhang KJ, Zhang HL, Zhang D, Wu J. Comments on "Wernicke's encephalopathy after laparoscopic Roux-en-Y gastric bypass: a misdiagnosed complication." *Obes Surg.* 2010;20(9):1329–1330.

50. El-Khoury J. The alcohol factor in Wernicke's encephalopathy post bariatric surgery. *Ann Surg.* 2010;251(5):992–993.

51. Lopez LI, Bronstein AM, Gresty MA, Rudge P, DuBoulay EP. Torsional nystagmus. A neuro-otological and MRI study of thirty-five cases. *Brain.* 1992;115:1107–1124.

52. Noseworthy JH, Ebers GC, Leigh RJ, Dell'Osso LF. Torsional nystagmus: quantitative features and possible pathogenesis. *Neurology.* 1988;38:992–994.

53. Morrow J, Sharpe JA. Torsional nystagmus in the lateral medullary syndrome. *Ann Neurol.* 1988;24:390–398.

54. Barton JJ, Cox TA. Acquired pendular nystagmus in multiple sclerosis: clinical observations and the role of optic neuropathy. *J Neurol Neurosurg Psychiat.* 1993;56(3):262–267.

55. Tilikete C, Jasse L, Pelisson D, Vukusic S, Durand-Dubief F, Urquizar C, Vighetto A. Acquired pendular nystagmus in multiple sclerosis and oculopalatal tremor. *Neurology.* 2011;76:1650–1657.

56. Averbuch-Heller L, Zivotofsky AZ, Das VE, DiScenna AO, Leigh RJ. Investigations of the pathogenesis of acquired pendular nystagmus. *Brain.* 1995;118(Pt 2):369–378.

57. Rucker JC. An update on acquired nystagmus. *Semin in Ophthalmol.* 2008;23:91–97.

58. Averbuch-Heller L, Tusa RJ, Fuhry L, Rottach KG, Ganser GL, Heide W, Buttner U, Leigh RJ. A double-blind controlled study of gabapentin and baclofen as treatment for acquired nystagmus. *Ann Neurol.* 1997;41(6):818–825.

59. Thurtell MJ, Joshi AC, Leone AC, Tomsak RL, Kosmorsky GS, Stahl JS, Leigh RJ. Cross-over trial of gabapentin and memantine as treatment for acquired nystagmus. *Ann Neurol.* 2010;67:676–680.

60. Starck M, Albrecht H, Pollmann W, Dieterich M, Straube A. Acquired pendular nystagmus in multiple sclerosis: an examiner-blind cross-over treatment study of memantine and gabapentin. *J Neurol.* 2010;257:322–327.

61. Cogan DG. Ocular dysmetria, flutter-like oscillations of the eyes and opsoclonus. *Arch Ophthalmol.* 1954;51(3):318–335.

62. Ellenberger C Jr., Campa JF, Netsky MG. Opsoclonus and parenchymatous degeneration of the cerebellum. The cerebellar origin of an abnormal eye movement. *Neurology.* 1968;18:1041–1046.

63. Leigh RJ, Zee DS. Diagnosis of nystagmus and saccadic intrusion. In: Leigh RJ, Zee DS, eds. *The Neurology of Eye Movements,* 4th ed. New York: Oxford University Press; 2006;Ch 10:475–558.

64. Anderson NE, Rosenblum MK, Posner JB. Paraneoplastic cerebellar degeneration: Clinical-immunological correlations. *Ann Neurol.* 1988;24:559–567.

65. Wray SH, Dalmau J, Chen A, King S, Leigh RJ. Paraneoplastic disorders of eye movements. *Ann N.Y. Acad Sci.* 2011;1233:279–284.

66. Bataller L, Dalmau J. Paraneoplastic neurologic syndromes: approaches to diagnosis and treatment. *Semin Neurol.* 2003;23(2):215–224.

67. Cher LM, Hochberg FH, Teruya J, Nitschke M, Valenzuela R, Schmahmann JD, Herbert M, Rosas HD, Stowell C. Therapy for paraneoplastic neurologic syndromes in six patients with protein A column immunoadsorption. *Cancer.* 1995;75(7):1678–1683.
68. Budde-Steffen C, Anderson NE, Rosenblum MK, Graus F, Ford D, Synek BJL, Wray SH. Post anti-neuronal autoantibody in paraneoplastic opsoclonus. *Ann Neurol.* 1988;23:528–531.
69. Luque AF, Furneaux HM, Ferziger R, Rosenblum MK, Wray SH, Schold SC, Glantz MJ, Jaeckle KA, Biran H, Lesser M, Paulson WA, River ME, Posner JB. Anti-Ri: An antibody associated with paraneoplastic opsoclonus and breast cancer. *Ann Neurol.* 1991;29:241–251.
70. Bataller L, Wade DF, Graus F, Stacey HD, Rosenfeld MR, Dalmau J. Antibodies to Zic4 in paraneoplastic neurologic disorders and small-cell lung cancer. *Neurology.* 2004;62(5):778–782.
71. Tsou JA, Kazarian M, Patel A, Galler JS, Laird-Offringa IA, Carpenter CL, London SJ. Low level anti-Hu reactivity: a risk marker for small cell lung cancer? *Cancer Detect Prev.* 2009;32(4):292–299.
72. Morad Y, Benyamini OG, Avni I. Benign opsoclonus in preterm infants. *Pediatr Neurology.* 2004;31:275–278.
73. Kinsourne M. Myoclonic encephalopathy of infants. *J Neurol Neurosurg Psychiat.* 1962;25:271–276.
74. Case 27–1995. Clinicopathological Conference. *New Engl J Med.* 1995;33:579–586.
75. Altman AJ, Baehner RL. Favorable prognosis for survival in children with coincident opsomyoclonus and neuroblastoma. *Cancer.* 1976;37:846–852.
76. Scudder CA, Kaneko CS, Fuchs AF. The brainstem burst generator for saccadic eye movements: a modern synthesis. *Exp Brain Res.* 2002;142:439–462.
77. Ramat S, Leigh RJ, Zee DS, Optican LM. Ocular oscillations generated by coupling of brainstem excitatory and inhibitory saccadic burst neurons. *Exp Brain Res.* 2005;160(1):89–106.
78. Ramat S, Leigh RJ, Zee DS, Optican LM. What clinical disorders tell us about the neural control of saccadic eye movements. *Brain.* 2007;130(Pt 1):10–35.
79. Shaikh AG, Ramat S, Optican LM, Miura K, Leigh RJ, Zee DS. Saccadic burst cell membrane dysfunction is responsible for saccadic oscillations. *J Neuro-ophthalmol.* 2008;28(4):329–336.
80. Shaikh AG, Zee DS, Optican LM, Miura K, Ramat S, Leigh RJ. The effects of ion channel blockers validate the conductance-based model of saccadic oscillations. *Ann NY Acad Sci.* 2011;1233:58–63.
81. Yee, RD. Nystagmus and Saccadic Intrusions and Oscillations. In: Yanoff M, Duker JS, eds. *Ophthalmology.* 2nd ed. St. Louis: Mosby; 2004:1350–1359.
82. Hotson JR. Convergence-initiated voluntary flutter: a normal intrinsic capability in man. *Brain Res.* 1984;294:299–304.
83. Ashe J, Hain TC, Zee DS, Schatz NJ. Microsaccadic flutter. *Brain.* 1991;114:461–472.
84. Foroozan R, Brodsky MC. Microsaccadic opsoclonus: an idiopathic cause of oscillopsia and episodic blurred vision. *Am J Ophthalmol.* 2004;138:1053–1054.
85. Selhorst JB, Stark L, Ochs AL, Hoyt WF. Disorders in cerebellar ocular motor control. II. Macrosaccadic oscillations. An oculographic control system and clinico-anatomic analysis. *Brain.* 1976;99:509–522.
86. Abadi RV, Gowen E. Characteristics of saccadic intrusions. *Vision Res.* 2004;44:2675–2690.
87. Herishanu YO, Sharpe JA. Normal square wave jerks. *Invest Ophthalmol Vis Sci.* 1981;20(2):268–272.
88. Shallo-Hoffmann J, Petersen J, Muhlendyck H. How normal are "normal" square wave jerks? *Invest Ophthalmol Vis Sci.* 1989;30:1009–1011.
89. Shallo-Hoffmann J, Sendler B, Muhlendyck H. Normal square wave jerks in differing age groups. *Invest Ophthalmol Vis Sci.* 1990;31:1649–1652.
90. Serra A, Leigh RJ. Diagnostic value of nystagmus: spontaneous and induced ocular oscillations. *J Neurol Neurosurg Psychiat.* 2002;73:615–618.
91. Fukazawa T, Tashiro K, Hamada T, Kase M. Multisystem degeneration: drugs and square wave jerks. *Neurology.* 1986;36:1230–1233.
92. Troost BT, Daroff RB. The ocular motor defects in progressive supranuclear palsy. *Ann Neurol.* 1977;2:397–403.
93. Averbuch-Heller L, Stahl JS, Hlavin ML, Leigh RJ. Square-wave jerks induced by pallidotomy in parkinsonian patients. *Neurology.* 1999;52(1):185–188.
94. Sharpe JA, Herishanu YO, White OB. Cerebral square wave jerks. *Neurology.* 1982;32:57–62.
95. Dell'Osso LF, Troost BT, Daroff RB. Macro square wave jerks. *Neurology.* 1975;25(10):975–979.

INDEX OF CASE STUDIES WITH VIDEO DISPLAYS

CHAPTER 1   HOW THE BRAIN MOVES THE EYES

CHAPTER 2   THE EYELID AND ITS SIGNS

CHAPTER 7 VERTICAL GAZE AND SYNDROMES OF THE MIDBRAIN

CHAPTER 8 DIZZINESS, VERTIGO, AND SYNDROMES OF THE MEDULL

CHAPTER 9 THE CEREBELLUM AND ITS SYNDROMES

CHAPTER 10 OSCILLOPSIA, NYSTAGMUS, AND SACCADIC OSCILLATIONS

INDEX